M I N A M A T A

Pollution and the Struggle for Democracy

in Postwar Japan

Harvard East Asian Monographs 194

M I N A M A T A

Pollution and the Struggle for Democracy

in Postwar Japan

Timothy S. George

Published by the Harvard University Asia Center and
Distributed by Harvard University Press
Cambridge (Massachusetts) and London 2001

Printed in the United States of America

The Harvard University Asia Center publishes a monograph series and, in coordination with the Fairbank Center for East Asian Research, the Korea Institute, the Reischauer Institute of Japanese Studies, and other faculties and institutes, administers research projects designed to further scholarly understanding of China, Japan, Vietnam, Korea, and other Asian countries. The Center also sponsors projects addressing multidisciplinary and regional issues in Asia.

Library of Congress Cataloging-in-Publication Data
George, Timothy S.
    Minamata : pollution and the struggle for democracy in postwar Japan / Timothy S. George.
        p. cm. -- (Harvard East Asian monographs ; 194)
    Includes bibliographic references and index.
    ISBN 0-674-00364-0 (cl : alk. paper) -- ISBN 0-674-00785-9 (paper : alk. paper)
        1. Mercury--Toxicology--Japan--Minamata-shi--History--20th century. 2. Public health--Japan--Minamata-shi--History--20th century. 3. Environmental health--Japan--Minamata-shi--History--20th century. I. Title. II. Series.

RA1231.M5 G46 2001
615.9'25663'095225--dc21   00-053944

Index by the author

☮   Printed on acid-free paper

First paperback edition 2002

Last figure below indicates year of this printing
11 10 09 08 07 06 05 04 03 02

Acknowledgments

One cannot study Minamata only by teasing truths out of musty documents in archives, nor can the scholar pretend to be a detached observer when he cries along with his subjects as they tell their stories. I could not have researched and written this book without a great deal of help. The people of the Minamata area, especially the victims of Minamata disease, welcomed an American researcher and his family into their tragically beautiful home. Hamamoto Tsuginori, the late Kawamoto Teruo, Ogata Masato, the late Onitsuka Iwao, Ishimure Michiko, and Hiyoshi Fumiko were especially generous, patient, and confident that I could understand.

At the Minamata Disease Center Sōshisha, Yoshinaga Toshio provided most of my introductions, Mochizuki Toshikazu supplied documents and help in reading names, and Ori Arisa helped in every way possible. The members of GAIA Minamata, especially Takakura Shirō and Yanagida Kōichi, shared their food, their homemade beer, and their experience. Mayor Yoshii Masazumi and Yoshimoto Tetsurō of the city government broadened my understanding of Minamata's history and environment, and Yamanaka Toshiharu opened the collection of the city's Minamatabyō shiryōkan to me.

Maruyama Sadami of Kumamoto University provided most of my documents by giving me full access to the Minamatabyō kenkyūkai Collection stored in his office. Two other Kumamoto University professors (both now retired) and members of the Minamatabyō kenkyūkai, Togashi Sadao and Harada Masazumi, improved my work with their confidence and insights. Matsuura Toyotoshi, proprietor of Karigari in Kumamoto and a member of the Minamatabyō o kokuhatsu suru kai, provided food, drink, conversation, and a congenial place to meet many helpful people.

Irokawa Daikichi of Tōkyō keizai daigaku (now retired) provided inspiration, encouragement, and suggestions from start to finish. Ui Jun of the University of Okinawa, Yahagi Tadashi of Urawa Junior College, Nakanishi Junko of Yokohama National University, Horikawa Saburō of Hōsei University, Gotō Takanori, and Jitsukawa Yūta provided essential guidance and materials. Aileen Smith helped me see Minamata as it was when she and W. Eugene Smith lived there. Members of the audience at my presentations at the University of Tokyo's Institute of Social Science, the Ph.D. Kenkyūkai at the International House of Japan, the Association for Asian Studies, the Edwin O. Reischauer Institute of Japanese Studies at Harvard University, the Graduate School of Oceanography at the University of Rhode Island, and the U.S. Environmental Protection Agency's National Health and Environmental Effects Research Laboratory in Narragansett, Rhode Island, gave me very helpful suggestions.

This book is an outgrowth of my 1996 Harvard Ph.D. thesis in history. Research was assisted by a Takahashi Zaidan grant from the Fulbright Foundation in Japan, a Dissertation Write-up Fellowship from the Joint Committee on Japanese Studies of the Social Science Research Council and the American Council of Learned Societies, and a Post-Doctoral Fellowship and two other grants from the Edwin O. Reischauer Institute of Japanese Studies. Research in Japan was also facilitated by an appointment as a Visiting Research Scholar at the Institute of Social Science at the University of Tokyo, for which I thank Banno Junji. Funding for photographs was provided by the Department of History and the College of Arts and Sciences of the University of Rhode Island. Robert Gutchen drew the maps.

John Dower of the Massachusetts Institute of Technology first suggested the topic of Minamata and helped me frame the issue in the context of modern Japanese history. Carol Gluck of Columbia University helped with grants, introductions, and interpretive context. Michael Reich of Harvard's School of Public Health, Margaret McKean of Duke University, and Frank Upham of the New York University School of Law were supportive from the early stages. Herbert Bix encouraged me to use the terminology—postwar democracy—most used in Japan. At Harvard, my advisers Albert Craig and Andrew Gordon improved this work immeasurably. My colleagues at the University of Rhode Island were encouraging as I did further research and rewriting.

This book is dedicated to my wife, Jane, and daughters, Emily and Sarah. They believed in me and in this project, tolerated long absences, late nights of work, and six moves in seven years, and taught me a great deal by making us part of the communities in which we lived in Japan.

T.S.G.

Contents

Tables, Maps, and Figures   xi

Note on Conventions   xv

Introduction   1

Part I: Background, 1907–1955

1 Town, Factory, and Empire   13
The Setting 13/   The Factory Comes to Minamata 16/
The Growth of Nitchitsu 18/   Nitchitsu, Minamata, and
Imperial Japan 21

2 Minamata Before the Disease   26
Nitchitsu and Minamata Society 26/   Defeat, Recovery,
and Boom 30/   Minamata Politics in the 1950s 35/   Life
in Minamata in the 1950s: Hamamoto Tsuginori 38

Part II: The First Round of Responses

3 Discovering the Disease and Its Cause   45

4 The First Solution, 1959   71
The Fisherfolk's Struggle for Compensation 71/   The
Victims' Struggle for Compensation 102/   "As Clean
as River Water": The Third Leg of the "Solution" 114

Part III: "Years of Silence"?

5 Maintaining the Solution   125
The Fishers 125/   The Patients 144

6 Change Undermines the Solution   154
   Changes in Minamata 154/   Changes in Japan 171

              Part IV: The Second Round of Responses, 1968–1973

7 Bringing the Issue to the Nation   179
   1968 179/   An End to Solidarity: Leave It up to Others,
   or Sue? 191/   Kawamoto Teruo and the Uncertified
   Patients 203/   New Forms of Action and a Broadening
   Base of Support 210

8 In and Out of Court: The Second Solution   222
   The Leaflet War in Minamata 222/   Direct Negotiations
   in Tokyo 228/   Defections and Confrontations 235/   The
   Mediation Group and the Forgery Incident 238/   The Trial:
   Proving Negligence 241/   After the Verdict: Negotiating from
   a Position of Strength 249

                            Part V: Since 1973

9 Minamata and the Tragedy of Japan's "Modernity"   261
   Remembering: Tales and Lessons of Minamata 261/
   Events Since 1973: Toward a More Complete Solution 263/
   Painfully Slow Healing 271

   Conclusion: Minamata and Postwar Democracy   280

   Epilogue: Restless Spirits   287

                             Reference Matter

   Notes   295
   Bibliography   339
   Index   365

Tables, Maps, and Figures

Tables

1 Brief chronology of the Minamata disease incident   xviii

2 Pollution effects on animals and seaweed in Minamata, 1949–1957   4

3 Declining fish catch in Minamata, 1950–1957   72

4 Mercury concentrations in hair, Minamata area and Kumamoto City, 1960–1961   146

5 Mercury concentrations in hair, Kagoshima prefecture areas near Minamata, 1960–1961   147

6 Japan's "Big Four" pollution cases   175

Maps

1 Minamata and the Shiranui Sea area   xx

2 Minamata   xxi

Figures

1 Products made from Chissolite and Chissoloid   19

2 Patents held by Nitchitsu in various countries   22

3 Chōsen Chisso's Hungnam factory in Korea   23

4 The Shōwa emperor Hirohito's visit to the Minamata factory, 1931   25

5 The fishing hamlet of Modō at low tide, 1960   28

6 Modō in 1994   29

7   The factory in Minamata   33

8   Itō Hasuo and Hosokawa Hajime   48

9   Sugimoto Eiko, 1962   52

10 The net surrounding Minamata Bay, 1977–97   54

11 Invasion of the factory by members of fishing cooperatives, 1959   91

12 The patients' Mutual Aid Society's set-in at the factory gate, 1959   109

13 Fisherman with little to sell and no customers, Minamata, 1960   129

14 The Minamata Fishing Cooperative meets to expel dissident
    members, 1960   135

15 An old woman in the fishing hamlet of Tsubodan, 1960   145

16 Congenital Minamata disease patients, 1962   159

17 The "Stable Wage Struggle" strike, 1962–63   165

18 Minamata disease patients' groups, 1957–73   194

19 A congenital Minamata disease patient with a summer
    gift from Chisso   195

20 The contorted hand of Funaba Iwazō   213

21 Congenital Minamata disease patient Sakamoto Shinobu   215

22 A certificate for 50 shares of Chisso stock, from the
    one-share movement   217

23 Patients confronting the Chisso president at the shareholders'
    meeting, 1970   221

24 Newly certified patients during their November 1971 sit-in at
    the factory gate   227

25 Kawamoto Teruo asking the Chisso president to sign a pledge
    in blood   230

26 Congenital victim Kamimura Tomoko   232

27 Kawamoto Teruo speaking with the Chisso president in the
    "Tokyo Negotiations," 1973   253

28 The director general of the Environment Agency visiting a
    Minamata disease patient   256

29 Stone statues on land reclaimed from the most polluted parts of Minamata Bay, 1996   262

30 Raising an octopus pot, 1994   265

31 Hamamoto Tsuginori speaking at the Minamata Disease Museum, 1994   273

32 Patients protesting remarks about "fake patients," 1979   274

33 The 1994 memorial ceremony at which the Minamata mayor apologized to the victims   279

34 The Minamata Tokyo Exhibition, 1996   288

35 *Utasebune* (sail-powered fishing boats) on the Shiranui Sea   290

Note on Conventions

Abbreviations

The following abbreviations are used in the text and notes (consult the Bibliography for complete information on the publications listed below):

EPA   Economic Planning Agency

JCIA   Japan Chemical Industry Association

JCP   Japan Communist Party

JNR   Japan National Railways

JSP   Japan Socialist Party

LDP   Liberal Democratic Party

MB   Tomita Hachirō (Ui Jun), ed., *Minamatabyō: Minamatabyō kenkyūkai shiryō*; an annotated collection of primary sources, mainly articles from newspapers and medical and scientific journals

MBJSS   Minamatabyō kenkyūkai, ed., *Minamatabyō jiken shiryōshū, 1926–1968*; an annotated collection of 841 documents dating from April 1926 to September 1968, selected from the Minamatabyō kenkyūkai Collection

MBKK   Minamatabyō kenkyūkai Collection; approximately 90,000 documents stored in the office of Professor Maruyama Sadami at Kumamoto University

MITI   Ministry of International Trade and Industry

NIH   National Institutes of Health (U.S.)

PVC   polyvinyl chloride

SKKS1   "Seiji ketchaku kankei shiryō I"; a collection of 68 documents
           related to the third "solution" to the Minamata disease inci-
           dent; in Minamatabyō kenkyūkai, ed., *Minamatabyō kenkyū*, vol.
           1, *Minamatabyō mondai no seiji kaiketsu*

Japanese Names

Japanese names are given in Japanese order: family name first, followed by
given name.

Table 1

Brief Chronology of the Minamata Disease Incident

Year	Event
1908	factory built in Minamata after successful campaign by local elite
1932	Chisso begins production of acetaldehyde using mercury catalyst

Round One

Year	Event
5/1/56	official discovery of Minamata disease
7/20/59	Kumamoto University research group announces probable cause is mercury
8/29/59	compensation agreement between Minamata Fishing Cooperative and Chisso
10/7/59	cat no. 400 develops Minamata disease after being fed factory waste in secret experiments at factory hospital
12/18/59	compensation agreement between Kumamoto Prefectural Alliance of Fishing Cooperatives and Chisso
12/19/59	Cyclator completed by Chisso, waste supposedly safe
12/30/59	*Solution #1*: solatium agreement between Chisso and Minamata disease victims: $889 for deaths, annual payments of $278 for adults and $83 for children; further demands prohibited
5/31/65	official discovery of Niigata Minamata disease

Round Two

Year	Event
1/12/68	Citizens' Council for Minamata Disease Countermeasures established
9/26/68	official government finding that Chisso's organic mercury causes Minamata disease (acetaldehyde production had ended 5/18/1968)
6/14/69	112 people (in 29 families) sue Chisso in Kumamoto District Court, other patients trust government to arbitrate compensation
10/71	new patients certified; some begin direct negotiations with Chisso, others accept government mediation
3/20/73	victims win suit against Chisso
7/9/73	*Solution #2*: compensation agreement with Chisso by both trial group and direct negotiations group; applied to all certified patients: one-time payments of $59,000–66,000, monthly stipends of $74–221 (later adjusted for inflation), medical coverage
6/16/78	Kumamoto prefecture begins issuing bonds to finance loans to Chisso so it can continue compensation payments; Chisso owes prefecture over $2.2 billion by 2001

Year	Event
12/15/1995	*Solution #3*: Cabinet approves plan to subsidize Chisso in paying $26,000 to each eligible uncertified patient and $51,500,000 to victims' groups. Prime Minister Murayama offers government apology. Nearly all victims' groups accept and agree to drop suits (some 2,300 had been suing over certification and government responsibility).
9/1/1997	net surrounding Minamata Bay removed after fish declared safe
4/27/2001	Osaka High Court decision in favor of 58 victims who rejected 1995 settlement: national and prefectural governments found guilty of allowing disease to spread; certification system found too strict (appealed to Supreme Court)
6/30/2001	2,265 victims of Kumamoto Minamata disease (830 living; 1,435 deceased) have been certified and compensated under 7/9/73 agreement (out of 19,376 applicants); 10,353 (9,438 living; 915 deceased) victims have been compensated under 12/15/95 plan, in return for agreement never to sue or request certification as patients

Map 1: Minamata and the Shiranui Sea Area

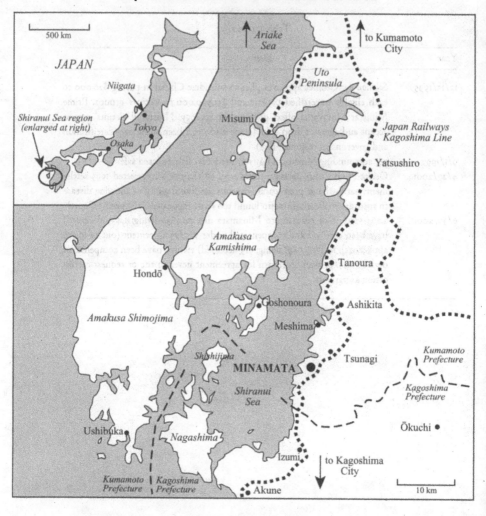

Map 2: Minamata

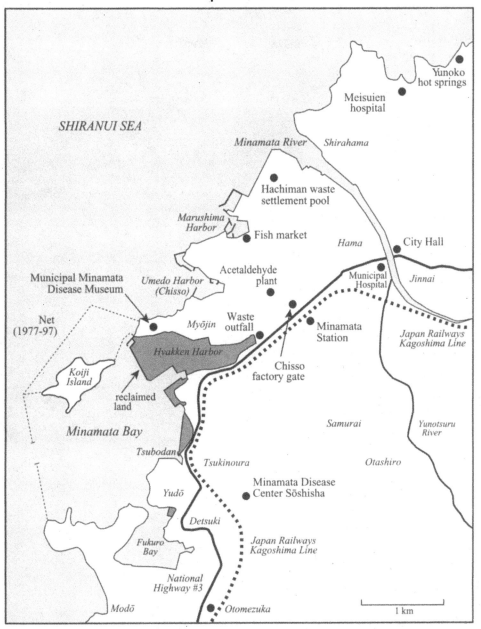

SHIRANUI SEA

Yunoko hot springs

Meisuien hospital

Minamata River   Shirahama

Hachiman waste settlement pool

Marushima Harbor

Fish market

Hama   City Hall

Acetaldehyde plant

Municipal Minamata Disease Museum

Umedo Harbor (Chisso)

Municipal Hospital   Jinnai

Net (1977-97)

Myōjin   Waste outfall

Minamata Station

Japan Railways Kagoshima Line

Hyakken Harbor

Koiji Island

Chisso factory gate

reclaimed land

Minamata Bay

Samurai

Yunotsuru River

Tsubodan

Tsukinoura

Otashiro

Yudō

Minamata Disease Center Sōshisha

Detsuki

Fukuro Bay

Japan Railways Kagoshima Line

National Highway #3

Modō   Otomezuka

1 km

MINAMATA

Pollution and the Struggle for Democracy

in Postwar Japan

Introduction

On a July day in 1955, Hamamoto Tsuginori was walking from his home in the Detsuki area of Minamata to the tiny inlet of Tsubodan, where his family kept their fishing boat. He was going to collect the previous day's catch of mullet from the traps they were kept in, kill them, and take them to market. Hamamoto had no reason to suspect that he and his family would never again lead comfortable lives.[1]

The road was bad, and going by the old highway took time, so I walked on the train tracks almost every day. Trains didn't come and go as often as they do now. If a train passed, no more would come for several hours. . . .

Then one day, walking off the crossing where the Detsuki bus stop is now, I tripped on a tie and fell.

I thought, "That's strange. Why would I trip on this and fall?" Then I fell again at the shore. Nakatsu Yoshio caught up to me from behind and said, "Tsuginori, are you feeling funny?" and it was then that I first realized that the numbness and shaking in my hands were serious.[2]

Nakatsu said he had similar symptoms and suggested they see a doctor. At a local clinic, a Dr. Ichikawa gave them injections and medicine, said they were exhausted from working in the heat, and ordered them to eat nutritious food and rest in the shade for a week. When they were asked to write their names and addresses, Nakatsu found he could not write at all, and Hamamoto could barely do so. They asked the doctor what he meant by nutritious food, and "he said there were all kinds of things, so we should just eat what we liked. I was a fisherman, and we could get fish, and I liked it, so every day I stuffed my belly with *sashimi* and rested."[3]

After a week Hamamoto's condition had gotten worse rather than better. The numbness had spread to his entire body. Nakatsu dropped a ten-yen coin on the bus and could not find it because his field of vision had become so narrow. Hamamoto and Nakatsu went from doctor to doctor for two months. Finally they returned to Dr. Ichikawa, who wrote them a letter of introduction to a wartime friend of his at the Kumamoto University hospital in the prefectural capital.

The doctor there nodded in understanding when he read the letter from Ichikawa. The two men were hospitalized and subjected to endless tests, with machinery the likes of which they had never seen in Minamata. They were given more injections and medicines, and their symptoms improved somewhat. Nakatsu was discharged, and then Hamamoto. His sister Fumiyo came to meet him and pay the bill, but had to borrow from relatives in Kumamoto since it was so much higher than she had expected.

Hamamoto returned to Minamata, carrying a letter from the university doctor to Ichikawa. The letter explained that since the tests had found nothing unusual, Ichikawa must have been correct in suspecting, as he had written in his letter of introduction, that the two young men were suffering from acetylene poisoning. The natural tendency of the effects of acetylene poisoning to wear off with time seemed to explain the patients' improvement. Hamamoto said to Ichikawa:

"I don't want to argue with you, doctor, but don't you think it's strange?"
"Why?"
"My father has fished with gas [acetylene lamps] for a long time; why do you think he hasn't gotten sick? I haven't used it for three or four years, since I graduated from school."
Then the doctor shook his head and said, "Hmm, that's right, isn't it. Well, uh, the university wrote that I should give you an injection of this, so let's give you the shot." So I went home after getting a shot and some medicine.[4]

The truth was that Hamamoto was suffering from mercury poisoning, contracted by eating fish that had absorbed and concentrated the organic mercury in the wastewater from the Shin Nihon Chisso Corporation (abbreviated as Shin Nitchitsu, later called Chisso) chemical factory in Minamata. Eating extra fish had increased his intake of mercury and worsened his symptoms. In the hospital in Kumamoto, he had eaten much less fish and improved slightly.

Hamamoto decided he could no longer fish and applied for work with Shin Nitchitsu. He passed the first test and then managed to pass the physical examination by making fists to hide his trembling. He began work in December 1955, for ¥270 ($0.75) per day, at the factory that was poisoning him.[5] Neither he nor anyone else realized that many other people were sick with the same disease and that the factory that was Minamata's main business and the source of its prosperity was causing the disease. Indeed, just the previous month, Maeda Eiki, leader of the effort to attract the factory to Minamata half a century earlier and still alive at age 79, had been given a special award by the city.[6]

Hamamoto Tsuginori was not the first person to contract the disease, nor were sick people the first indication of environmental problems in the sea around Minamata (see Table 2). Hamamoto had noticed that the water was getting dirty around 1951, but at first only around Hyakken Harbor, where the factory's waste entered the sea. He found fish floating on the surface more and more often and took them if they were alive. Kawamoto Teruo, who lived near Hamamoto, remembers complaints in the neighborhood young people's group (*seinendan*), which he headed, about the factory's "bad water" (*akusui*) beginning in 1952 or 1953.[7] Crows and seabirds, too, were dying.[8] Even earlier, pine trees near the shore in the fishing hamlet of Modō had turned brown and died.[9]

In 1952, in response to several complaints from the Minamata fishing cooperative, Kumamoto prefecture requested data from the company and then sent Miyake Reiji, chief clerk of the fisheries section in the prefectural government's economics division, to investigate Shin Nitchitsu's effluent and its effects. Miyake reported that the company was uncooperative, but that it appeared that factory waste was affecting the area from Hyakken Harbor to Koiji Island and causing a reduction in fish catches. He recommended that the contents of the factory's wastewater be analyzed and concluded that it was "necessary to consider both the immediate damage and the long-term cumulative damage caused by the wastewater."[10] Yet nothing was done. Production and pollution increased. One of the first chances to prevent or limit the coming tragedy had been missed.

Something was having horrible effects on cats; they would often "dance" crazily before dying. Three of the Hamamotos' cats died in 1953 and 1954, along with some of their chickens.[11] Cats were invaluable in preventing damage to fishing nets from mice, and in 1954 the *Kumamoto nichinichi shinbun* reported that a resident of Modō asked the city's hygiene section for help in controlling the mice, whose population had exploded as the cats died. In this hamlet of 120 households, around 100 cats had died in two months. New

Table 2

Pollution Effects on Animals and Seaweed in Minamata, 1949–1957

Date	Fish	Shellfish	Seaweed	Birds	Cats, Pigs
1949–50	Some fish float in the bay and can be caught by hand	Barnacles do not cling to boats anchored near factory waste outfall	Some seaweed in the bay floats to the surface near the factory		
1951–52	More fish float in the bay	Noticeable increase in the number of empty shells	Seaweed color fades; roots break and seaweed drifts; amount of seaweed only 1/3 of normal	Crows fall from the sky; seabirds can be caught easily	
1953–54	Fish float further south than Minamata Bay; fish swim crazily in Yudō Bay	Shells die along Tsukinoura coast; cockleshells within 1,000 m off shore die	Amount of drifting seaweed increases	More birds fall, as far west as Modō; crows crash into sea and rocks	One cat dies in Detsuki, 1953; many more, over a wide area, go crazy and die in 1954: pigs die in Detsuki and Tsukinoura
1955–57	Fish float over a wider area, including Minamata River and Yunoko	Powerful smell of dead shellfish along seashore	Edible seaweed disappears from Minamata Bay	Number of affected birds increases	Number of affected cats increases

SOURCE: Minamatabyō kenkyūkai, Minamatabyō ni iai suru kigyō no sekinin, p. 193.

cats brought in by the residents soon began to gyrate wildly and then died, just as those native to Modō had. This first media report on Minamata disease foreshadowed some of the debates that would soon follow concerning the cause of the disease, noting that "since there are no rice fields in the area, there seems to be no connection with agricultural chemicals."[12] Kumamoto University researchers later reported that 50 of 61 cats kept by the families of Minamata disease patients died between 1953 and 1956.[13] The sickness was affecting people too, of course, although like Hamamoto they were all misdiagnosed before April 1956. A neighbor of the Hamamotos in Detsuki, Mizoguchi Toyoko, developed problems walking and talking in 1953 and died at the age of eight in March 1956.[14] She was by no means the first person to get the disease or to die from it, but when the first patients were officially designated on December 1, 1956, she was listed as patient no. 1 since she had contracted the disease earlier than any of the other patients known at the time. Because of the stigma traditionally attached to disease, especially to debilitating diseases such as this, Mizoguchi and many other early victims were kept hidden at home.[15] Local doctors saw several patients with unexplained symptoms in 1954 and 1955, the year that Hamamoto and Nakatsu were sent to Kumamoto University's hospital for examinations. Yet it was not until two young sisters fell ill in April 1956 that Minamata's best doctor realized there was an epidemic of a strange new disease.

Five-year-old Tanaka Shizuko was brought by her mother to the pediatric department of Shin Nitchitsu's hospital from their home in Tsubodan on April 21, 1956. Shizuko had difficulty walking and talking and was hospitalized April 23. Her two-year-old sister Jitsuko developed similar symptoms two days later and was hospitalized on April 29. The girls' mother told the doctors that a five-year-old neighbor, Egoshita Kazuko, seemed to have the same disease. The doctors investigated and soon had hospitalized eight patients. On May 1, hospital director Dr. Hosokawa Hajime sent Dr. Noda Kaneyoshi to report to the municipal public health office that "there is an epidemic of an unknown disease of the central nervous system."[16]

Itō Hasuo, who headed the public health office, reported the outbreak to the prefecture on May 4, but the prefectural government waited until August 3—by which time it knew of eighteen patients, including three deaths—to notify the Ministry of Health and Welfare.[17] Arita Shigeo, head of the prefectural public health department, visited Minamata in the fall, speaking with patients in their homes and with city officials. He later recalled: "I reported to Governor Sakurai that the [sea]water seemed to be the cause. When I did, I was banned [from going there again] when Vice-Governor Mizugami [Nagayoshi] said: 'Mr. Arita, from now on you'd better not go south of Yatsushiro [a city between Kumamoto and Minamata].'"[18]

The disease was terrifying. Egoshita Kazuko's gait and speech became unnatural around April 28, and she was unable to grasp things well.[19] By May 9, when given water to drink, she choked and spilled it. On May 10 she became completely unable to walk, and by May 17 she could no longer swallow, and her legs and arms had become rigid. On May 21 she developed pneumonia and convulsions and lost consciousness, and on May 23 she died. Every single member of her family got Minamata disease, three of them in May and June 1956. W. Eugene Smith and Aileen Smith open their book *Minamata* with a description of Kazuko's parents bringing her body home:

Mr. and Mrs. Egoshita were forced to walk home from the Minamata city hospital. . . .

They walked the railroad tracks, avoiding the roadways—wanting no recognition.

Mr. Egoshita walked a few steps ahead. On his back he carried the autopsied body of his daughter. . . . She had died of the "strange disease" in Minamata that could not be explained, a disease which conjured such fears of contagion that the victims and those close to them became outcasts, stigmatized and degraded, frequently even in their own eyes.

That was years ago.[20]

On August 17, 1956, Hamamoto Tsuginori's father, Sōhachi, overslept, something he virtually never did. Tsuginori and his mother, Matsu, woke him with great difficulty. He seemed disoriented, unable to speak clearly or to understand what they said, and had great trouble getting to the door, getting his feet into his wooden *geta*, and going out to the toilet. They immediately feared he had the disease. When Tsuginori said he should stay home while they went out to fish, Sōhachi angrily refused, mumbling: "If I don't go, what can you do?" He walked as if drunk on the way down to the boat, and they had a hard time getting him in it. When their boat was rocked by a passing boat's wake, Sōhachi fell in the water. Tsuginori brought his father home, and on the way Sōhachi mumbled to a neighbor: "I've . . . got . . . that . . . strange . . . disease . . . that's going . . . around . . . that . . . fashionable . . . disease [*hai kara byō*]."[21]

Within a few days Tsuginori, who had been scheduled to be rehospitalized, and his father were in Kumamoto at the university's isolation hospital with several other victims of the "strange disease." Before long, his father was suffering convulsions and bleeding from his fingertips where he had ripped off his nails by scratching the walls. It took four or five people to hold him down and try to feed him, but soon he was unable to swallow. The films of Sōhachi in the hospital are some of the most horrifying ever made of Minamata disease patients, showing a strong man as he wastes away, and his shaky attempts to smoke and drink. Soon Matsu came down with the disease and moved in with her husband and son. Sōhachi died on October 5, after being moved to a separate room so his wife would not have to watch. Tsuginori and his elder brother, Kazunori, persuaded the other family members to allow an autopsy, hoping the results might help the patients who were still living. Kazunori watched the autopsy and told his family Sōhachi had been "cut up like a fish."[22] Although the doctors in Kumamoto had assured the Hamamoto family the disease was not contagious, Minamata city officials disinfected their home soon after Sōhachi's death. Tsuginori's sister Fumiyo, then 29, nursed their mother for three years until she died and believes she thereby gave up any chance of getting married.[23]

This book describes three rounds of responses to Minamata disease. The first began with the discovery of the disease in 1956 and ended with a partial settlement in 1959. The potentially inconvenient and embarrassing dispute over the disease—inconvenient and embarrassing not only to the company but also to the Ministry of International Trade and Industry and national leaders about to enshrine high growth as *the* project of postwar Japan—was kept in the hands of the local elite, out of the courts and off the national stage. The "solution" concluding the first round of responses consisted of "sympathy" payments to victims, meager compensation to fishing cooperatives, and waste treatment facilities that did not remove mercury. This ended a period characterized by efforts of scientists to find the cause, of the company to hide it, of victims to gain compensation, and of government to sweep the incident under the rug. The story was almost never brought to the attention of the nation as a whole, and for some time after this first settlement the only funding for continued research came from the United States.

Virtually all the themes that run through the Minamata case appeared in this first period. Minamata is a story not just of the environmental and human costs of rapid "modernization," but also of a callous and murderous corporation hiding its guilt; of the collusion and confusion at all levels of government and society, including the scientific community and the media, that allowed the tragedy to happen and then to be covered up; of powerful pressures against speaking out and taking action; of stigmatization and ostracism in the local society of a company town; of popular politicization and grass-roots movements; of the social constraints on these movements and on individuals; and of the persistence and adaptation of "traditional" uses of language and religion and concepts of moral economy.

After 1959, dramatic changes in Minamata and Japan—a lessening of the city's loyalty to the Chisso corporation, Japan's rapid economic growth, the development of the New Left and citizens' groups, and the appearance of other diseases caused by pollution—undermined the first settlement and suggested new patterns of organization and action. In the late 1960s and early 1970s, partly because of Minamata and the other frightening environmental diseases that appeared in Japan and the belated government admission that mercury from the Chisso plant caused Minamata disease, it became both possible and virtuous for citizens to be politically active. Minamata was brought to center stage through a nationwide network of support, separate from the established opposition parties and without an official center or hierarchy. In this second round of responses, some of the victims, along with their supporters, forced a more complete and just settlement. Some sued Chisso; others forced "direct negotiations" with company executives. Together, they won both monetary compensation and legal recognition of the company's responsibility.

Yet problems remained—many victims were uncertified and therefore ineligible for compensation, the question of government responsibility remained unsettled, and social discrimination against the victims and scapegoating of them continued. A third "full solution" to the Minamata disease incident, agreed to in 1995 and 1996, compensated many uncertified patients, but this one, too, assigned no legal blame to the government and left some victims uncompensated.

Minamata is a peripheral factory town far from Japan's political, economic, and cultural center in Tokyo. But these events, especially those in the second and third decades after World War II, raise questions central to an understanding of democracy in postwar Japan. In the context of Japanese history, Minamata is more than the site of one of the world's worst cases of industrial pollution. It is also the locus of the development of new forms of civic action; of contending and evolving relationships among society, corporations, and the state; and, most important, of an ongoing redefinition of citizenship and democracy in postwar Japan.

Japan is the first non-Western industrial democracy, and it is still a young one. The Japanese changed from imperial *subjects*, whose rights could be limited, to *citizens* in a constitutional democracy when the current constitution, imposed by the American Occupation, took effect on May 3, 1947. The constitution took sovereignty away from the emperor and handed it to the people. One question we can ask of this process is how they subsequently defined and redefined citizenship and democracy, in practice, for themselves. The responses to the tragic mercury poisoning discovered in Minamata in 1956 can help us answer this question.

It is a question too rarely asked in descriptions of postwar Japan, which often manage to analyze and explain the operation of a supposedly democratic system of government without saying much about the populace, the *demos*. For the most part,[24] these studies have been carried out by political scientists interested in the policymaking process and high politics, and few have made the reciprocal relations between the state and civil society their central focus.[25] Interestingly, though, several of the most important of these studies of postwar political history identify a significant turning point in the late 1960s and early 1970s. They find that the power elite expanded, changed complexion, and became more responsive to pressures from outside and below.[26] It is no coincidence that this was the decisive period for the Minamata issue as well: the kind of citizen politics represented by the movement surrounding Minamata at this time deserves a large share of the credit for the changes at the elite policymaking level.

The Japanese polity, I argue, is defined socially as well as politically. Citizens themselves, as much as do the legislature and the courts, determine the meaning of citizenship. This is by no means a uniquely Japanese phenomenon, as the civil rights movement in the United States illustrates. In both Minamata and the United States, the established legal and political institutions moved only when pushed to do so by social action. Yet in every society, including Japan, the context, process, and results are in many respects particular to that society and to that time.

A society's responses to an environmental disaster say a great deal about it. What resources are mobilized to find and halt the cause? What allies and powers do the perpetrators have if they attempt to impede this search or to avoid punishment? How many of the victims are found, and how fairly are they compensated? And particularly relevant for Minamata, what resources do the victims have in their attempts to obtain justice? What historical legacies do they draw on, what support do they have, and how do these responses change over time?

Minamata is more than a symbol of the dark side of high growth and the flowering of the citizens' movement, more than a morality play of poor victims fighting a corporation and a state whose concerns were power, profits, growth, and the stability that guaranteed them. It is not just a reminder of the social costs of modernization—we know those well now—but also a story of a struggle to define equality and justice. Minamata is the best example of how the Japanese people have constantly tested and redefined the limits and meaning of what they call not citizenship, civil society, or public space, but simply postwar democracy. Democracy is a process, most of the time, of evolution more than revolution, and this has certainly been the case in Japan since the Occupation reforms ended. It is better therefore to ask not *whether* Japan is democratic—I believe it is—but *how* democratic it is, how its democracy is constrained, and how its democracy is changing. The responses to Minamata illuminate three key chapters in the tale of Japan's postwar democracy.

The Minamata story *is*, in many ways, the history of postwar Japan. It enables us to look at this period from the bottom up, and from the periphery toward the center, and to put it in historical context. And as a human drama and an intensely personal tragedy, it compels us to begin with the experiences and actions of individuals and communities rather than policies, parties, and theories. It shows that power and policy in postwar Japan depend on more than just the relative strengths of politicians and bureaucrats, that the "economic miracle" is not the whole story of postwar Japanese history, and that citizenship and democracy have been contested and continually redefined by the patterns of organization and action among ordinary Japanese citizens.

PART I

Background, 1907–1955

ONE

Town, Factory, and Empire

The Setting

Minamata has always been far from Japan's centers of power. Travelers to Minamata—an area even now conspicuously absent from travel guides despite its beauty and its history—have usually approached from the north. On the Hayabusa overnight train from Tokyo, one wakes up near Hiroshima in the western part of Japan's main island of Honshū, before the train passes through the undersea tunnel to Kyūshū and turns south toward Kagoshima, the last stop on this longest train run in Japan. The train enters the tunnel near Dannoura, site of the 1185 A.D. offshore battle that led to the founding of the first of the shogunates, the military governments that would rule Japan for the next seven centuries.

The train emerges from the tunnel in Kitakyūshū, a smoggy city of the smokestack industries promoted by the Meiji period leaders who overthrew the last shogunate in 1868, "restored" the emperor to "power," and transformed the new imperial Japan into a world-class industrial and military power in a few decades. The industrial city includes Yawata, at which Japan's greatest steel mill began producing steel in 1901 for the railroads and weapons so crucial to Japan's rise to great power status.

Farther south a train line branches off toward the port of Nagasaki on the lobe of Kyūshū extending toward Korea. Slightly farther on is Ōmuta, whose Miike coal mines helped fuel Japan's industrial revolution and were the scene of the bitter, protracted strike in 1960 that sealed the fate of radical unionism and marked the decline of the coal industry in postwar Japan.

The train next passes through the rich agricultural plain around Kumamoto City, where the traveler might catch a glimpse of Kumamoto Castle, one of Japan's three greatest castles. Here and there the rice fields have been displaced by semiconductor factories.

After the smelly paper mills of Yatsushiro, the landscape suddenly changes. The flat land disappears, and the mountains run right down to the sea. There are a few terraced fields, a few pomelo groves on the hillsides, and a few small fishing villages. The train line, only single-tracked here, runs close to the sea—close enough, along one stretch, that one could literally dive in from the train.

The beauty of the calm Shiranui Sea, glimpsed in shimmering flashes on the right side of the train between tunnels, attracts the traveler's attention as it has throughout recorded history. Emperor Keikō, returning from subduing the tribes of southern Kyūshū (according to legend, in 88 A.D., but actually several centuries later), is said to have seen mysterious glowing lights across the sea at night and commanded his lost helmsman to steer toward them to reach the shore. He asked whose fire it was, but no one could answer, so the sea was given the name Shiranuikai, "Sea of Unknown Fires."[1]

The Shiranui Sea is a rich, gentle, inland sea, with only a few narrow outlets to the East China Sea. On a clear day one can see across to the active volcano Unzen on the Shimabara peninsula. It was at Shimabara in 1638 that 37,000 peasant and samurai rebels, some of them Christians, were defeated with Dutch assistance in the last serious challenge to the Tokugawa shogunate, which unified Japan in 1600 and isolated it from most foreign contact for two and a half centuries. In the nearer distance are the Amakusa Islands, home to many "hidden Christians" while their religion was banned by the Tokugawa, and source of many *karayuki-san*, the women who worked in the brothels that accompanied imperial Japan's commercial and military expansion in East and Southeast Asia. The Amakusa Islands also provided many immigrants to Minamata, especially after the factory was built.

Abruptly, after the track runs slightly inland and emerges from a tunnel, the traveler finds himself looking ahead and down at Minamata, a small city crowded between mountains and sea on the first flat land in many kilometers. This is the delta of the Minamata River, which enters the sea just after its junction with the Yunotsuru River. This southernmost part of Kumamoto prefecture (also known as *Hi no kuni*, or "Land of Fire") was brought under the control of the Yamato court by the fifth or sixth century. Until the twentieth century, the isolated village of Minamata had little contact with government except through tax collectors, although it was the site of battles in the late sixteenth century preceding Japan's unification under the

Tokugawa and in the Satsuma Rebellion of 1876–77, the last domestic military challenge to the Meiji government.

The earliest historical mention of Minamata records its clever dealings with the distant central authorities.[2] A rare white turtle with red eyes was discovered in 768 and sent to Empress Shōtoku. The empress was pleased, and exempted the area from two types of taxes. Two years later two more white turtles were sent to the court, and Emperor Kōnin, who had only recently ascended the throne, changed the era name to Hōki, meaning "treasure turtle." After two more years, a third turtle was sent, and to this day the turtle remains the official symbol of the city.

Minamata, it is often said, has been governed by three local rulers (*tonosama*; "feudal lords"): the Sagara family from the thirteenth to the sixteenth century, the Fukami family from the sixteenth to the nineteenth century, and the Nitchitsu factory in the twentieth century. Sagara Nagayori was appointed land steward (*jitō*) of Hitoyoshi, well inland from Minamata, by the Kamakura shogunate in 1205.[3] He soon expanded his control to the Ashikita area—Minamata and the coastal areas to its north—and the Sagara family governed the region for the next three and a half centuries. They were dislodged in the tumultuous Warring States period preceding the establishment of the Tokugawa shogunate, when many of Kyūshū's powerful daimyo of the sixteenth and early seventeenth centuries—the Ōtomo, Ryūzōji, Shimazu, Katō, Konishi, and Hosokawa—fought over and sometimes controlled the area. This area was the location of the southernmost fighting in the successful campaign by Toyotomi Hideyoshi, the second of Japan's three great unifiers, to subdue the powerful Shimazu and push them south to their home province of Satsuma (now Kagoshima prefecture). The Fukami family assisted Hideyoshi in these battles in 1587, and a Fukami was appointed intendant (*daikan*) of Minamata under the Hosokawa, who were assigned to be daimyō of Higo (Kumamoto prefecture) by the Tokugawa in 1631. Such chains of indirect rule, using local notables where possible, were typical of Japan's political structure before the Meiji period.

The Fukami family dominated Minamata for the rest of the Tokugawa period and well into Meiji (1868–1912), holding the post of *daikan* until it was abolished in 1870. There were a number of peasant rebellions, including four in the eighteenth century, with one in 1747 involving 7,000 to 8,000 persons, but none of these displaced the Fukami.[4] Neither were they or the other powerful local samurai families immediately displaced by the Meiji Restoration of 1868. A 1634 list of local samurai (*jizamurai*) includes nearly all the important families in Meiji period Minamata.[5] The first and fifth mayors of the village of Minamata (in office 1889–97 and 1904–10, respectively) were named Fukami.[6] Because of this continuity of control by the leading families from the Tokugawa period, Irokawa Daikichi suggests that Minamata's Meiji Restoration came only at the very end of the Meiji period, in 1908, when Noguchi Shitagau built his factory in the town.[7]

The Factory Comes to Minamata

> "There is probably no place in the world that changed as much as Minamata from the late Meiji period to the Taishō years."
>
> —Saiki Shigeru, Minamata, born 1901[8]

In 1907 Minamata was a town facing economic disaster. Its residents' two main sources of employment, other than small-scale farming, fishing, and shipping, had been salt production and the transport of coal. There were few other sources of cash income. Over 200 families had been involved in making salt, an enterprise begun in 1667 under Hosokawa sponsorship as a source of revenue for the domain.[9] The salt was shipped mostly to Amakusa, Shimabara, and Saga, and noodles (produced using the salt from Minamata), tiles, and pottery were imported in return. Since the Bakumatsu (late Tokugawa) period, the salt pans had been extended farther out to sea. In 1905, however, the central government decided to monopolize and rationalize salt production and sales to help cover the huge costs of the Russo-Japanese War (1904–5). By 1910, salt making in Minamata was ended.[10]

Over 400 carts had been used to transport coal, shipped from Ōmuta to Minamata, into the mountains to the gold mines at Ōkuchi and Ushio.[11] There it was used to provide energy and light. The carts returned laden with lumber and charcoal, which was shipped to Nagasaki and northern Kyūshū. The same mountains that held gold were also rich potential sources of hydroelectric power. The Sōgi Electric Corporation was established in 1906 to provide power to the mines; it also put carters and dockworkers out of business.

A group of leading figures (*yūshi*) of Minamata came up with a plan to save the village by turning its problems into advantages. In so doing, they were not only following in the creative footsteps of their forefathers who sent the white turtle to Empress Shōtoku in 768, they were also creating a model for local industrial policy in twentieth-century Japan.

The hydroelectric power that put Minamata's carters out of business was a new and growing industry in turn-of-the-century Japan. It also made possible other new industries, one of which was electrochemicals.[12] Noguchi Shitagau, a brilliant engineering graduate of Tokyo Imperial University, was making plans to build a calcium carbide factory south of Minamata, at Komenotsu in Kagoshima prefecture. Maeda Eiki, a member of a Minamata samurai family, formed a group of leading citizens determined to lure Noguchi and his factory to Minamata.[13] They argued that Minamata had a good harbor at Umedo and promised to provide cheap land, available in abundance near the mouth of the river as the salt industry disappeared. They even agreed to donate the poles for the two extra *ri* (about eight kilometers) of power lines needed to bring electricity to Minamata rather than to Komenotsu. Noguchi, "touched by their enthusiasm" (according to the official city history), decided on Minamata and set up a temporary office in Maeda's home.[14] The Nihon Carbide factory was completed in 1908; later that year Noguchi merged Nihon Carbide with Sōgi Electric to form Nihon chisso hiryō K.K. (Japan Nitrogenous Fertilizers, Inc.; usually referred to as Nitchitsu).

The successful *yūshi* may not have realized that this marked the end of their domination of Minamata. Many others did and refused to allow the power poles to be placed in their fields. Some landlords, like the town fathers in Sashiki, the village to the north, feared that laborers would no longer be available to work their fields.[15] It is clear from oral histories that many servants and poor tenant farmers were in fact glad to leave their old work for the factory, even though the factory paid less than the going wage (25 or 27 sen versus 35 sen per day).[16] Since they were considered desperate, having come from the lowest status jobs, those who took jobs at the factory were looked down on for some time.[17] Yet factory work was steady and in some ways liberating for servants and tenants.

No one could have imagined in 1908 that Nitchitsu would be at the forefront of high technology in imperial Japan, that it would grow to become one of the "new *zaibatsu*" and Japan's third largest manufacturer, and that it would industrialize northern Korea.[18] None could have dreamed that it would inflict on their town and the world the single worst long-term, man-made industrial pollution disaster in history.

The Growth of Nitchitsu

For Noguchi and for most people in Minamata, the future of both town and company looked bright in 1908. The main use of carbide at first was to produce acetylene, which fueled lamps on bicycles, at festivals, and in the coal mines where some from Minamata found work. In Minamata, acetylene lamps made possible the growth of night fishing. (Ironically, some early Minamata disease victims such as Hamamoto Tsuginori were later to be misdiagnosed as suffering from acetylene poisoning.) Electricity was supplied to the town long before most other rural areas in Japan. In 1909, Noguchi bought the rights to the German Frank-Caro calcium cyanamide process, in which calcium carbide was used to produce nitrogen fertilizer, absorbing nitrogen from the air. In a country with limited arable land and a great deal of small-scale tenant farming, and in which the most efficient farming practices were already widely diffused, fertilizer was seen as the best way to raise productivity.

In the following decades, Nitchitsu became a leader and model for Japan's chemical industry, just as Sony and Honda became models for postwar technological entrepreneurs. Although fertilizers were its main product for many years, it also used calcium carbide to produce acetic acid, ammonia, explosives, and butanol. It continued to develop new products, to import and improve on new processes and equipment, and before long to win its own patents and order its equipment in Japan.

Minamata grew with the company, reaching a population of 20,000 in 1921, 30,000 in 1941, 40,000 in 1948, and a peak of 50,000 in 1956.[19] The village became a town in 1912, and the town became a city in 1949. As early as 1920, 29.8 percent of Minamata's work force was employed by industry and only 50.7 percent was in agriculture; in all the rest of Kumamoto prefecture industry employed only 11.8 percent of the work force, and 63.8 percent were engaged primarily in agriculture.[20]

Even before its overseas ventures in Korea and elsewhere, government contacts were essential to Nitchitsu. From the start, it had to get water rights to build its dams. In September 1918 its president, Nakahashi Tokugorō, resigned to become minister of education. Partly at Nakahashi's urging, the ban on fertilizer exports was ended, bringing large profits for Nitchitsu on exports to Southeast Asia because World War I had cut off European supplies.[21]

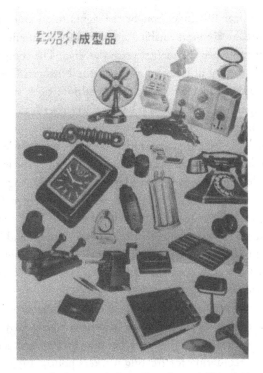

Fig. 1 Products made from Chissolite and Chissoloid,
from a 1937 Nihon Chisso publication.

Domestic sales skyrocketed as well, as imports of ammonium sulfate
dropped from 112,000 tons in 1913 to 1,000 tons in 1918, and the price on
the Japanese market rose from ¥151 ($74) to ¥372 ($191) per ton.[22] Ammonium sulfate sales grew from ¥1,865,117 ($933,000) in 1916 to ¥7,538,801
($3,807,000) in 1919, and total sales rose from ¥2,140,782 ($1,070,000) to
¥7,884,082 ($3,982,000) and Nitchitsu's share of Japanese production rose to
67 percent.[23] In 1914 Nitchitsu's new plant in Kagami, Kumamoto prefecture, produced Japan's first ammonium sulfate made using the nitrogen-
fixation method, and in 1918 a new facility at the Minamata factory began
using the same process, producing ammonium sulfate for around ¥70 per
ton and selling it for five and a half times cost. The corporation's annual net
profits exceeded 35 percent of its total worth in both 1918 and 1919.[24]

When prices plummeted after the war with the return of foreign competition, these profits saved Nitchitsu by enabling it to invest in new technology to lower its production costs. In 1921 Noguchi traveled to Europe, and at

the end of that year Nitchitsu bought the rights to an ammonia synthesis process that within five years enabled it to produce ammonium sulfate at a cost of ¥30 per ton when the market price was ¥150. The company also pursued a parallel strategy of lobbying through the Nitrogen Council (Chisso kyōgikai) for protection from foreign competition; tight restrictions were imposed on imports of ammonium sulfate in December 1931.[25]

The company grew steadily, and Noguchi continued to invest his profits in new technology. Nitchitsu expanded both horizontally and vertically, continuing to develop spin-off products, and remained at the leading edge of technological development in imperial Japan. The Nitchitsu group included 48 companies by April 1941.[26] It became what is known in Japanese as a *kontserun* (from the German *Konzern*), and one of the "new *zaibatsu*" (*shinkō zaibatsu*), along with such conglomerates as Mori, Nissan, and Nihon Soda. Noguchi came to be called "one man" in recognition of his power and management style, and was dubbed one of the "Four Heavenly Kings" along with other new *zaibatsu* leaders.[27]

Even as it grew into a massive conglomerate, Nitchitsu in its first half-century never lost its reputation as an innovative, technology-driven company, run by scientists and engineers rather than bankers and accountants. It also retained its reputation for treating workers poorly. Noguchi is said to have declared, "Don't think of workers as people; use them like cattle and horses."[28] Nitchitsu was one of the first companies in Japan to introduce the eight-hour day, but this was not done out of concern for the workers. It was difficult and unprofitable to shut down a large chemical factory. Three eight-hour shifts could keep the factory running nonstop; two ten-hour shifts could not.[29]

After the company began making ammonium sulfate through nitrogen synthesis at its Nobeoka plant in 1924, using what were then extremely high temperatures and pressures, Hashimoto Hikoshichi, one of the most important figures in Nitchitsu history, helped convert the Minamata factory to the new process. He went on to win numerous patents for producing organic chemicals from carbide.[30] One of these was acetaldehyde, which the factory began producing in 1932 using Hashimoto's new method, in which acetylene gas became acetaldehyde when blown over mercuric sulfate. Acetaldehyde had been produced in Germany since 1912 using what was known as the "excess acetylene method"; Hashimoto's technique became known as the "reaction liquid circulation method."[31] Both methods used mercury as a catalyst. Acetaldehyde production in Minamata peaked at 9,159 tons in 1940, a level not matched after the war until 1955, but by 1960 it was quintupled to 45,200 tons, 39 percent of the total produced in Japan.[32] The mercury used in producing this acetaldehyde was the cause of Minamata disease. Ironically, after rising to head the factory during World War II, Hashimoto went on to serve four terms as Minamata's mayor (1950–58 and 1962–70), a post he held when the disease was discovered.

Nitchitsu, Minamata, and Imperial Japan

Growth required new factories and new products. If land, power, and labor could be acquired cheaply, Nitchitsu could continue the innovation on which its growth was based.[33] Noguchi had been attracted to Kyūshū because of its hydropower potential and relatively low land and labor costs. By the 1920s, Korea offered similar advantages—on a far greater scale.

Korea became a Japanese protectorate in 1905 after the Russo-Japanese War and was annexed in 1910. By the 1920s control had been consolidated, and with its profits continuing (although not at the exceptional levels of 1915 through 1920), Nitchitsu had the capital to consider large-scale projects. To innovate, to keep costs down, and to expand his markets, Noguchi realized he needed to take advantage of the opportunities offered by Japan's colonial empire. The greatest of these, for him, was the vast hydroelectric potential of the rivers of northern Korea. Noguchi was not the first to recognize this potential, but the established *zaibatsu* hesitated to make the huge investments necessary to produce large amounts of electricity for which they saw little use. Noguchi was far more bold and soon was called the "entrepreneurial king of the peninsula."[34]

Nitchitsu established Chōsen chisso hiryō (Chōsen Nitrogen Fertilizers), which completed the first part of its huge chemical factory at Hungnam (Kōnan in Japanese) in 1929. What had been a small fishing village was soon home to 45,000 factory employees, and the city's total population reached 180,000 near the end of World War II.[35] In 1931 the electricity required to produce one ton of ammonium sulfate cost Chōsen chisso ¥12; the cost for Nitchitsu in the home islands was ¥21.[36] In 1933 the value of Chōsen chisso's fixed assets was eight times that of Nitchitsu's.[37] Nitchitsu sent its most talented workers, scientists, and managers to Korea, and everyone in the company came to see service in Korea as the best way to get ahead.[38]

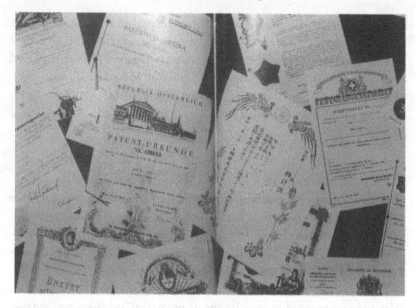

Fig. 2 Patents held by Nitchitsu in various countries, from a 1937 Nihon Chisso publication.

During the war, a number of Koreans also worked at the Minamata factory, beginning at least as early as 1942. Some, who had been working in the Chikuho coal mines to the north, came to Minamata for the higher wages. In 1980 one Korean former worker claimed that in 1942, when he began working at the factory, he earned ¥3.5 per day, and that as the labor shortage became more severe he and other Koreans were able to negotiate raises to ¥5, ¥8, and then ¥10.[39] These wage rates seem highly unlikely, given that in 1942 one senior worker, hired in 1909, earned ¥3.14, and another worker hired in 1940 earned ¥1.62.[40] Yet the facts that there were Koreans in Kyūshū who were not forced laborers but freely changed jobs in search of higher pay and that they negotiated raises as labor supplies became tighter during the war are worth noting.

Noguchi cultivated close ties with Japan's government officials in Korea, including General Ugaki Kazushige, governor-general from 1931 to 1936. While Noguchi was building a hydroelectric generating plant on the Changjin River, Ugaki built a vacation villa there. A meeting in this house in September 1936, attended by Ugaki and General Koiso Kuniaki, former head of Japan's Guandong (Kwantung) Army in Manchukuo, helped secure permission for a massive project on the Yalu River, the boundary between

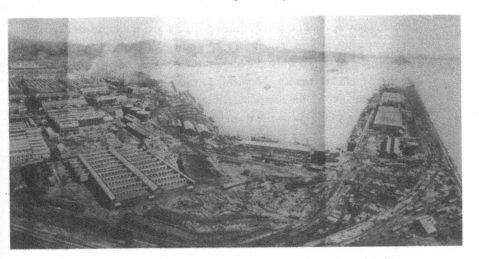

Fig. 3 Chōsen Chisso's Hungnam factory in Korea, from a 1937 Nihon Chisso publication.

Korea and Manchukuo.[41] The project began in October 1937 and used the world's largest crane to build the world's second largest dam (after Grand Coulee), for which some 100,000 residents of the area had to be moved.[42] As of 1942, 27 percent of all capital invested in Korea had come from Nitchitsu.[43]

Nitchitsu came to play an important role throughout Japan's empire. During the war it had operations in northern China (producing ammonium sulfate in Taiyuan), Taiwan (manufacturing explosives), Hainan Island (mining iron ore), and Southeast Asia (producing electricity, calcium carbide, aluminum, and soda). It planned but never built dams in Vietnam, but much of the development of hydroelectric power in Southeast Asia after the war, partly financed by Japanese reparations, was planned and supervised by Nihon kōei, a corporation formed in 1946 by former executives of Nitchitsu-affiliated companies in Korea and Manchuria.[44] Nitchitsu was Japan's largest civilian manufacturer of munitions and even produced synthetic fuel.[45] Its synthetic fuel plant, the world's third, operated at a loss for its first five years, but Noguchi explained that the only question was "what next will be the enterprise most useful to the nation."[46] What was good for the nation was good for Nitchitsu as well: at its founding in 1908 it was capitalized at ¥1 million ($493,000; paid-in capital); by 1945 this had increased to ¥3.5 billion.[47]

The company symbol on all Nitchitsu products was the Japanese flag, a red circle on a white field. Nitchitsu's importance to imperial Japan was publicly recognized in 1931 when the Shōwa emperor, Hirohito (r. 1926–89), visited the Minamata factory. Noguchi, as tour guide and host, walked ahead of the emperor, to the side of his red carpet. The author Ishimure Michiko, who was a young girl at the time, has written about the visit.[48] A policeman came to her house to explain that her blind, insane grandmother would be removed to Koiji Island in Minamata Bay during the visit, along with all beggars, lepers, and insane persons from the town. The benevolent authorities (_okami_, "those above") would provide food while watching that their charges did not attempt to swim off the island. Ishimure's father insisted that his mother was harmless and promised to lock her in the house, swearing that he would commit _seppuku_ (ritual disembowelment; less commonly called _hara kiri_) if she caused any trouble. The policeman relented, and the emperor's visit went smoothly.

The company's 1940 official history and description of the company explains the importance of Nitchitsu to the war effort in a section entitled "The Holy War and Nihon chisso":

Under His Majesty the Emperor, the people of Japan are now pressing onward with all their might toward the completion of the greatest enterprise since the founding of the nation....

Modern wars are total wars requiring the strength of the whole nation, and they are scientific wars. And industry is one component of military strength. Many sectors of the chemical industry are especially directly related to war; such products as gunpowder, explosives, and poison gas are foremost among these....

Nihon chisso is our nation's largest producer of explosives.

The book goes on to explain that Nitchitsu was unlike other manufacturers of explosives because it produced all the chemicals used in its explosives, such as ammonia, acetic acid, and glycerin. It boasts of the large amounts and high quality of these chemicals. The descriptions of the artificial fuel produced in Korea and the capacity of its generating stations there are heavily censored. The work concludes by saying: "In this holy war Nihon chisso should not be seen as a profit-making company; it should be called a huge chemical combine that is a national policy corporation. Nihon chisso's mission is truly important and great. All 70,000 employees are united in carrying out their important duties day and night."[49]

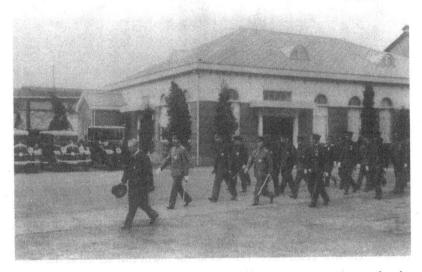

Fig. 4 The Shōwa emperor Hirohito's visit to the Minamata factory, 1931. Company founder Noguchi Shitagau is in the lead, followed by the emperor. © The Mainichi Newspapers.

Nitchitsu's fortunes rose and fell with the empire to which it was so intimately tied. All its overseas possessions were lost with the defeat in 1945, and its factories in Japan were bombed heavily. Noguchi Shitagau, who suffered a brain hemorrhage in 1940 and died in 1944, did not live to see his empire collapse along with Japan's.

TWO

Minamata Before the Disease

Nitchitsu and Minamata Society

After the Nitchitsu factory was built in 1908, Minamata rapidly became a company town under the third of its historical rulers. It was often referred to as Nitchitsu's "castle town" (*jōkamachi*; the towns that served as the headquarters of the *daimyō* in the Tokugawa period), with the company as "feudal lord" (*tonosama*). The replacement of the old samurai and landlord families by a large modern corporation did not make Minamata society any less hierarchical. If anything, it strengthened the hierarchy, widened the gap between top and bottom, and intensified the discrimination and prejudice against those on the lower rungs.

Like other companies, Nitchitsu drew a sharp line between its blue-collar workers (*kōin*; literally "factory persons") and its white-collar engineers and managers (*shain*; "company persons").[1] The former were paid a daily wage that started at 40 sen (¥0.4) in 1918, an amount that would yield annual earnings well below that year's average per capita consumption of roughly ¥148. Middle-school-graduate, white-collar workers began at a salary of ¥18 per month; university graduates got ¥45. The annual bonus for factory workers in 1916 was 5 days' pay; regular *shain* received 3 months' and higher executives 10 months' pay.[2] Blue- and white-collar employees were strictly separated, both on the job and at lunch. The laborers carried their lunches from home, and servants ("boys," *bōi*) delivered boxed meals to the white-collar workers who chose not to eat in the Shiranui Club, the dining hall open only to *shain*. White-collar employees and their families, it was said, were served first at stores, restaurants, and doctors' offices, and schoolteachers were said to favor their children.[3]

What made the gap broader than those in many other companies was the fact that at this factory so far from Tokyo, engineers and managers were graduates of elite schools and universities in the capital and had difficulty understanding the workers's dialect. Virtually all the *kōin* were from the Minamata area and the Amakusa islands, and few had been educated much beyond elementary school. Until 1947 Japan's education system was two-tracked beyond elementary school, with higher elementary schools leading to vocational or normal schools, and middle schools leading to higher schools and then universities. There was no higher elementary school for boys in Minamata until 1935, although one for girls was built in 1911.[4] Since the factory saw little need for advanced education for its workers, neither did the town.

Outside the factory, one could judge a person's rung on the social ladder simply by knowing where he or she lived.[5] In Minamata, as in other former castle towns, the segregation of the social classes in different districts remained evident. In Jinnai, at the foot of the hills where Minamata castle had once stood, the old native upper class was joined by the factory managers and high executives. Across the river from Jinnai is Hama-chō, the former merchants' and craftsmen's quarter. On the northern bank of the mouth of the river is Shirahama, also called Sarugō ("Monkey Village") or Tonton-mura. This was the home of the lowest strata of society, of the crematorium, and of the isolation hospital to which many early Minamata disease sufferers were confined. Ishimure Michiko lived in Shirahama and remembers neighbors' strategies to "reduce the number of mouths" (*kuchiberashi*) to be fed: girls were sold into prostitution; others went to Chikuhō (northern Kyūshū) to work in the mines or to factories in the Kansai or Kinki regions.[6]

Across the river was Funatsu, whose inhabitants were said to have immigrated from somewhere across the sea. Stories were told of children in Funatsu with three eyes. Its inhabitants supposedly spoke a dialect so different it was nearly a foreign language, and parents in other parts of town warned their children they must never associate with—or, heaven forbid, marry—anyone from Funatsu.

Moving south from the Minamata River, on the other side of the factory is the old farming village of Tsukinoura. Next is Detsuki, which branched off from Tsukinoura and was therefore one rung lower in social standing. Most families there combined farming and fishing. Following the coast farther south, one passes through the fishing hamlet of Yudō to Modō, on the

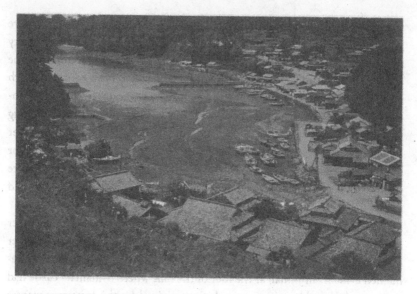

Fig. 5 The fishing hamlet of Modō at low tide, 1960. © Kuwabara Shisei.

border with Kagoshima prefecture. As one travels from Tsukinoura to
Modō, there is less and less farmland; in Modō most families depend on
fishing for their living. Along this same stretch, the percentage of families
who migrated to Minamata from Amakusa over the past three or four generations also increases.

The historian Irokawa Daikichi has analyzed the "social pathology" resulting from this geography of status.[7] The elite from Tokyo scorned the
crude country bumpkins of Minamata, the descendants of samurai looked
down on the commoners, executives looked down on blue-collar workers,
townspeople looked down on those in outlying farming and fishing hamlets,
farmers looked down on fisherfolk, and the native born looked down on
immigrants. This "pathology" greatly complicated the responses to Minamata disease (most of whose early victims were from fishing families in the
hamlets on the southern fringes of Minamata) and was effectively used by
the company to protect itself. The hierarchy of status in Minamata was
challenged only after World War II, in union attempts in 1953 to eliminate
discrimination against blue-collar workers, in the 1959 riots at the factory by
fishermen, and in the bitter, divisive factory strike in 1962–63.[8] By the late

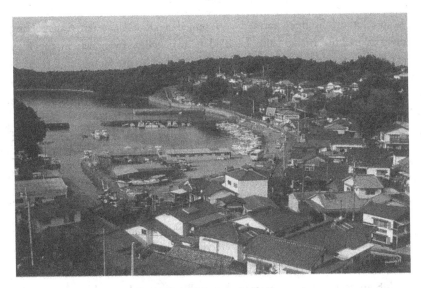

Fig. 6 Modō in 1994. © Timothy S. George.

1960s, the struggle by and for disease victims was to many people equally a struggle against what they considered an oppressive, "feudal" structure of discrimination. The strength of this structure (although I would not call it feudal in the 1960s) and the dominant role of the company help explain why effective action came so slowly in Minamata, compared to the sites of other major pollution incidents in Japan.

At its peak the company employed over a tenth of the population of Minamata, and there were few families without a *kaisha-yuki* (literally, someone who "goes to the company") relative. From Izumi, just south of Minamata, to Tsunagi in the north, elementary schools would recommend their top ten graduates each year for the Nitchitsu examinations, rumored to be more difficult than the middle-school entrance examinations. In 1932 Nitchitsu hired 11 of the 489 boys who took the tests.[9]

One who took a job at the factory was Onitsuka Iwao.[10] The Onitsuka family has lived for generations in the steep hills not far inland from the factory, in the hamlet of Samurai (pronounced "Samune" by its residents) on the Satsuma *kaidō*, the road used by the *daimyō* of Satsuma for their trips between Edo and their powerful domain at the southern end of Kyūshū.

Iwao's father, Shinpei, farmed and pulled a *jinrikisha*, often transporting doctors making house calls; he died in 1939 when Iwao was in the fifth grade.[11] In 1943, at the age of 14, Iwao was hired by the factory as a second-class *kōin* at a daily wage of 70 sen. His mother's response to the news was to admonish him never to urinate facing the factory. He retired in 1983 at the age of 55 (at the time, still the normal retirement age in Japan).

Chemical factories can be dangerous places to work. The residents of Minamata grew accustomed not only to the smells but also to the frequent explosions. Onitsuka recalls:

"When I first started, there was an explosion every three or four days, or every week. If there were no explosions for a while, we'd fear it was about time for another. . . . The company talked about 'safety, safety,' but that was just putting a fig leaf over their production first policy, telling everyone to produce just one more ton. . . . Where was the famous 'Chisso technology'?"[12]

Job applicants had to attest to their willingness to brave these dangers. In the first Minamata disease trial, longtime worker (1932–65) Chō Michiaki testified that in his job interview (by then–production manager Hashimoto Hikoshichi and others), he was asked: " 'There may be explosions; can you accept this?'. . . By leaving home and coming to take the exam, I had already decided to risk my life, so I answered: 'Yes, I'm willing to die.'"[13] In 1952, 18 percent of the factory's employees were injured on the job.[14] The Shin Nitchitsu factory was actually a bit safer than others, since the overall injury rate for the chemical industry in 1952 was 24 percent.[15]

Defeat, Recovery, and Boom

During the war, Nitchitsu's Minamata factory was administered by the military and renamed "Kumamoto Factory #7042." It made products for the army and navy ranging from explosives to bulletproof glass. At the end of the war, its 4,151 employees included 620 students and 100 members of "women's volunteer corps" mobilized to keep the factory fully staffed.[16] Soldiers from Korea, the "Arirang Brigade," were brought in as forced laborers to dig a network of cave shelters large enough to hold all 4,000 factory workers during air raids.[17] After bombings, the Koreans were assigned to dig out of the rubble the bodies of those who had not made it to the shelters.[18] Onitsuka Iwao was one of the workers assigned to purge the acetylene gas tanks when the air raid sirens sounded and could not take shelter until the job was done. This left no time to reach the large tunnel shelters dug by the Koreans, and he and his coworkers had to huddle in tiny three-man holes known as "octopus pots."[19]

The city was bombed thirteen times between March 29 and August 11, 1945.[20] It was hit with high explosives, cluster bombs, and then in early August with firebombs (napalm). Most but not all of the bombs were aimed at the factory, and much of the city was burned. The last attack was a strafing of company housing in Jinnai by P-38s. When the war ended on August 15, the factory was almost completely destroyed, at least 69 people had been killed, and 1,500 homes had been destroyed.[21] On that day, it was announced that all those in the factory were to assemble in front of the air raid shelters. There they heard the emperor's radio broadcast announcing the end of the war. The sound quality was so poor and the language so strange that Onitsuka was not sure what had happened until he saw women crying and heard people saying "We've lost the war. They've dropped a parachute bomb on Nagasaki." Others called it a "light bomb." Only much later did he learn that it had been an atomic bomb.[22]

On August 22, a seven-member American survey team arrived to study the effectiveness of the bombing and investigate the capacity of Japan's chemical industry. Factory manager Hashimoto served them *sukiyaki* at his home and then gave them a tour of the factory.[23] They reported that 49 tons of bombs had hit the plant and that "incendiary machine gun bullets were reported by the Japanese as being especially effective in setting fire to wooden buildings." They estimated that factory repairs would require 972,200 man-hours. "So far as is known," they wrote, "only one other chemical plant, the Kawasaki Plant of the Shōwa Electrical Industry Co., was hit by a higher tonnage of high-explosive bombs."[24]

After August 15, Onitsuka spent the next week or ten nights on guard duty at the factory gates. There was little left to guard, however, and with the end of the war Nitchitsu, like the Japanese empire, lost all of its vast overseas assets. Within a few years the Occupation's *zaibatsu*-busting program deprived the company of its domestic holdings except for the Minamata plant itself.[25]

The Mission on Japanese Combines submitted a report to the U.S. State and War departments in 1946 dealing with Nitchitsu and eighteen other *zaibatsu*. The description of the company in the "Edwards Report" would seem to be a recommendation against harsh punishment:

The company's growth has consisted chiefly in starting new plants and new subsidiary companies, not in acquiring control of going concerns. . . . Nippon Chisso's
growth has been based primarily upon the exploitation of Korea rather than the
expansion of Japanese war industry. . . . The war actually reduced the rate of capital
expansion. . . . Since . . . the foremost 10 stockholders have less than 21% of the
total stock issue, it appears improbable that the company is controlled by any one
combine.

Yet Nitchitsu was broken up. The report goes on to say that:

Nippon Chisso has submitted a voluntary dissolution plan. According to this proposal, claims based upon overseas properties, which it estimates at more than 80% of
the total investment by itself and its subsidiaries, are to be retained by Nippon
Chisso. However, the part of the combine which is in Japan is to be broken up.[26]

Nitchitsu did have some important assets left, and these enabled it to recover even before the U.S. procurements of supplies and services for the Korean War that are often credited with jump-starting Japan's postwar economy. Like Japan as a whole, only more so, Nitchitsu had an inexpensive,
capable labor force. Its technological knowledge and its cadre of skilled,
creative scientists and engineers meant that Nitchitsu, unlike many other
factories, had no immediate need to buy foreign technology. This would
have been financially and politically difficult just after the war. At its inception, some in the Occupation envisioned a Japanese economy based on agriculture, and overall the Occupation authorities showed little interest in
helping factories rebuild and modernize.

Nitchitsu's dams and power stations in the mountains of Kyūshū had
sustained little damage during the war, and production at the Minamata
factory was resumed less than two months after the defeat. The country
suffered from a food shortage and its farmers needed fertilizer, and in the
early days factory workers traded fertilizer and salt to farmers for food. In
1949 the Occupation permitted Nitchitsu to resume production of polyvinyl
chloride (PVC).

That same year, as part of a tour of Kyūshū during which he also visited
the Yawata Steel complex and the Mitsui Miike coal mine, the Shōwa emperor visited the Nitchitsu factory for the second time.[27] Nitchitsu symbolized the strong belief in postwar Japan in science and technology, a belief expressed in a letter the emperor had written in September 1945 to his
son, Crown Prince Akihito, to explain why Japan had lost the war: "Our

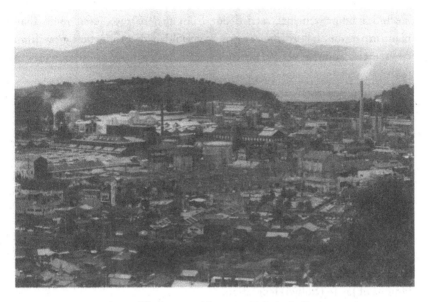

Fig. 7 The factory in Minamata. © Onitsuka Iwao.

people put too much faith in the empire and made light of the British and Americans. Our military gave too much weight to spirit and forgot about science."[28]

In 1950, the year after the emperor's visit, production matched its prewar peak, and the company was reorganized as Shin Nihon chisso hiryō K.K. (New Japan Nitrogenous Fertilizers, Inc.), capitalized at ¥400 million ($1.1 million). By 1955 this had been tripled to ¥1.2 billion ($3.3 million), and the amount doubled the next year to ¥2.4 billion ($6.7 billion).[29] The PVC plastic market grew rapidly in the 1950s, and Shin Nitchitsu, still called the "head temple" (*sōhonzan*) of the chemical industry, did well.[30] It gained a virtual monopoly on the production of dioctyl phthalate (DOP, produced from octyl alcohol), an essential ingredient in the production of film, electric wire insulation, and other products made from PVC. In 1952 Shin Nitchitsu built Japan's first octyl alcohol production facility, producing octyl alcohol from acetaldehyde, which was an intermediate product in making PVC as well.

When the rest of Japan suffered a short slump in 1957–58 after the Jinmu Boom (1955–57), Shin Nitchitsu kept right on booming. The factory newspaper reported in the spring of 1957 that Shin Nitchitsu could not keep up with the skyrocketing demand for vinyl chloride, DOP, and octanol.[31]

Technical improvements carried out from 1951 to 1956, even more than plant expansion, helped the company's acetaldehyde production grow from 5,000 metric tons per year in 1950 to 10,000 in 1955 to a peak of 50,000 tons in 1961.[32]

A union was established at the factory in 1946, but it was decimated in the Red Purge that began with Supreme Commander for the Allied Powers Douglas MacArthur's criticism of the Japan Communist Party in May 1950, just before the beginning of the Korean War. The Occupation, which was by then pursuing Cold War objectives rather than its early anti-*zaibatsu* policies, encouraged the Japanese government to purge communists instead of the militarists who had been the focus in the first years of the Occupation. At Shin Nitchitsu, 25 factory workers and three others were purged.[33] Everyone else quit the union. In 1951 the union was reorganized as part of the Japanese Federation of Synthetic Chemistry Workers Unions (known by its abbreviated name, Gōka Rōren) in the new General Council of Trade Unions of Japan (Sōhyō) federation.

Shin Nitchitsu's union was somewhat late, and achieved mixed results, in joining Sōhyō's "workplace struggles" (*shokuba tōsō*), which Andrew Gordon has called the "early postwar surge of organizing and collective action [in which] blue-collar workers gained 'citizenship' in the enterprise and a measure of control over it."[34] In August 1953 the union finally demanded an end to the strict blue collar–white collar (*kōin-shain*) status system that had already been eliminated in many other companies and went on strike for 40 days. This struggle for the first time turned many workers into activists and made them concerned with discrimination inside and outside the factory— changes in worker consciousness that were to have important repercussions in the divisive strike of 1962–63 and again in the movement on behalf of victims of Minamata disease after 1968.

After the 1953 strike, the company agreed to designate all employees *shain* when the new fiscal year began in April 1954, but there was no immediate agreement on the pay system. In 1955, pay for blue-collar workers at Shin Nitchitsu ranked eleventh out of the twelve companies in its field, but pay for department and section heads was second from the top.[35] However, beginning in 1958 all employees were paid under a combination of the daily wage and monthly salary systems. The retirement age, which had been 55 for white-collar and 50 for blue-collar employees, was fixed at 55 for all employees after July 21, 1958.[36]

Despite these victories, the union never gained significant control over the operations of the factory and company, as happened at least temporarily in some other companies. An example close to Minamata was Mitsubishi's Miike coal mine. Workers there went on strike for 113 days in 1953 and, between 1953 and 1960, had rather striking success in "democratizing" control of working conditions.[37] The Minamata union's inability to follow suit is usually explained as a result of the company tradition, begun by Noguchi, of taking a hard line against workers. This tradition was supposedly intensified by the colonialist attitudes brought home by the executives repatriated from Korea, who by the early 1950s had forced aside many of the managers who had remained in Minamata.[38] This is an important part of the explanation, but not all of it. Another part is the fact that close central observation and control of the work process is both easier and more necessary in a chemical factory than in industries such as mining or shipbuilding in which workers gained more autonomy.

Minamata Politics in the 1950s

A further reason for the success of Shin Nitchitsu's hard line was the company's political prominence in its "castle town," a dominance far greater than was common even in other company towns. This dominance was strengthened in the residents' consciousness by the geographic isolation of the city. Minamata is surrounded by mountains on three sides. From the city, no place beyond Minamata is visible except for the Amakusa islands across the sea—and rather than offering an escape hatch for the people of Minamata, they had long been the main source of newcomers seeking jobs in Minamata.

In fiscal year 1954, Shin Nitchitsu and its employees accounted for 45.5 percent of the city's total tax income. Because of the strike over the blue collar–white collar status system, individual taxes paid by workers were lower than usual; 37.4 percent of the total paid by all city residents. The previous year Shin Nitchitsu employees had paid 51.2 percent.[39] In 1960 the company's taxes made up 48 percent of total municipal tax receipts.[40] That same year Shin Nitchitsu and a subsidiary, Shin Nihon kagaku, accounted for 19.2 percent of the 19,819 persons employed in Minamata, and 85.3 percent of those in manufacturing. Primary industry (fishing, farming, and forestry) and secondary industry (manufacturing and construction) each employed just over 30 percent of all workers, and tertiary industry (wholesale and retail sales, finance, transportation, service, and government work) took just under

40 percent. If Shin Nitchitsu's suppliers are included, it was probably responsible for creating a quarter of all jobs in Minamata.[41]

Mayoral politics provide some insight into the complex effects of Shin Nitchitsu's presence.[42] Ui Jun once suggested that "the actual lord of this castle town is industrial capital, and the mayor is the intendant (*daikan*) appointed by the lord."[43] One might expect, then, that the Liberal Democratic Party (LDP), Japan's most conservative and business-oriented party, would dominate local politics. Yet since this was not always the case, at first glance it might not seem that the company's influence was decisive. The mayor from 1950 to 1958, and again from 1962 to 1970, was aligned with progressive forces, particularly the Japan Socialist Party (JSP). In fact, however, this ostensibly progressive mayor was Hashimoto Hikoshichi, the former Nitchitsu engineer who devised the mercury catalyst method for producing acetaldehyde in 1932. Hashimoto, the factory manager during the war, was later forced out by executives repatriated from Chōsen chisso in Korea. He was elected mayor as a reformist, with broad union support.

With the company union constituting by far the largest voting bloc in the city, it was difficult to be elected without its backing. It also elected many of the city council members. The union was ostensibly JSP-affiliated, but supporting its members' interests often meant supporting those of the company. Some in Minamata therefore reversed the first two characters of the name "Socialist Party"—Shakaitō—and called it the Kaishatō ("company party").[44]

Mayor Hashimoto's efforts on behalf of the company gave little hint of any resentment he might have felt against the executives who had taken his place. He worked hard to get Minamata's Hyakken Harbor dredged, rebuilt, and declared an international trade port. The port, originally built in the 1930s by the prefecture, had been silted in by factory sludge and become unusable, but the company was not asked to contribute to the costs. The reopened port cut Shin Nitchitsu's freight costs by two thirds, and 99 percent of the imports and exports passing through it were Shin Nitchitsu's.[45]

Mayor Hashimoto became less progressive over the years. Local politics in Minamata, however, boiled down to a competition not so much between progressives and conservatives as between, on the one hand, the interests of the company and its union and, on the other, the agricultural and fishing areas on the fringes of the city, which provided more support for the LDP. Much of the debate in the city council concerned incorporating adjacent areas into the city, which would have benefited the LDP most. Local LDP leaders, however, received so little support from prefectural and national party officials that they privately called their party not the Jimintō (Liberal Democratic Party), but the Jibuntō ("on-your-own party").[46]

Both sides in Minamata politics were internally divided and ideologically confused and frustrated. Independent shopkeepers and business people were torn between the two. They aspired to the status enjoyed by Shin Nitchitsu executives but did not share their cosmopolitan background and elite education. They had little sympathy for union activists or farmers and fisherfolk. At the same time they felt squeezed by the company's economic domination of the city, symbolized by Suikōsha, the cooperative department store for Shin Nitchitsu employees, which sold everything from soy sauce and kerosene to radios, clothing, and groceries, taking away much of the benefit Minamata businesses might have gained from Shin Nitchitsu employees' consumption.[47] Suikōsha was founded as an employees' cooperative in 1920, and in 1981 it became a regional cooperative open to anyone. That year saw the opening of the Kotobukiya department store, its first real competition. As late as 1985, however, Suikōsha still accounted for a third of Minamata's retail sales, a quarter of its retail floor space, and one-seventh of its retail employees.[48] The political fragmentation and economic weakness of those parts of the community not affiliated with Shin Nitchitsu slowed and restricted the responses of Minamata and its government to Minamata disease after its official discovery in 1956.

Newspapers were a potential counterweight to the dominance of the company, as Ui Jun has noted.[49] But this potential was not realized until 1968 and later, in the second round of responses to the disease. In the first round, the national papers largely ignored Minamata. The regional and local papers did little investigative journalism and usually took a detached, "neutral" stance, which tended to benefit the company more than its victims.

The newspapers read in Minamata included the *Kumamoto nichinichi shinbun* (Kumamoto daily newspaper), based in Kumamoto city; the *Nishinippon shinbun* (West Japan newspaper), with headquarters in Fukuoka; and national dailies such as the *Asahi shinbun* and the *Mainichi shinbun*. There were also smaller regional papers, such as the *Minami Nihon shinbun* (South Japan newspaper) from Kagoshima and the *Amakusa minpō* (Amakusa people's report) and *Amakusa shinbun* from the Amakusa Islands. Perhaps most interesting were two small Minamata papers. The *Minamata jiji shinpō* (Minamata current events news) was generally sympathetic to the company, whereas the *Minamata taimusu* (Minamata times), a carefully handwritten paper whose motto was "the big events in a small town," proved to be more sympathetic to fishers and Minamata disease victims. The company pushed its own line in the *Minamata kōjō shinbun* (Minamata factory newspaper), later renamed *Chisso Minamata*.

Life in Minamata in the 1950s: Hamamoto Tsuginori

Socially and materially, life in Minamata in the early 1950s was similar to that of two decades earlier. Although it was an industrial city, Minamata was quite rural in character outside its small center. Few residents were without relatives working for the company, but at the same time there were few who did not do at least a little farming or fishing. Of the company's 4,063 employees in March 1950, 44 percent engaged in farming as a secondary occupation. The proportion is even higher—68 percent—if employees living in company housing are excluded.[50] For many residents of Minamata, fishing and farming continued to set the patterns for daily life, even if they came to mark these patterns with the factory whistle and the passing trains as much as with the sun and the tides.

Hamamoto Tsuginori and his family, living in the hamlet of Detsuki, illustrate many of the common patterns of life in Minamata.[51] They engaged in fishing, farming, forestry, and factory work. Tsuginori's father, Sōhachi, moved the family to Minamata from Amakusa around 1934. He had fished there as a net owner (*amimoto*), hiring assistants (*amiko*) to help him use his nets (*ami*) to fish for sardines.[52] Looking for a better life, he sold his house, nets, and boat and moved to Minamata. There he worked as a construction worker building the new harbor at Hyakken and as a miner in the Chikuhō area. Working for others did not suit him, however, and since the money was not as good as he had hoped, he went back to fishing.

The eldest son, Kazunori, was a good student and went to middle school. He worked at Nitchitsu before going off to war, and his boss promised he could have his job back if he returned. He did come back, but since he thought the company's prospects after the war were poor and considered its wages too low, he took a series of jobs in Osaka factories. Kazunori was wrong about the company's future, but leaving Minamata saved him from the disease that struck the family members who stayed.

Tsuginori was born in 1936. As the war progressed, air raid drills took up more and more time in elementary school, and he and other children went after school to the local shrine or the neighborhood meeting hall for extra tutoring. He remembers the bombings of the factory vividly but had little knowledge at the time of what the factory made.

After the war, from about the time he was in sixth grade, Tsuginori helped row the family's four-meter fishing boat. The Hamamotos' staple diet consisted mostly of fish and sweet potatoes. They grew about three months' supply of dry-field rice, but like most people living in the rural outskirts of Minamata, they did not eat rice every day. They rented small fields, paying as rent the seeds from the *haze* (Japan wax) trees that bordered or were scattered through the fields. With the coming of land reform after the war, they and other tenants gained ownership of their fields. However, controversy and a lawsuit resulted in Minamata when the former landlord (a wax company) claimed it still owned the trees. The suit dragged on from 1951 to 1967, when the company won, and the farmers had to pay it a total of ¥10,000,000 ($27,800) for the trees. Onitsuka Iwao's family paid ¥23,677 ($66).[53]

In the winter, Hamamoto Tsuginori and his father supplemented their income by cutting wood in the hills for charcoal. Areas were assigned by lot, and the woodcutters were paid according to the amount they cut. The two of them could earn ¥12,000 to ¥16,000 ($33 to $44) in two months of work. The family also raised calves to earn money. Tsuginori's sister Fumiyo worked in the fields and sold fish door to door or at the market. To transport the fish in Minamata, the family had one cart with wooden, iron-banded wheels and another with bicycle wheels. They occasionally took mullet by train to Kumamoto, where the price was higher.

In 1951, when Tsuginori finished middle school, the Hamamotos bought a boat with an engine and built what is still the family home for ¥100,000 ($280). The new boat put them in a rather elite group: even three years later, in 1954, only 106 of Minamata's 497 fishing boats had engines.[54] The financial strain meant that Tsuginori did not attend high school, but helped with the fishing and other work full time. Shrimp netting became popular, and he remembers making up to ¥10,000 ($28) in a single night. Several years later, when he took his first paying job, he was shocked to earn only around ¥8,000 ($22) per month. This was the first time, he says, that he realized the value of money and the need to work hard for it.[55]

Hamamoto says that "books on Minamata disease say 'many fishing families were poor,' but my family was not very poor."[56] As farmers and fishers, they were probably better off than most city dwellers in the first few postwar years. Well into the 1950s, they rarely used much cash. They had yet to be left behind by the high growth that was just beginning or to be exposed to the rising expectations and consumerism that both fueled and were fueled by that growth. And they had yet to discover that they were being exposed to the toxic mercury that also helped catalyze Japan's growth.

Minamata from 1907 to 1955 condensed much of the experience of Japan's century of modern development that began in the mid-1800s. At the beginning of the twentieth century, the village was still an isolated backwater politically, governed by the same families that had held power for several centuries. Within a few decades it was intimately tied to Japan's empire and rewarded with a visit from the emperor. Before the coming of the factory, it had an active but preindustrial economy. Minamata's leaders, in a model of local industrial policy, lured to the village a company that made it not only an industrial city but also in some ways an internal colony.[57] Minamata served as the home base of a company that was active throughout the Japanese empire and symbolized the leading edge of technological and industrial development. In 1945, Nitchitsu lost its overseas empire, and its Minamata factory was virtually flattened. But drawing on its technology and labor force and the growing market for its products, the company and its city recovered and boomed even faster than Japan as a whole.

Yet not everything in Minamata reflected conditions throughout the nation, and some of these peculiarities were decisive in conditioning responses to the disease that was discovered in 1956. Minamata was even more of a company town than the steel-producing city of Kamaishi or Toyota's Toyota city.[58] Land reform, intended by the Americans to help democratize Japan, strengthened the position of the company by weakening landlords as rivals for economic, social, and political power.[59] Residents of all backgrounds, throughout the area, worked at the factory. Nearly everyone saw the company and the city as one unit, a "community sharing a single fate" (*unmei kyōdōtai*).[60] When demands for compensation for Minamata disease seemed likely to harm the company, many citizens would rally to defend it in order to defend their city.

Although the city's fate was considered inseparable from that of the company, community ties in the outlying fishing hamlets from which most of the first and worst disease victims came were relatively weak compared with those in many other rural areas in Japan, and getting weaker. Fishing requires less community cooperation than rice farming, and many of the residents of these areas were recent immigrants to Minamata. Factory work and the slow spread of a cash economy also served to weaken the traditional community.[61] Institutions such as the young people's associations were disappearing in the early 1950s, as were many local festivals and rituals. The traditional hierarchy of prejudice and discrimination, however, was not weakened but perpetuated by the changes the coming of the factory brought. Finally, although fishers did well into the 1950s, they were soon to be overtaken by the tremendous economic transformation of Japan's second and third postwar decades, becoming symbols of the life the nation had left behind. These same decades saw Shin Nitchitsu fall from the top ranks of Japanese corporations. Its last appearance on the list of Japan's 100 largest corporations was in 1955, when it was ranked 99th.[62] With its cohesion weakening and its hierarchy hardening, Minamata was sick before it was struck by Minamata disease. Yet its problems before the disease differed mainly in degree—due to the exceptionally powerful presence of the factory—from those of many other rural industrial cities in Japan.

The First Round of Responses

PART II

The First Round of Responses

THREE

Discovering the Disease and Its Cause

The unknown disease that afflicted Hamamoto Tsuginori was officially "discovered" on May 1, 1956. On the same day, Minamata was designated an official foreign trade port, and the city inaugurated a three-year plan to make itself a "city of health and welfare." The reality of the next few years could not have betrayed the plan more cruelly.

Three stories unfolded. The first was the search for the cause. This began with remarkable cooperation among medical and scientific specialists and local government officials, but then stalled in the face of obstacles thrown up by the company and the central government. The second was the struggle by fisherfolk in Minamata and throughout the Shiranui Sea to survive economically by obtaining compensation for the income they lost, as catches and prices declined and demand for fish from Minamata disappeared. Finally, there were the efforts by the victims, struggling with painful disease, ostracism, persistent false rumors, and financial disaster, to obtain compensation for their suffering and losses. Woven through all of these are the efforts of the company to prosper and evade responsibility, and of many groups in the city to protect the company in order to protect Minamata, as well as the reluctance of the government to jeopardize the industrial growth that was already the centerpiece of its policies. Japan's "economic miracle" was bought at the price of citizens' health and lives and communities.

The events of these years show a criminally irresponsible corporation achieving remarkable success at covering up its responsibility and the huge volume of poisons it discharged and at promoting false explanations for the disease. Government at all levels was responsible as well, and for a time research funding had to come from the United States. The city, the prefecture, the Diet and cabinet, the Ministry of International Trade and Industry (MITI), the Economic Planning Agency (EPA), the Ministry of Health and

Welfare—all failed to prevent or limit the tragedy. Minamata emerged at precisely the moment when major development policies were about to be promoted, and it could not be allowed to delay or derail them. The government disbanded a research group in 1959 and did not announce that discharges of mercury from the factory were causing the disease until 1968— condemning hundreds or thousands more people to the disease. And unlike the corporation, which was forced by victims' lawsuits to accept legal responsibility for the disease in 1973, the local and national governments have managed to avoid accepting legal responsibility. Scientists, doctors, and members of the media also contributed to the problem in this first round of responses, intentionally and unintentionally and through their inability to withstand social pressures. The resulting sense of guilt caused some of them to act differently a few years later.

The many names used for the disease soon after its discovery testify to the confusion surrounding it. The most common name was "strange disease" (*kibyō*), but it was also called "Tsukinoura disease," "dancing cat disease" (*neko odori byō*), "sauntering disease" (*burabura byō*), and "fashionable" or "stylish disease" (*hai kara byō*).[1]

In the eight months after Dr. Hosokawa Hajime reported the disease on May 1, 1956, effective cooperation at the local and prefectural levels went a long way toward discovering the cause. After January 1957, however, progress slowed to a crawl as investigators attempted to identify the heavy metal causing the disease and prove exactly where it came from. Inter-ministerial disputes at the national level, and above all Shin Nitchitsu's effective diversionary tactics, meant the cause was not conclusively proven to be organic mercury until 1959, the mechanism and location of the creation of organic mercury were not explained until 1961 (and not reported in newspapers until 1963), and the final riddles of why Minamata disease appeared where and when it did were not solved until 1998. The company continued to deny responsibility and promote other explanations until the government finally announced its official findings in September 1968—over twelve years after the disease was discovered and four months after the company stopped producing acetaldehyde in Minamata.

Ui Jun uses a four-stage model to describe Minamata and Japan's other major pollution incidents.[2] First, people become aware of the pollution. Second, in order to determine the proper countermeasures, a search for the cause begins. Although one might expect this to be a rapid process, it takes a great deal of time to link cause and effect conclusively since the balance of power and information favors the polluter. (This assumes, as was the case in Minamata and many other major pollution incidents, that the polluting company knows itself to be the source of the problem.) In the third stage, countertheories are issued or sponsored by the polluter, and with so many explanations from which to choose, the public becomes confused and unable to tell fact from fiction. This is the fourth stage, a sort of limbo in which all the theories "neutralize" each other. Between 1956 and 1959, the Minamata disease incident progressed through the first three of these stages, and then it stalled in the fourth for nearly a decade.

The early efforts to understand what was happening in Minamata were led by two men, Hosokawa Hajime and Itō Hasuo, head of the municipal health department. Both were exceptionally capable, sympathetic, approachable, and highly respected on all sides, especially by victims of the disease. Their efforts, especially those of Hosokawa, still loom large in narratives of the Minamata story as examples of what could and should have been done by others and of the overwhelming pressures on conscientious authorities. Hosokawa kept relatively quiet for many years after his research suggested the factory was the cause of the disease. Why Hosokawa, who finally broke his public silence by testifying from his deathbed in 1970, remains so universally respected by patients and activists is one of the most fascinating, puzzling, and important questions of the entire Minamata disease incident.[3] He was a good man, and a good doctor, who kept silent for many years because of the difficulty of transgressing social restraints. Patients respect him for the compassion he showed them and sympathize with him for the pressures he faced from the company and the city.

Hosokawa Hajime had headed a hospital in Korea (built by Chōsen chisso for him) and served as an army doctor during the war. After the war he studied the diseases of southern Kyūshū, becoming an expert on Japanese encephalitis—which was the diagnosis given in some early cases of Minamata disease. He headed the Shin Nitchitsu hospital, the only general hospital in Minamata until the municipal hospital was built in 1953, and was generally considered the best doctor in town. He was scheduled to retire in the fall of 1956 but stayed on because of Minamata disease.

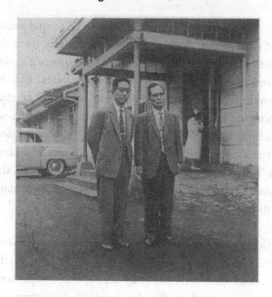

Fig. 8 Itō Hasuo (left), head of Kumamoto prefecture's public health office in Minamata, and Hosokawa Hajime (right), at the Shin Nitchitsu factory hospital, headed by Hosokawa. Photo courtesy of Miyazawa Nobuo.

Itō, whose hobbies were fishing and eight-millimeter movie making, was an unusual bureaucrat.[4] He wrote and performed comedy skits (*manzai*) to explain and promote family-planning policies. Before Itō sent Hosokawa's report of the strange disease to the prefecture's public health section on May 4, he visited the factory hospital to see the patients, and he testified later that their "symptoms were so severe, I had to turn away."[5]

The city quickly created a Strange Disease Countermeasures Committee (Kibyō taisaku iinkai), bringing together the doctors' association, the municipal and factory hospitals, and the public health department.[6] The members of the group cooperated well and worked quickly. Dr. Noda Kaneyoshi of the Shin Nitchitsu hospital, along with other young doctors, bicycled daily to the fishing hamlets at the southern end of town and completed a house-to-house survey within two months. They discovered many more patients and produced a report of their findings. At the same time, the committee examined doctors' records for the past several years and discovered other patients, some already dead, who had been misdiagnosed with diseases ranging from Japanese encephalitis to alcoholism. The doctors' honesty in admitting their mistakes is admirable and rare, as Ui Jun notes.[7]

Although the strange disease often struck several members of the same family, or several families living near each other, Hosokawa soon suspected it was not contagious. Since the city authorities felt they could not afford to do nothing, however, they disinfected the victims' homes. This fed fear of the disease, even among nurses; so Hosokawa and Itō put patients in the city's isolation hospital in July and asked Kumamoto University and the Ministry of Health and Welfare to test for bacteria and viruses.

The university researchers concluded in November, after examining the patients and their well water and food, that the disease was not contagious, and that it was caused by a heavy metal, probably from the factory's effluent, in fish consumed by the patients.[8] But isolating the patients and disinfecting their homes had contributed to the spread of the persistent but false view, still held by some to this day, that the strange disease was contagious. This increased the social isolation of the victims and the discrimination against them. Many, including Tanaka Asao, mother of Shizuko and Jitsuko, tell tales of being forced at shops to put their money into a bamboo basket and watch the shopkeeper disinfect it.[9]

The Ministry of Health and Welfare's National Institute for Public Health (Kokuritsu kōshū eiseiin) sent two doctors to Kumamoto University and Minamata from late November to early December. One of them, the epidemiologist Dr. Miyairi Masato, submitted a report laying out plans for studies using the methods of "medical ecology."[10] At Itō's urging, the city's Strange Disease Countermeasures Committee had already done much of this type of research, particularly in its house-to-house survey, but after 1956 little more was done for many years. Had such fieldwork been carried out, the nature and extent of the disease would have been understood much better and much earlier. Patients with less severe symptoms would have been discovered much sooner, and the realization that the disease was widespread might have prompted earlier and stronger efforts to halt the cause.

Instead, after the results of the research coordinated by the municipal, prefectural, and national governments were compiled and reported by January 1957, the focus of investigation shifted away from the patients themselves. One reason is that the municipal committee had done its work so well that it seemed there was little more to be done. On December 1, 1956, it designated the first 52 official victims of the disease, seventeen of whom had already died. Its report describing the symptoms and course of the disease remained the basis for diagnosis and official certification until 1971. For most people, even today, the early victims of acute Minamata disease still represent the typical image of patients. Patients who had less severe or less typical symptoms, or who lived outside the areas initially studied, were consequently rarely certified until fifteen years after the discovery of the disease.

A report compiled by Hosokawa and other doctors at the factory hospital in January 1957, probably for submission to a meeting held that month by the National Institute for Public Health in Tokyo, summarizes some of their findings:

Location

The vast majority of the patients are from coastal areas of the bay inside Koiji Island. There are a few from other areas, but none who do not catch fish in the bay. Those from Yudō, Detsuki, and Tsukinoura predominate; 61 percent of the cases have appeared in these areas.

Concentration in Families

Patients come from a total of 41 families, and nine of these families include two or more patients. The largest number of patients in a single family is four; there is one such family. It is also especially noteworthy that there are cases of patients not only from the same family but also from families that have close contact, such as immediate or near neighbors, those that are related, and those that are friends.

Relation of This Disease to Animals

In the regions where patients have been found, cats have died in large numbers. In some hamlets cats have virtually disappeared. Furthermore, there are many patients' families whose cats have gone into convulsions and died. It is believed that the onset of the disease in cats precedes that in human patients by several weeks to several months.

In addition, two pigs, one dog, and one rabbit kept by patients' families have died.

Relation to Fish

Fish such as gray mullet, shrimp, octopus, and crabs can be caught in Yudō Bay. Many of the patients still eat fish such as these, and many eat them in large amounts. In the areas in which the disease has appeared, there are many poor families who eat large amounts of fish they catch themselves. However, there are one or two exceptions.

The report goes on to note a narrowing of the field of vision as a characteristic symptom.[11] This would later become a key to diagnosing the disease.

The second reason for the shift of emphasis in research from the patients to the laboratory in 1957 was the need to discover the agent causing the disease, a task for which the necessary knowledge and equipment were not available in Minamata (except perhaps in Shin Nitchitsu's research division). A research group formed by the Ministry of Health and Welfare, consisting mostly of researchers from Kumamoto University, also submitted a report to the January 25, 1957, meeting at the National Institute for Public Health. Soon after the meeting, the group's conclusion that the disease was probably caused by a heavy metal in fish and shellfish became known in Minamata.[12] The city council discussed the connection between fish and the disease as early as December 1956, and Itō later commented to reporters: "I'm worried too, so I'm eating only canned fish."[13]

In 1957 and 1958, the search for the cause was carried on mostly in the laboratories of the Kumamoto University Medical School rather than in the fishing hamlets and doctors' offices of Minamata. The suspicion that people and fish were being poisoned by factory waste made cooperation on the local level more difficult, and the results of the work done in 1956 made it seem less necessary. The focus on laboratory work diverted attention from the fact that more and more people were getting sick. Those who could still fish saw their catches continue to decline and found their fish difficult to sell.

While the research continued, the disease continued to affect more people. Sugimoto Eiko came home one day in 1958 to find her mother, Toshi, sitting outside their home in Modō surrounded by matches, trying to light her pipe but succeeding only in burning her face. Eiko's father, who was one of four *amimoto* in this hamlet of 160 families, took his wife to the municipal hospital. Their neighbors shunned the Sugimotos when they heard on the radio that Toshi had the "manganese disease" (*mangan byō*), and Toshi was put in the isolation hospital. Eiko's father had had 30 *amiko* working for him. Toshi had fed them, and from the time Eiko entered first grade, it had been her job to feed the *amiko* children and then walk them to school. Yet when Toshi developed Minamata disease, none of the *amiko* offered to help the family; none would even come near them.[14]

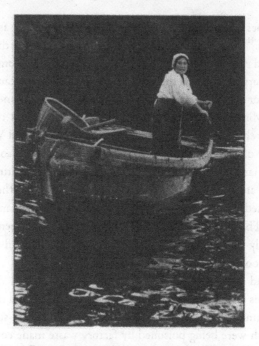

Fig. 9 Sugimoto Eiko, 1962. © Kuwabara Shisei.

Discovering which of the many heavy metals in the sludge of Minamata Bay was causing the disease was a daunting task. It was made even more difficult by the lack of cooperation from the company. Even with the advantage of hindsight, it is difficult to see how researchers could have concluded sooner than they did that the cause was mercury. Takeuchi Tadao of Kumamoto University began by making a list of 64 possible poisons.[15] His list included mercury, but attention focused first on manganese, partly because of similarities between the Minamata case and a well-known case of manganese poisoning in well water in Hiratsuka (in Kanagawa prefecture near Tokyo) in 1939.[16] The researchers, nearly all from the Medical School, did not know what substances were used in the factory and had little contact with those in the science and engineering departments who might have a better idea of the processes used in the factory. They initially assumed the factory, if it used mercury, would not throw away such a valuable substance, and they were unaware of the few articles in European medical journals concerning organic mercury poisoning.

The Shin Nitchitsu factory claimed it operated under MITI supervision and therefore could not provide the university with samples of its waste without written permission from MITI.[17] The university researchers managed to get the proper document from MITI, but the company then refused to let them enter the factory to collect samples and insisted on providing them itself. As a result, the researchers could never be sure of the authenticity and exact source of the samples.[18]

In April 1957, Mayor Hashimoto put forth the first of the many counter-theories that would emerge in the next few years in opposition to Kumamoto University's heavy metal theory. He informed the Ministry of Health and Welfare that the disease must have been caused by pesticides and fertilizers washed into the sea by a typhoon that flooded Minamata in 1953, and that it was possible no new patients would appear.[19] On May 25 the *Minamata taimusu* printed a story with one subheading reading "Strange Disease Cause a Political Issue" and suggested that "political and other pressures" were being brought to bear.[20]

On August 13, the *Kumamoto nichinichi shinbun* reported:

In early July at a public health conference, the general conclusion regarding the cause of the strange disease in Minamata was that it is dangerous to eat fish and shellfish from Minamata Bay. For this reason, out of concern for public health, the prefecture will decide to "ban the taking of fish in Minamata Bay for the purpose of selling them," under Article 4 of the Public Health Law. This will be announced in the name of the governor within two or three days.[21]

In fact, however, such a ban was never issued (although Kumamoto University researchers had recommended it in February 1957), perhaps because the Fisheries Law would have required that fishers be compensated. The prefectural government consulted the Ministry of Health and Welfare, which replied that while "we would like you to continue to advise against consumption," a ban under the Food Sanitation Act was not possible because "no clear basis can be found [for concluding that] all fish and shellfish in the designated area in Minamata Bay are poisoned."[22] Instead, the prefecture banned only the *sale* of fish from Minamata Bay. Hoping to make its fish marketable, the Minamata Fishing Cooperative decided on a policy of "self-restraint," under which its members promised not to catch fish in the bay. The self-restraint policy continued until the governor declared the bay's fish safe 40 years later, in 1997. Not once has fishing in Minamata Bay ever been legally prohibited.

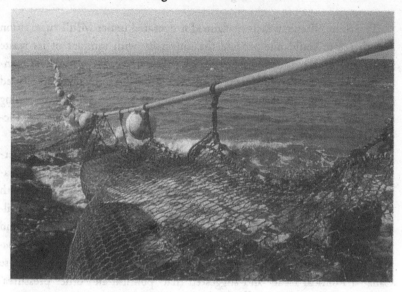

Fig. 10. The net that surrounded Minamata Bay from 1977 to 1997. It was important mainly for its symbolic value, since fish swam through and under it and through the opening left for ships. © Timothy S. George.

While Shin Nitchitsu's stance hardened, Dr. Hosokawa continued his work.[23] He consulted with Itō, treated patients in the hospital and visited them in their homes, and regularly dispatched young doctors from the factory hospital to work with researchers at Kumamoto University. It was at this time that Minamata-born poet and critic Tanigawa Gan prevented his Minamata cell of the Japan Communist Party from branding Hosokawa a "running dog" of the company.[24] Tanigawa also suggested that Hosokawa read Ibsen's *An Enemy of the People*, a play about a small-town doctor ostracized for pointing out that the town's hot springs, on which its tourist industry depended, were polluted.[25] The parallels with Hosokawa's difficult position were obvious to Tanigawa, who in 1956 had telephoned his former professor Hidaka Rokurō in Tokyo to tell him of the disease and his suspicion that Shin Nitchitsu was the cause.[26]

In 1958 the factory conducted a horrible human experiment by switching the discharge of the acetaldehyde plant's wastewater from Hyakken Harbor to the mouth of the Minamata River. Hyakken Harbor and Minamata Bay form a sheltered area within the Shiranui Sea. From the river mouth, the waste was much more rapidly circulated throughout the Shiranui Sea. The factory managers must have hoped the waste would be sufficiently diluted to be harmless—and therefore must have already suspected that it was causing the disease. In fact, as had happened in Minamata Bay, the sea did the opposite of what they expected: instead of being diluted, the mercury was concentrated in the food chain. In "solving" the problem this way, the managers were repeating what they had done earlier with the carbide tailings that had been dumped in Minamata Bay until complaints (due to pollution and the silting up of the bay) had forced them to begin piping the tailings as slurry to the Hachiman (sedimentation) Pools at the mouth of the Minamata River in 1951. Now in 1958, the acetaldehyde waste was piped to the Hachiman Pools, from where it flowed into the river and then the sea.[27]

That spring Douglas McAlpine, a British neurologist visiting Kumamoto University, examined 22 patients in Minamata and at the university hospital. In an article published in the British medical journal *Lancet* in September, he noted, in speculating on the cause, that their symptoms resembled those of methyl mercury poisoning (Hunter-Russell syndrome) as described in articles in medical journals in 1940 and 1954.[28] This hint helped the Kumamoto University researchers find the cause, but not before they had worked their way through several other theories.

Kitamura Shōji of Kumamoto University suggested selenium caused the disease, and his colleague Miyagawa Kuheita suggested thallium.[29] Mc-Alpine, too, had proposed thallium as the most likely cause, and although experiments failed to prove this, Miyagawa stuck doggedly to his belief until his death in September 1960, when his theory died with him. In the meantime, reflecting standard practice in Japanese academia, over twenty papers had been written in support of the thallium theory by researchers working under him.[30] Working in their mentor's laboratory, they unfortunately had little choice of research subjects.

Another possibility, that the fish were being poisoned by a red tide, was suggested by Bruce Halstead of the Tropical Research Institute in California. Halstead visited Minamata in September 1958 with Leonard Kurland, chief of the Epidemiology Branch of the National Institute of Neurological Diseases and Blindness at the National Institutes of Health (NIH), who was studying multiple sclerosis in Kumamoto.[31] Once mercury was found to be present, Halstead abandoned his theory, but Shin Nitchitsu continued to promote it. Kurland tried to buy fish in Minamata to bring back to the United States for analysis, but Shin Nitchitsu forestalled him by buying up all the fish in the markets. Kurland was forced to get samples from the public health office.[32] At the NIH, Kurland and others replicated the symptoms of Minamata disease in cats to which they fed seafood samples from Minamata. They later discovered methyl mercury in the samples when the Kumamoto researchers alerted them to its presence.[33]

A notice sent by the Ministry of Health and Welfare to other ministries on July 7, 1958, and Shin Nitchitsu's defensive response, foreshadowed the controversy that was to mark the year 1959. Two days later, the ministry's suspicions became public knowledge, when the *Kumamoto nichinichi shinbun* published a story headlined "Minamata Disease Cause Is Shin Nitchitsu's Waste, Ministry of Health and Welfare Scientific Group Infers."[34] Based on the conclusions of the scientists assembled by the ministry to study Minamata disease, headed by Matsuda Shin'ichi of the National Institute for Public Health, Public Health Bureau chief Yamaguchi Masayoshi wrote in this notice that "waste from the Shin Nitchitsu factory pollutes the sludge of the bay and harbor, and fish, shellfish, and migratory fish become poisonous due to a substance identical in type to a chemical poison in the waste. Eating large amounts of these causes the disease, it is believed."[35] The ministry was still uncertain what the chemical culprit might be and suspected the waste might undergo some sort of change in the fish and shellfish that made it poisonous. It asked the relevant ministries and local governments to help solve the puzzle. This document was perhaps the first instance in which the central government linked Shin Nitchitsu in writing to Minamata disease.

The company responded within the month with the first in a series of pamphlets it was to issue in 1958 and 1959. "This Company's View of the Strange Disease in Minamata" ("Minamata kibyō ni kan suru tōsha no kenkai") explained why the company was not satisfied with the findings of the Ministry of Health and Welfare. The company asserted that it was cooperating fully and wanted the cause discovered as soon as possible. It dismissed the selenium, thallium, and manganese theories, said there was no proof yet that the disease was seasonal, and speculated that the cause was probably "a complex organic poison."[36]

The year 1959 saw the dramatic climax in the first round of responses to the disease, including a major turning point in the search for its cause. After two years with little progress, in 1959 the Kumamoto University researchers began to focus on organic mercury as the cause of the disease. Takeuchi Tadao, who had been pursuing his mercury theory since the previous year, published an article in March 1959 showing the similarities between the symptoms of Minamata disease and organic mercury poisoning.[37] However, he did not yet know whether organic mercury was found in the bay. Experiments at the Medical School showed that methyl and ethyl mercury, two types of organic mercury, produced Minamata disease in cats. The researchers discovered that the factory used inorganic mercury in producing vinyl chloride and acetaldehyde. They still could not explain how the inorganic mercury could become organic but guessed that it happened in seawater or in the fish.

To solve the puzzle, they wanted to do on-site research in Minamata during the university's summer vacation. Eight days before they were to announce their theory and request funding at a meeting concerning the research budget, the *Asahi shinbun* published a report on their tentative conclusions in one of the biggest journalistic scoops of the entire Minamata disease incident. The *Asahi* article revealed that Professors Tokuomi Haruhiko, Takeuchi Tadao, and Kitamura Masatsugu would announce that they had "virtually confirmed" organic mercury as the cause through "scientific analysis, clinical experiments, and pathological observations."[38] They believed, the article said, that the mercury was dumped into the sea by the Shin Nitchitsu factory and was transformed into organic mercury in fish and shellfish.

Kitamura's tests of sludge in the bay clearly showed that the amount of mercury increased as one approached the factory's Hyakken waste outlet. Near where the waste emptied into the bay he found 2,010 parts per million (ppm), such a shockingly high concentration that he repeated his tests several times.[39] This number translates into 0.2 percent, or 2 kilograms per ton—twice the amount needed for a viable mercury mine. The company in fact later established a subsidiary, Minamata kagaku (Minamata Chemical), to reclaim mercury from the sludge in this area.[40]

Ui Jun describes an emergency meeting of factory executives held in response to the *Asahi* report.[41] Despite explanations of the Medical School researchers' studies by Hosokawa Hajime, all but one refused to believe the university scientists' explanation could be correct. They decided to marshal arguments to refute it. The first salvo was fired by plant manager Nishida Eiichi on August 5, when he and six other company officials and researchers were called to a meeting of the prefectural assembly's Special Committee on

Minamata Disease Countermeasures (Minamatabyō tokubetsu taisaku iinkai):

The organic mercury theory is not only fraught with the same problems as the manganese, selenium, and thallium theories. In addition, looking at it from the point of view of scientific common sense, it is based on assumptions and contradicts the facts. At this stage it would be premature to immediately conclude that organic mercury is the cause of Minamata disease. Even linking it to the Minamata factory's waste would be jumping to conclusions.[42]

Ui uses the shifting stance of the *Kumamoto nichinichi shinbun* to illustrate the effectiveness of the company's counterattack. On August 5, just before Nishida's testimony to the assembly committee, the newspaper editorialized: "Because it is a fact that the Minamata factory uses mercury as a catalyst, and that it is discharged in its effluent, we believe there is no doubt that the cause of Minamata disease is the factory's effluent."[43] Two weeks later, the same newspaper wrote in another editorial: "At the present stage, it has not been determined that the Shin Nitchitsu factory is the cause of Minamata disease."[44]

The company produced four pamphlets between July and October 1959 in an attempt to discredit the organic mercury theory.[45] The two main tactics were to assume an air of scientific superiority casting doubt on the ability of the university scientists, and to lay out every possible argument against the mercury theory, even if some of these contradicted each other. The first of these tactics involved reminders that Kumamoto University had suggested other substances before mercury and then dropped them, and that some at Kumamoto University still believed thallium was the cause. The logical inconsistency of some of the company's arguments is exemplified by three of its assertions. (1) Although the factory does discharge small amounts of inorganic mercury, this cannot become organic. (2) Organic mercury is not found in the bay's fish and shellfish. (3) There are other more likely sources of organic mercury, such as agricultural chemicals.[46] Another argument was that although plants in many other countries used similar processes, there were no reports of similar diseases. In fact, though Chisso has never admitted to knowing of them, articles had been published by Swiss and German researchers in 1930 and 1933, respectively, describing the poisoning of workers by organic mercury created as a by-product of acetaldehyde production.[47]

The company's second pamphlet added another argument, one first put forth by Mayor Hashimoto in 1956: the disease could be caused by ordnance dumped into the bay by the Japanese military in 1945 at the end of the war. Hashimoto soon thereafter switched to the pesticide theory, but the explosives theory was ably promoted by the "Ōshima Report" issued by the Japan Chemical Industry Association (Nihon kagaku kōgyō kyōkai; JCIA) in the name of its director, Ōshima Takeji.[48] According to Ōshima, the bombs had deteriorated and begun to leak their poisonous contents in 1956. The report offered no evidence to support its thesis, but the university and prefecture were forced to spend a great deal of time and effort to disprove it.

The Imperial Japanese Navy had in fact built a storage facility in Modō during the war. The man responsible for disposing of the materials in question submitted signed testimony to the prefectural public health department stating that all the explosives stored at the facility had been transported by horse cart, under close supervision by Occupation forces, to Minamata station. From there, the Americans told him, they were to be taken to Misumi, loaded on ships, and dumped far at sea.

That is what happened. We did not dispose of any of them around Fukuro Bay or dump any in the water.

Shin Nitchitsu came to ask me about this too, and I told them clearly exactly what I have just said, but now they are saying I did not tell them a thing. I suspect this is because it puts them in a difficult position.

The Minamata police came too, and I told them the same thing.[49]

According to Ui, the company's third pamphlet was criticized by a scientist so severely that it never went beyond draft form.[50] It was revised and issued as the fourth pamphlet in late October 1959. One of its arguments was that no Minamata disease had appeared near any of the many other factories in Japan making acetaldehyde and vinyl chloride. (In less than five years, a "second Minamata disease" appeared in Niigata prefecture downriver from an acetaldehyde plant.) The pamphlet also asserted, correctly, that the Kumamoto University researchers could not show how the inorganic mercury from the factory could become organic in the sea. This was quite true, but the university researchers were to prove by 1961 what at least some in the factory had known since 1950—that organic mercury was created *inside* the factory, in the production process itself.[51]

The pamphlet's final argument was that organic mercury was not found in cats fed factory wastewater or sludge from the bay containing mercury, and that these cats did not develop Minamata disease. Moreover, "there is no link between the factory wastewater and organic mercury, and the relationship between organic mercury and Minamata disease is dubious."[52] The pamphlet cites data from Dr. Hosokawa's cat experiments to back this up— but omits the data that would show it knew the cause of the disease. The company already knew, from Hosokawa's experiments, that the wastewater from its acetaldehyde plant caused Minamata disease.

Hosokawa had announced his suspicions that the cat and human diseases were related as early as October 1956, at a meeting of the Kumamoto Medical Association (Kumamoto igakukai).[53] The first successful cat experiments were begun by Itō Hasuo, head of the city health department, in March 1957. Since researchers at Kumamoto University had difficulty getting fish from Minamata and keeping them fresh, they asked Itō to conduct experiments. He fed Minamata Bay fish and shellfish, some of which he caught himself, to cats, and filmed them with his eight-millimeter movie camera when they became sick. By July, autopsies showed that five of seven cats had Minamata disease. He and Hosokawa Hajime assumed that the mystery of the disease was close to being solved.[54]

Hosokawa conducted his own experiments with cats, and began giving them wastewater taken from various locations inside the factory in June 1959.[55] After workers in the company's research labs helped him collect and analyze the samples, they were ordered to stop assisting him. He continued the experiments with samples he collected himself but could only guess at their mercury content. His notes explain what happened with the famous "cat #400":

Experiment I Acetic acid factory wastewater given directly to cats
•Concentration of mercury under 100 ppm
•Cat experiment #400—From July 2, 1959, 20 grams per day added to food and fed to cat. On October 7, suffered loss of consciousness and convulsions. Minamata disease confirmed through autopsy and clinical examination.[56]

Hosokawa planned follow-up experiments, but when he reported his results to the factory manager and the head of the research department, they ordered him to halt all experiments with factory waste. A year later, under a new head of the research department, Hosokawa was allowed to resume his experiments with waste from the acetic acid factory but required to keep them secret and to conduct them jointly with the research department. He had already passed the retirement age, and the company may have feared that if they did not let him resume his experiments, he would leave and announce his findings.[57] Hosokawa finally did resign in April 1962, and several other doctors left with him, but he did not make his knowledge public. He later told Ishimure Michiko that he had gone to work with his letter of resignation in his pocket for some time before he resigned.[58] Around the same time cat #400 developed Minamata disease, the research department discovered organic mercury in a factory drain, but this was also kept secret.[59]

After issuing its anti-mercury pamphlets and halting Hosokawa's experiments, Shin Nitchitsu found indirect approaches more effective in evading blame for Minamata disease. It found help from outside scientists, industry, and the government.

On November 12, 1959, the Food Hygiene Investigation Committee (Shokuhin eisei chōsakai) submitted its interim report to the minister of health and welfare. The committee's report was based on the work of its Minamata Food Poisoning Subcommittee (Minamata shoku chūdoku bukai), composed mostly of Kumamoto University faculty members. The committee report concluded that "Minamata disease, which results from the consumption of large quantities of fish and shellfish from Minamata Bay and the surrounding areas, is a food poisoning that attacks mainly the central nervous system. The main cause is an organic mercury compound."[60] The Ministry of Health and Welfare, under pressure from the Diet after the November 2 fishermen's riot at the factory (described below), was expected to announce its official conclusion soon after receiving the report.

Instead, this move was blocked by well-timed maneuvering by Shin Nitchitsu, Governor Teramoto Hirosaku of Kumamoto, and the Ministry of International Trade and Industry under its head Ikeda Hayato. On November 11, the day before the Ministry of Health and Welfare received its committee's report, Teramoto traveled to Tokyo and visited the head of the ministry's Environmental Sanitation Section (Kankyō eiseibu). Teramoto informed the ministry that Shin Nitchitsu's president Yoshioka Kiichi had agreed to accept the governor's mediation in talks with the fishing cooperatives. Teramoto was quoted as saying the section head "sympathetically replied 'If that's so, maybe it would be best if we just sat on the Food Hygiene Investigation Committee's conclusion.'"[61] In fact, Teramoto's announcement of Shin Nitchitsu's acceptance was premature. The company did not agree to mediation until November 13, and then only out of fear that the prefectural assembly would order it to halt its dumping of waste and in the face of rumors that fishermen would dynamite the factory.[62]

On November 10, the day before Teramoto arrived in Tokyo, MITI had sent a questionnaire to Shin Nitchitsu President Yoshioka concerning the factory's waste and its use of mercury in the acetaldehyde and PVC monomer production processes. The accompanying letter noted that the Kumamoto University mercury theory was "gaining acceptance," but said the fact that Minamata disease had not occurred near any other factories making the same products was "the biggest problem with the theory that mercury is the cause." It said that the survey form was being sent to all these factories, and "since the Minamata strange disease problem is becoming a political issue now, this survey is being carried out confidentially. We ask your understanding of this, and hope you will take proper care in your handling of it [to keep it confidential] not only from those outside the company, but also within the company."[63]

The next day, while Governor Teramoto visited Tokyo, MITI distributed a hastily prepared pamphlet by Kiyoura Raisaku of the Tokyo Institute of Technology (Tokyo kōgyō daigaku) rebutting the mercury theory.[64] Kiyoura's argument carried weight because he was one of the best known of Japan's few water-quality engineers. The main point of the paper, based on his measurements of mercury content in fish and sea water in Minamata and other parts of Japan, was that Minamata disease could not be caused by mercury since it did not appear in other areas with even higher concentrations of mercury. He implied that these higher levels elsewhere showed Minamata's levels were not so unusual, but stacked the deck by making his measurements in areas near mercury mines (in Hokkaidō and central Honshū) and factories using mercury (on Ise Bay and the Naoetsu River).

The Ministry of Health and Welfare accepted its committee's interim report on November 12 and disbanded the Minamata Food Poisoning Subcommittee the same day. The pressure it was under was clear at a cabinet meeting the next day when Minister of International Trade and Industry Ikeda Hayato upbraided Minister of Health and Welfare Watanabe Yoshio, and insisted that it was too soon to conclude that the mercury came from the Shin Nitchitsu factory. Minister of Agriculture and Forestry Fukuda Takeo (like Ikeda, a future prime minister) suggested solving the problem by helping the fishers switch to producing pearls.[65] No official government announcement regarding the cause of Minamata disease was made until nine years later, just after the factory stopped using mercury. There is no way of knowing how many of the victims of Minamata disease—and the total number of patients is undoubtedly much larger than the over 13,000 deemed eligible for compensation—contracted the disease during these nine years.

In late 1959 Ikeda and MITI desperately needed to avoid harming the chemical industry and Shin Nitchitsu. The nation's economic growth depended on increasing the international competitiveness of Japanese industry. MITI was particularly concerned with avoiding dependence on imported chemicals and with financing the transition to more efficient processes. In 1959, even though Japan's octanol production increased 50 percent over 1958, four tons of octanol had been imported. DOP, a plasticizer for vinyl chloride, was made from octanol, and octanol was made from acetaldehyde. Shin Nitchitsu produced most of Japan's octanol and a third or more of its acetaldehyde. It was one of the target companies for the second phase, beginning in 1960, of MITI's plan to guide the switch to petrochemicals, and had submitted its plans to MITI in July 1959. It was essential for Shin Nitchitsu to continue its profitable acetaldehyde production to finance the construction of a new petrochemical plant and to keep imports to a minimum. Such considerations overrode any concerns for the victims and determined policy regarding Minamata. The problem had to be contained and "solved" without harming the company or the rest of the chemical industry.[66]

Bureaucrats in the Ministry of Health and Welfare, too, were persuaded of the need for high growth, even if it required some sacrifices. Hashimoto Michio, who played a leading role in the ministry on environmental issues beginning in 1961 and headed its Environment Section when it was established in 1964, considered growth essential to providing health insurance, sewage and water systems, and pensions for a population living longer and longer.[67]

On November 20, 1959, Kumamoto University president Wanibuchi Takeshi and Medical School dean Sera Kansuke held a news conference. They said it was "regrettable" that the committee was "dissolved at a critical stage in its research because of turf wars between ministries."[68] They criticized the company for blocking research by refusing to allow collection of wastewater samples. They suggested that many of the children in Minamata diagnosed with cerebral palsy might actually have Minamata disease and promised to quickly prove how inorganic mercury became organic in fish. Leonard Kurland published articles in both the *Asahi* and *Mainichi* on December 8 supporting the Kumamoto scientists' conclusion that mercury caused the disease. On December 10, Kurland wrote Takeuchi Tadao of Kumamoto University: "I have the impression that factory management has not been as cooperative with the Kumamoto University scientists as they should have been but, on the other hand, we can appreciate how concerned they are since the very existence of the factory may be at stake."[69] The U.S. National Institutes of Health, for which Kurland worked, funded the Kumamoto University Medical School research on Minamata disease for the next three years, since Ministry of Health and Welfare funding ended.

Yet few voices from the public, the media, or the Diet protested the dissolution of the committee and the burying of its findings. At the end of 1959, the public, if it cared about Minamata at all, was not convinced that the cause had been proven to be mercury, and the countertheories sponsored by the company confused the issue even further. In this "neutralization" (to use Ui Jun's term) of the Kumamoto University conclusions, Shin Nitchitsu was assisted by industry, the medical establishment, and the government.

The industry journal *Mizu* (Water) wrote in its December 1959 issue that "if only the wastewater issue had been dealt with before it became a big problem, not by a hick university like the Kumamoto University Medical School but by scholars from the center, who were true authorities," the problem never would have gotten so bad that the factory was invaded by fishermen, as it was in the summer and fall of 1959.[70] This line of attack—that scientists from the "center" could be trusted over those from "hick" universities on the periphery—was epitomized in an interview with Dean Sera of the Medical School, published in the February 1960 issue of *Mizu*:

Q: Selenium, manganese, thallium . . . the average layman just doesn't trust you any more. Why have you changed your minds three or four times?

A: The main thing for us is discovering the cause of the disease; we're not trying to oppose the factory. It can't be helped if the result is harmful to the factory. As for our coming up with three different theories, when you do research that's what happens; there's no need for me to defend this. . . .

Q: Won't you just change your minds a fourth time and come out with another theory?

A: That won't happen. . . .

Q: Maybe not, but why does Kumamoto University confuse laymen by putting out all these haphazard theories?

A: They're not haphazard. That's just the way the research happened to turn out. . . .

Q: When you can't give a satisfactory explanation to a layman like me, I can't help thinking yours really is a country university. Scholars from the center are much better. . . .

A: I have made something of a name for myself in forensic medicine.

Q: And forensic medicine in the postwar period has been divided over opposing theories since the Shimoyama Incident.[71]

A: (Laughs, does not reply.)[72]

Kiyoura Raisaku, just the type of "authority" from the "center" so highly praised by *Mizu*, put out another paper in April 1960.[73] In this article he put forth his "amine thesis," which asserted that Minamata disease was caused by poisonous amines that were produced as fish spoiled. No one who has spent much time with fishing families would find it credible that they poisoned themselves by eating rotten fish, but perhaps Tokyo "authorities" who got their fish in shops and sushi restaurants were more gullible. In his experiments, Kiyoura injected rats with extracts from fish and shellfish from Minamata Bay. He reported that when he used extracts containing mercury, the rats survived; if the extracts contained poisonous amines (produced when the fish and shellfish were left to spoil in lukewarm water), the rats died of symptoms resembling Minamata disease.

Kiyoura's experiments were rather crude and outside his own specialty. More sophisticated support was soon forthcoming from Tokita Kikuji, a pharmacologist at Tōhō University. In a 67-page article published in 1961, Tokita and twelve other researchers described their experiments, in which some cats were fed fish and shellfish from Minamata Bay and others were fed mercury. The cats were observed, their hearts and brains were monitored, their blood and urine were analyzed, and they were autopsied. Those fed a soup made from spoiled fish went mad, like the cats with Minamata disease. The very tentative conclusion to these meticulous experiments was that it seemed likely the causative agent was some sort of amine in the fish. As Ui Jun notes, however, Tokita never proved that organic amines caused Minamata disease or even that his cats had Minamata disease at all.[74] As in the case of Miyagawa Kuheita of Kumamoto University and his thallium theory, none of the scientists working with Tokita continued research on the amine theory after Tokita's death. One thing that is clear from Tokita's acknowledgments at the end of his article is that his research, in contrast to that at Kumamoto University, was assisted by Kiyoura Raisaku, MITI, Shin Nitchitsu, the JCIA, and Tamiya Takeo, head of the Japan Medical Association.

In Ui's metaphor, just as an acid and an alkali can neutralize each other only if they are poured into the same beaker, these countertheories required a "location" in which they could "neutralize" the truth.[75] The media, in uncritically reporting all the theories out of a desire to be balanced and fair, provided one such location. Two prestigious national committees provided another.[76] One, directed by the EPA and billed as a replacement for the dissolved Minamata Food Poisoning Subcommittee of the Food Hygiene Investigation Committee, was the Minamata Disease General Investigation and Research Liaison Council (Minamatabyō sōgō chōsa kenkyū renraku kyōgikai). The other was the Japan Medical Association's Minamata Disease Research Consultation Group (Minamatabyō kenkyū kondankai), better known after its chairman as the Tamiya Committee. Both were created in 1960, met in private, and disappeared without issuing public reports.

The EPA committee had ten members: six from Tokyo universities (including Kiyoura Raisaku), only two from Kumamoto University (Kitamura Shōji and Uchida Makio), one from Kyūshū University, and one from the National Hygiene Laboratory (Kokuritsu eisei shikenjo). There was also an observer from Shin Nitchitsu, although he was not on the list of members.[77] Of its six staff members, two were from MITI, two from the EPA, one from the Ministry of Health and Welfare, and one from the Fisheries Agency. The committee met four times from February 1960 to March 1961 and distributed over ¥10 million ($27,800) in research funds, but announced no new findings.[78] Many of the discussions consisted of attacks on the Kumamoto University mercury theory and Kiyoura's promotion of his amine theory. But one member of the committee, Han'ya Takahisa of Tokyo toritsu daigaku, later stated that the results of many of the committee members' investigations clearly supported the November 1959 conclusions of the Minamata Food Poisoning Subcommittee, which the EPA committee replaced. His own research confirmed mercury pollution throughout not only the Shiranui Sea but also the Ariake Sea to its north. At its March 6, 1961, meeting, the committee decided to hold another meeting to discuss submitting a report. No more meetings were ever held, although Han'ya was never informed that the committee had been dissolved. He and the others were told they could never publish their research results, and he was convinced that the committee's meetings were halted because its conclusions would have differed from those the government desired.[79]

The Tamiya Committee of the Japan Medical Association was established in or before March 1960.[80] All seven regular members of the committee were from universities in Tokyo, including Kiyoura Raisaku and Tokita Kikuji. It submitted an interim report (never made public) in May 1962 and was dissolved after Tamiya died in July 1963.[81] According to Ui, Dean Sera of the Kumamoto University Medical School was asked by Tamiya to join the committee, but refused because in return for research funds, he would have been required not to make the results of the research public. Tamiya is said to have apologized to Sera through an intermediary just before his death.[82] Ui also believes the Tamiya Committee was actually created at the behest of Ōshima Takeji and JCIA, citing as evidence the JCIA's journal *Geppō*:

Since the issue of Minamata disease is a major problem, in order to make a fair judgment as to whether the opinion announced by Kumamoto University Medical School is correct or not, . . . this association has commissioned seven people from the medical field, who have now begun research.[83]

As for industrial pollution, under the Industrial Wastewater Committee (Yasunishi Masao, chairman) [president of Shōwa denkō, the company that caused Niigata Minamata disease], a Vinyl Chloride and Acetaldehyde Special Committee has been established, and attached to this is Professor Tamiya's committee.[84]

In addition, the JCIA drew up a draft plan for the Tamiya Committee and later testimony by Ōshima confirmed the JCIA's role.[85]

Although the committee was ostensibly connected to the Japan Medical Association through its chairman, it was in fact, as the JCIA's *Geppō* stated, attached to the JCIA's Vinyl Chloride and Acetaldehyde Special Committee. This meant that Shin Nitchitsu was the largest source of its funds.[86] And it is clear that the company felt that, with the help of these committees, its strategy for making the issue go away was succeeding. According to Ōshima, at the end of 1961 the JCIA was planning to announce that the committee had found nothing to support the mercury theory but canceled the announcement at Shin Nitchitsu's request. The company, he said, told him: "We're no longer suspected, no more patients are appearing, we're paying solatium money, and [making such an announcement] would only encourage Kumamoto University, so please don't."[87]

While these committees were accomplishing little, the work continued at Kumamoto University. The *Kumamoto nichinichi shinbun* reported in February 1963 that Professor Irukayama Katsurō had shown that organic mercury was created inside the factory in the acetaldehyde production process.[88] This meant that the efforts the researchers had spent trying to show how inorganic mercury—what the company insisted it used and discharged—became organic in fish and shellfish had largely been wasted. Irukayama had found test tubes left over from samples taken in 1959 and 1960 and brought to Kumamoto University by Dr. Kojima Akikazu of the factory hospital, whom Hosokawa Hajime had sent to do research at the university. The article reported Irukayama's announcement of his findings to the first meeting of the university's Minamata disease research group in over a year, but Irukayama was in fact summarizing a report submitted to the *Kumamoto Medical Journal* in October 1961 and published in June 1962.[89] Perhaps because Irukayama's article was published in English (possibly since the research was funded by the U.S. NIH), its conclusions were not reported in the press until Irukayama announced them in Japanese at the February 1963 meeting.

Researchers at the factory, hearing of Irukayama's findings, conducted their own tests. They reported to the head of the research section that organic mercury was indeed created in the acetaldehyde production process, and rats and cats got sick and died when given fish that had absorbed this mercury. They did not say conclusively that the animals had Minamata disease, and neither did Hosokawa and the research department head in reporting on their own experiments with cats, since Professor Saitō Morisuke of the University of Tokyo lost the cats sent to him by Hosokawa for autopsy.[90] Company executives kept the reports secret, as they had Hosokawa's experiment with cat #400.

Ui Jun, who was visiting Kumamoto at the time of the media reports on Irukayama's findings, was told by a factory executive, "I've just had a telephone call from the Medical School dean apologizing for the trouble they caused us when an interim report was leaked."[91] Sera had by this time been replaced as dean of the Medical School by Kotsuna Masachika, under whom relations with Shin Nitchitsu and its allies were much improved. Kotsuna agreed to participate in the Tamiya Committee, and the committee began supplying research funds to the university around September 1961. A few months earlier the company had donated ¥1 million to fund the university's research, and some of this money helped pay for trips by faculty researchers to international conferences.[92] In 1966, when the Kumamoto University researchers published a volume collecting their research reports, Kotsuna, the editor, contributed a chronology of his faculty's research on Minamata disease but did not mention two of their most important accomplishments: the confirmation that organic mercury was created in the factory, and the confirmation of the existence of congenital Minamata disease.[93]

The writer of the *Kumamoto nichinichi shinbun* article on Irukayama's discovery also included a comment by the public prosecutor for Kumamoto, who said that his office had not been able to do anything up to that point, "but if a conclusion is reached in the medical research, then we'll have to pay a great deal of attention to this issue." The prosecutor was soon transferred to Chiba prefecture, near Tokyo. In August 1963 Sera urged the public prosecutor to investigate the company, but nothing was done.[94] No criminal charges were brought against company executives until 1975.

And no further breakthroughs in explaining the source of the organic mercury were announced until 1998, despite the riddles that still remained after Irukayama's discovery. Why, if acetaldehyde production using mercury as a catalyst began in 1932, were severe cases of Minamata disease not noticed until over two decades later? If the acetaldehyde production levels of 1938–44 were not regained until 1954, why is it easy (in hindsight) to confirm a number of cases of the disease in 1952 and 1953, but difficult to find much evidence of the disease a decade earlier? Why did Minamata disease appear at only one of the six other acetaldehyde factories nationwide using similar processes, and there not until 1964?

In 1998 the answer finally became known: an August 1951 technical innovation that speeded the production process led to the production of vastly greater amounts of organic mercury waste. The pieces of the puzzle were assembled by Okamoto Tatsuaki, a former factory union head who obtained internal company data on the production process, Nishimura Hajime, a chemical engineer who explained what had happened by combining this data with information gathered by Kumamoto University researchers, and Akagi Hirokatsu, a specialist in chemical analysis who re-created the factory's production process on a small scale to confirm Nishimura's explanation.[95] In August 1951 the oxidizer used in the process was changed from manganese oxide to nitric acid. The nitric acid, partly because it was recycled from other factory processes and not very pure, frequently resulted in the production of a foam that was discarded. The foam contained a large amount of organic mercury. Also, the water used by the factory was taken from near the mouth of the Minamata River and was therefore slightly salty. This salt resulted in the production of a highly soluble type of organic mercury that was discharged with wastewater into the bay. In less than two years, the amount of organic mercury in the factory's waste increased from under 10 to over 50 kilograms per year. By the end of the decade, it approached 100 kilograms per year.

Even as early as 1963, however, when the *Kumamoto nichinichi shinbun* announced Irukayama's findings, the source of the organic mercury was treated as merely an academic question. The national and prefectural governments took no further steps in response to this confirmation that the organic mercury came from the factory, even though Dean Sera reported it to the prefecture and the Ministry of Health and Welfare and even though other factories were using similar processes.[96] As described in the following chapter, the agreements the company made with fishing cooperatives and patients, and its installation of waste treatment facilities, had supposedly "solved" the problem at the end of 1959. Similar patterns were repeated in other pollution incidents elsewhere in Japan. The Toyama cadmium poisoning case (*itai-itai byō*, or "ouch-ouch disease"), for example, also featured ineffective government committees, countertheories, and research funding from the U.S. National Institutes of Health.[97] In retrospect, these events are discouraging: too many scientists seem to have been in the service of money and power. Too many in the media saw it as their duty to be "neutral" by uncritically reporting every theory, rather than investigating who sponsored them and whether they were backed by solid evidence. Too many government officials seem to have been willing to sacrifice poor fisherfolk on the altar of high growth.

FOUR

The First Solution, 1959

At the end of 1959, Minamata witnessed a three-part "solution": the payment of compensation to fishing cooperatives, the awarding of sympathy money to patients, and the construction of pollution control equipment (which failed to remove the mercury). This was a victory for Shin Nitchitsu, as well as for the government authorities, who would not be willing to pay, or to make companies pay, the costs of high growth for another ten years. Acetaldehyde production, the pending switch to petrochemicals, and, most of all, the plans for economic growth were too important to be jeopardized.

The victims' defeat highlights their extreme weakness, politically, economically, socially, and physically. They were failed by the Left, by the media, and by their own leaders, and they were opposed by a "united front" of nearly all other organizations and citizens in Minamata. They failed to take their struggle out of Minamata in an effort to seek national support. The conclusion to this first round of responses to the Minamata disease highlights the persistent contradictions between Japan's democratic constitution and its political attitudes and practices. The differences between this round of responses and the second, which began a decade later, illustrate the important changes that occurred during Japan's second and third postwar decades.

The Fisherfolk's Struggle for Compensation

By 1959, fishing families in the Minamata area were in dire straits. Some fishers were sick and unable to fish. Fish populations had declined drastically, as had prices, and fish from Minamata were nearly impossible to sell (see Table 3). The city government was providing welfare payments to 144

Table 3
Declining Fish Catch in Minamata, 1950–1957
(*in kg and as percentage of 1950–53 average*)

Average, 1950–53	1954	1955	1956	1957
32,656 (100%)	19,871 (61%)	12,253 (38%)	6,798 (21%)	2,884 (9%)

SOURCE: Minamata-shi, "Minamata-shi gyohōdaka chō," 1957, in *MBJSS,* I: 366–73.

fishing families (366 people). In 1953 only four fishing families had received a total of ¥296,997 ($825) in welfare payments, but in the first half of the fiscal year 1959 (April through September), the city paid a total of ¥1,692,468 ($4,700) to fishing families. In 1960 the city covered 28 percent of these costs from its own coffers; the rest presumably came from the prefectural and national governments.[1]

The fishing families' desperate condition, the growing evidence that the company was to blame, and the company's denials finally pushed the fishing cooperative to take action. Action escalated from petitions and demands to protests, demonstrations, and even violence. The violence brought belated attention from politicians and the media and forced Shin Nitchitsu and the Kumamoto prefectural government to deal with the fishers' plight. The fishers won partial compensation for their losses, but not through the courts. Instead, mediation committees, whose membership favored the company's interests, dictated settlements that the fishers were forced to accept for lack of other alternatives. Lack of cooperation between the Minamata Fishing Cooperative and the other cooperatives in the Shiranui Sea area further weakened their position. In contrast, an effective alliance of nearly all other groups in Minamata was formed to "protect" the city from the dangers that would result from harm to the company.

The Minamata Fishing Cooperative had negotiated directly with the company for compensation for damage to fishing on several occasions before the outbreak of Minamata disease was recognized.[2] As early as the Taishō period (1912–26), the co-op had demanded compensation for damages to fishing caused by the factory's waste, and the company's response set the tone and pattern for later disputes. On the condition that the co-op would "never again lodge complaints," the company paid the co-op a "solatium," or sympathy payment (*mimaikin*), of ¥1,500 ($704) on April 6, 1926.[3] This condition became a standard part of agreements the company made with those who demanded compensation. The characterization of the money as a sympathy payment meant that the company did not accept responsibility. It also implied a vertical relationship of status and power, in which the superior showed proper benevolence toward the inferior in return for humility, gratitude, and acceptance of the hierarchical relationship. Similar relationships and "legal" responses to such situations continued through the 1940s and 1950s and beyond.

A new agreement between the fishing co-op and the company was signed in January 1943. Fukami Yoshitake signed twice: as chairman of the co-op, he was a party to the agreement, and as mayor, he was an official observer. The other official observer was the head of the Minamata police station. The co-op was paid ¥152,500 (meaningful conversion of 1943 yen into dollar equivalents is difficult) as compensation for all past and future damage to fishing; in return the company gained the fishing rights to two areas. The ability of the fishers to win such a settlement in wartime from the "lord of Minamata," despite the clause in the earlier agreement banning new demands, suggests that damage to fishing was already severe.[4] Yet the co-op had to recognize in the agreement the factory's "extremely important position for the existence of the state, in both peacetime and war," as well as the factory's "importance to the prosperity of Minamata" and "the need to cooperate so as not to harm its operations."[5]

The old cooperative was dissolved and a new one formed in 1949. The pollution issue resurfaced, but factory manager Maeda Kōzō wrote in 1950 to Fuchigami Sueki, head of the co-op, that the company would entertain no further requests for compensation because they were prohibited by the 1943 agreement.[6] Why Nitchitsu's response was different in 1950 is impossible to say, but perhaps the hard line was related to ongoing management struggles between returnees from Korea and the executives who had remained in Minamata through the war. The company argued that the co-op's complaints were unscientific and unsupported by evidence. In fact, says Harada Masazumi, since they "were based on the fishers' experience and on facts, they must be considered quite scientific."[7] The facts were that "catches were declining, nets were being damaged by carbide sediment, barnacles dropped off boats anchored near the factory wastewater outlet, and fish put in water from Hyakken Harbor died."[8]

In 1951 Shin Nitchitsu gave the fishing co-op an interest-free loan of ¥500,000 ($1,390) in return for promises not to ask for further damages and to sell fishing rights when the company wanted to create more landfills in the future to build new settlement pools.[9] In the summer of 1952, the Kumamoto prefectural government investigated damage to fishing in Minamata at the fishing co-op's request. Two years later the company bought the co-op's fishing rights to the Hachiman area so that it could extend its landfill. As part of the agreement, the co-op received ¥400,000 ($1,110) per year to cover past and future damage to fishing, with the familiar proviso that "in the future, absolutely no further demands for damage compensation or other reasons shall be made."[10] Further discussions and exchanges of notes, involving requests that the company stop discharging polluted water, install pollution equipment, and raise the annual payments under the 1954 agreement from ¥400,000 to ¥4 million ($11,100), were held from January 1957 to February 1959, when they ended without agreement.[11]

The company maintained that there had been no change in its waste in recent years, and that its waste had no connection to the disease or the damage to fishing. Yet researchers had already suggested that a heavy metal was causing the disease, and until around the time the disease was discovered the only waste Shin Nitchitsu dumped in Minamata Bay was from its acetaldehyde and vinyl chloride plants, which used a total of 64,020 kilograms of mercury in 1956. Nishida Eiichi, who became factory manager in 1957, later told police that executives were concerned that mercury might be the cause. In 1957, the company devised and then canceled a plan to reduce the amount of mercury being lost.[12]

On September 1, 1958, the Minamata Fishing Cooperative voted to demand that the prefecture ban fishing in Minamata Bay and also to request (1) compensation of fishers, (2) rapid determination of the cause of Minamata disease, (3) national government payments to cover patients' medical costs, (4) solatium payments to patients and their families, (5) cleanup of polluted fishing grounds, and (6) economic assistance for the recovery of the fishing industry. These demands were incorporated into a petition by the city council's Minamata Disease Countermeasures Committee (chaired by Fuchigami Sueki, who was concurrently head of the Minamata Fishing Cooperative) to prefectural governor Sakurai Saburō on September 12, but there was no response.[13]

There could hardly have been a greater contrast in the Japan of 1959 than that between the fairy-tale wedding in Tokyo of Crown Prince Akihito to Shōda Michiko, the "commoner" daughter of a wealthy businessman, and the fishing families of Minamata, where rumors abounded of struggling fishermen selling their daughters into prostitution or being abandoned by their wives.[14] Television and supermarkets were appearing in the cities, and the gap in living standards between Tokyo and the countryside, especially the countryside of southern Kyūshū, was becoming enormous.

In Minamata, even fish caught outside the bay were difficult to sell, for both fishers and fish shops. Signs such as this one were common:

Notice

This inn and sushi restaurant absolutely do not use fish caught in Minamata Bay, which are linked to Minamata disease, and you may eat here without fear. This is our firm, firm promise.

The Manager[15]

By June 1959, several fish shops had gone out of business.[16] Some 100 people from the Minamata Fish Retailers' Cooperative and the Minamata Fish Market paraded through the city on June 20, in an attempt to ease the fears that lowered prices and made fish difficult to sell. Through loudspeakers mounted on four cars, they proclaimed: "By agreement of the cooperative, fish shops in the city sell only fish from the fish market. We absolutely do not sell fish caught off Minamata or that are suspect. Please eat our fish with confidence."[17]

Still the customers stayed away, and the fish sellers' next step in attempting to save their businesses finally pushed the members of the fishing co-op into taking action to save theirs. On July 14 the *Asahi shinbun* broke the news of the Kumamoto University Medical School research team's mercury theory. On July 31, the 80 fish sellers in Minamata, whose sales had dropped by two-thirds, notified the fish market that as of August 1 they would not purchase fish caught by Minamata fishers or caught in the Minamata area.[18] The fishing co-op's 297 members begged them to delay, promising not to catch fish in dangerous areas, to expel any members who did, and to send out patrol boats to enforce this. The fish sellers refused, saying that the fishing co-op delayed enforcing its policy prohibiting fishing in the bay too long. In any case, they added, designating and monitoring unsafe areas would be meaningless if Shin Nitchitsu did not install pollution-control equipment soon.[19] This last point was a reminder that the disease was spreading—cats had been dying of Minamata disease in Tsunagi, north of Minamata, since 1957—and that the company, not the fish sellers, was responsible for the problem. Understandably, though, the fish sellers felt that any potential benefits from cooperating with the fishers, rather than distancing themselves from them, would be too long in coming to be worth gambling on.

The fishing co-op had petitioned the city for help, but got nothing beyond a promise to study the situation. With no other options available, they attempted to negotiate directly with the company again. This was a difficult time to do so, since the company was feeling embattled and beginning its counterattacks. It had issued the first of its 1959 series of anti–mercury theory pamphlets in July, and factory manager Nishida testified to the prefectural assembly's Special Committee on Minamata Disease Countermeasures on August 5.

The next day 400 members of the fishing co-op and the fish sellers' co-op began a "zigzag demonstration" through the city at 8 A.M.[20] They entered the factory gate shouting "*wasshoi, wasshoi*" (as if carrying a portable shrine in a festival), occupied the hallway outside the General Affairs Section, broke windows, and shouted, "Bring out the factory manager." Factory manager Nishida soon appeared with two assistant managers and the head of the General Affairs Section. Negotiations began in a meeting room with Fuchigami Sueki, head of the fishing co-op (and now also speaker of the city council), and fifteen other co-op representatives. Outside, a unit of police watched the situation from in front of the train station, facing the factory gate. The demonstrators moved back and forth between the gate and the entrance to the General Affairs Section, where they occasionally tussled with company employees.

The fishermen (although women fished, I have found no evidence that they participated in these violent incidents) explained their plight and demanded that the company "show sincerity" (*seii o shimese*) and state whether it would pay compensation. The executives' reply was: "Because the cause of Minamata disease is not yet confirmed, we cannot give a final answer, but we are sincere about compensation for your damages." The fishermen then made their first concrete proposal: ¥100 million ($278,000) in compensation for fishing losses, not for Minamata disease. The company responded by offering an "emergency solatium payment" of ¥500,000 ($1,390) in return for the rights to 6,612 square meters of Hyakken Harbor for landfill. They promised to reply to the demand for ¥100 million by August 12, after consulting with company headquarters in Tokyo. The fishermen agreed to accept the ¥500,000 solatium and threatened that if the company offered to pay only half of the ¥100 million compensation they demanded, they would force further negotiations until they received the rest and might then make even further demands. They insisted that the ¥500,000 solatium agreement be put in writing. Fuchigami read it aloud to the demonstrators outside and got their approval. They dispersed at 5:30 P.M.

This first encounter established a pattern for the Minamata Fishing Cooperative and Shin Nitchitsu. The company would negotiate only when forced. It would not acknowledge responsibility for Minamata disease but was quite willing to pay off the members of the co-op by compensating them for some of their lost income. The co-op was willing to set aside the issue of Minamata disease and its cause. Although it might request an end to the pollution and a cleanup of the bay, these were side issues: settlement of its dispute with the company required agreement only on the amount of compensation. Refusing to press the company directly on the disease may have helped the co-op in the short term, but it marginalized the co-op, prevented an alliance with patients' groups, and enabled the company to pursue a "divide and conquer" strategy.

On August 12, 300 co-op members pushed their way into the factory again to hear the company's reply.[21] It offered ¥3 million ($8,330) but only as a "solatium." The company refused the co-op's request that it clean up the sludge in the bay, on the grounds that the bay was "public water" and the company had no right to "arbitrarily deal with it on its own"—rather interesting logic since it did claim the right to dump its waste in the bay. In response to a request that it treat its waste before dumping it, the company promised that part of the treatment facilities then under construction would be completed in October.

The co-op reiterated its demand for ¥100 million, saying the 1,600 people in its member-families could not possibly live on ¥3 million. The company promised to reply by the next afternoon, but then about 80 fishermen forced their way into the meeting room from outside. Nishida said that he realized the fishers needed more; the company could not possibly pay ¥100 million but would respond in good faith by the next afternoon. The discussion ended at 2 A.M. on August 13, after a written agreement was drawn up stipulating that the ¥3 million would be paid as part of the compensation to be negotiated. The fishermen remained at the factory all night.[22]

When the talks reopened on the afternoon of August 13, Shin Nitchitsu raised its offer to ¥10 million ($27,800), promising that if the fishing co-op accepted this amount and agreed never to demand further compensation for fishing losses incurred from 1954 to that date, the money would be paid promptly.[23] In one week, then, the company had raised its offer from ¥500,000 to ¥10 million, and was leaving open the possibility of future payments for future damages. The fishermen still refused to compromise, and the two sides agreed that (1) they would jointly investigate fishing conditions in the bay on August 15, (2) henceforth negotiations would be conducted in an orderly manner, and (3) they would meet again on August 17, when the company would make a new offer based on the August 15 survey.

Opening the meeting on the seventeenth, Nishida announced:

As a result of the joint survey by the fishers and the factory on August 15 of conditions in polluted fishing areas in the bay, we recognize that there are areas in which fishing operations are impossible, but we believe ¥10 million is appropriate compensation. However, since we strongly desire a full solution, we will add ¥3 million [$8,330] to this amount, but this is our final offer.[24]

The fishermen flatly rejected the offer. Some 100 fishermen stormed into the building and up to the second-floor meeting room. Two company employees and one fisherman were injured by broken glass. Nishida called a halt to the talks, the fishermen temporarily retreated, and a detachment of riot police arrived. The chief of police asked the fishermen to refrain from violence and allow the negotiations to proceed. The fishermen agreed, but the company officials said negotiating in such a situation was impossible. The fishermen camped outside the door, refusing to leave or to allow the company officials out.

The next morning, August 18, Nishida formally requested that he and the other hostages be released.[25] The fishermen answered that they could not give an official reply because co-op leader Fuchigami had gone to Kumamoto to petition the governor. The fishermen attempted to enter the building and were stopped by about 150 riot police in a struggle that injured five policemen, nine fishermen, and one company guard. The fishermen then set up tents in front of the meeting room and the factory gate. Just before noon, there was another fight when some of the riot police attempted to exit the gate. From then on, the Minamata police, who had previously tried to stay out of the dispute, were in regular contact with Shin Nitchitsu and rapidly responded to its requests for assistance.[26]

Fuchigami and six other co-op delegates, accompanied by Mayor Naka-mura Todomu and three prefectural assembly representatives from the Minamata area, met Governor Teramoto Hirosaku on the morning of August 18.[27] Complaining of "being sacrificed for the factory's development," they asked the governor to (1) mediate a resumption of negotiations, (2) aid fishermen who were out of work because they could not sell their fish, and (3) shut down the polluting factory. The governor responded that he hoped (1) to certify fish caught outside the affected area as safe, in order to make them marketable, and (2) to apply the Welfare Protection Law to those in need. He insisted the hostages must be released to make negotiations possible. Finally, he asked Mayor Nakamura to mediate the negotiations.

The violence, which had brought in the police and attracted media attention, had made the problem one the local and prefectural authorities could no longer ignore. The mayor had been forced by the governor to get involved. That night he formed a committee stacked in favor of the company, in a pattern typical for "mediation" between powerful and weak local interests. The committee consisted of the mayor himself, the vice-mayor, two prefectural assembly representatives, and five city council members. Three of these committee members were Shin Nitchitsu employees, and all were well aware of the city's dependence on the company. None was a member of the Minamata Fishing Cooperative.[28] By the afternoon of August 19, both sides had agreed to accept mediation and reopen negotiations.

The two sides met in the presence of the mediation committee on August 20, while 150 fishermen conducted a sit-in demonstration at the factory gate.[29] Shin Nitchitsu had sent an executive director, a Mr. Ikeda, for the negotiations. Factory manager Nishida began by explaining how the factory had calculated its offer of ¥13 million ($36,100). The fishing co-op had requested in December 1958, he said, that the 1954 agreement be readjusted to require the company to pay ¥4 million per year. For the five years since 1954, this would make a total of ¥20 million. Assuming that half of this was probably intended as compensation for Minamata disease left ¥10 million to cover damage to fishing, the issue now under negotiation. A bonus of ¥3 million had been added as an incentive to finalize the solution. Nishida announced that he was now adding ¥2 million for fishing rights to a larger area the company wanted to claim in Hyakken Harbor, for a total of ¥15 million.

Adding to this the ¥400,000 per year already paid under the 1954 agreement, the co-op would receive a total of ¥17 million ($47,200) for damage to fishing since 1954.

The co-op rejected the company's calculations, saying its request for ¥4 million per year had been for damage to fishing only in the area around Koiji Island. Pollution now extended as far as Hachiman at the mouth of the Minamata River, and in any case the company had rejected the demand as "unfair" when it was first made. Ikeda announced: "Considering the company's financial situation, we cannot pay more than ¥13 million." The co-op replied that if the company was still offering only ¥13 million, Nishida could do the talking; they expected a better offer from an executive director. The meeting ended, and the committee conducted separate discussions with the company and the co-op over the next few days.

The mediation committee summoned the two sides to hear its decision on the afternoon of August 26.[30] As compensation for damages to fishing since 1954, specifically excluding Minamata disease, the company would be required to make a one-time payment of ¥20 million, set up a ¥15 million fund to promote fishing recovery, and pay the fishing co-op ¥2 million per year in perpetuity under the 1954 agreement. It would also have to reclaim 6,600 square meters of land in Hyakken Harbor within three years and give the land to the co-op. This proposed agreement, said the committee, was not open to negotiation. The two sides had to accept or reject it, as presented, by 10 A.M., August 29. If either side refused, the committee would end its mediation.

The fishing co-op decided to ask for amendments, despite the mediation committee's ultimatum.[31] First, it wanted to add a provision requiring the company to dredge the polluted sediment from fishing areas. Second, it asked that the yearly payments of ¥2 million be increased to ¥4 million until the company completed its pollution-control facilities. Finally, it wanted to ensure that the land it would receive was not reclaimed with polluted sediment dredged from the fishing grounds and demanded the company pay a penalty of ¥5 million per year if it failed to hand over the land within three years. The committee, true to its word, refused to consider these or any other changes to its proposal. On the night of August 28, fishing co-op members assembled in their respective hamlets to hear co-op representatives explain the agreement.

Company executives met in Tokyo on August 28 and 29 and concluded that the agreement and the pollution-control facilities they were installing would soon put an end to their troubles. The one-time payment of ¥20 million and the recovery fund of ¥15 million together equaled nearly 1.3 percent of the company's capitalized value. The ¥20 million amounted to an average payment of ¥12,500 ($35, or 8.7 percent of per capita annual GNP) per person for the 1,600 people in co-op members' families.[32] This was a paltry sum, even in 1959, for people in such straits to receive from the company that had ruined their livelihood.

The two sides presented their replies just before the deadline on August 29.[33] Fishing co-op secretary Nakamura entered the mayor's office at 9:50, and Ikeda and Nishida arrived five minutes later. Mayor Nakamura opened and read the coop's decision first: "In order to end the anxiety of the citizens, we swallow our tears and accept." Next he read Shin Nitchitsu's reply: "Although parts of it are difficult to bear, because of the great efforts of the members of the mediation committee, and in order to achieve a full solution, we accept the mediated agreement." Ikeda remarked: "This is a big sacrifice for the factory, but since we do not want any more trouble, it was unavoidable. We now want to get along well as fellow citizens."

The fishing cooperative formed a committee to determine how to distribute the money, all of which the company paid by September 10.[34] Eight members received ¥230,000 ($638) each, about 40 "members in name only" received ¥10,000 ($28) each, and the others received ¥160,000 ($444), ¥130,000 ($361), ¥110,000 ($306), or ¥40,000 ($111). Most of those who depended exclusively on fishing for their livelihood used the money to repay loans. According to the co-op, most net owners (*amimoto*), who hired others to work for them, had debts exceeding ¥2 million ($5,560); the largest award of ¥230,000 did not even cover the interest on their debt.

The company's hope that the agreement would end its troubles and allow it to get along with its neighbors was not realized. Its troubles had just begun. The day after the settlement, the *Kumamoto nichinichi shinbun* wrote: "Since the problem of compensation for fishing losses related to Minamata disease was fully solved on August 29, the focus from then on has been narrowed to aiding Minamata disease patients and to reducing the number of new patients."[35] In fact, the company was about to encounter even worse troubles over compensation for fishing losses, and the disease was spreading. The same *Kumamoto nichinichi shinbun* article noted that two new patients had appeared in the area around the mouth of the Minamata River, and that cats were dying of Minamata disease in the Ashikita area to the north and in Izumi, Komenotsu, Shishijima, and Nagashima to the south.

The *Kumamoto nichinichi shinbun* described the rippling of problems outward from Minamata.[36] On August 17, the Ashikita Village Fishing Cooperative, whose sales had dropped 30 percent, issued a statement saying the fish it sold were safe. Fish shops in the town of Yunoura had tried bringing in sardines and mackerel from far away, but no customers could be found for anything but whale meat. In Tanoura people were afraid to eat not only fish but also chicken and pork. In Tsunagi, closest to Minamata, many people were eating only canned fish and meat.

On September 23, Funaba Tōkichi was diagnosed as the first Minamata disease patient from outside Minamata.[37] This 35-year-old fisherman from Tsunagi had eaten only fish from Tsunagi Bay, over seven kilometers north of Minamata Bay. Some 310 of the 1,611 households in the village of Tsunagi fished, and fishing provided about 30 percent of the town's total income.[38] The village council met on September 24 and 25 and decided to petition the prefecture, asking that the cause be discovered quickly and that aid be provided to the fishing families. The Tsunagi Village Fishing Cooperative met on September 28 and decided to ask the prefecture for help and to negotiate with Shin Nitchitsu for compensation.[39] On October 2, the Tsunagi Village Women's Association began collecting rice to distribute to fishing families, some of whom were playing the *shamisen* in the street to survive, and the 55-member village government employees' union donated ¥40,000 ($111) to the fishing co-op.[40]

The prefectural government ignored the requests of the village. As was evident earlier, it seemed its inertia could be overcome only by much greater pressure than that exerted by petitions. That pressure was soon to be brought to bear on both the prefecture and the company, from both above and below. On October 14, Funaba Tōkichi's father, Iwazō, developed Minamata disease.[41] One week later, Tōkichi died. That very day, Itō Hasuo's eight-millimeter films, including footage showing the shocking physical effects of the disease on Funaba Tōkichi, were shown to Diet members in Tokyo by representatives of the Kumamoto Prefectural Alliance of Fishing Cooperatives. Eight days later, on October 29, the Diet decided to send a delegation of Diet members and officials from various ministries and agencies to investigate the situation in Kumamoto and Minamata from November 1 to November 3.

The Diet's decision was prompted, and then in turn intensified, by what was later called the "Shiranuikai Fishing Dispute." This was a larger version of the dispute between the Minamata Fishing Cooperative and Shin Nitchitsu, which came to be called the "First Minamata Fishing Dispute." The Shiranuikai Fishing Dispute was between the Kumamoto Prefectural Alliance of Fishing Cooperatives and Shin Nitchitsu. It repeated much of the earlier pattern. Fishermen assembled, petitioned the government, and demanded negotiations with the factory. There were small fights, negotiations were broken off, fishermen forced their way into the factory, and the police intervened. In the end, a committee of local notables was formed to mediate and dictated a settlement. In comparison with the earlier struggle, this one involved more people, more violence, a larger total (but not per person) settlement, and far more media coverage. The company's agreement with the Minamata co-op came six weeks after the Kumamoto University mercury theory was made public, and its agreement with the regional alliance of fishing cooperatives came five weeks after the Ministry of Health and Welfare received the interim report of the Food Hygiene Investigation Committee and disbanded its Minamata Food Poisoning Subcommittee.

The Shiranuikai Fishing Dispute began on October 17, 1959.[42] A group of 1,500 fishermen from the Kumamoto Prefectural Alliance of Fishing Cooperatives approached the factory in about 60 boats, demanding an end to the pollution. They then held a general meeting and resolved that Shin Nitchitsu must halt its dumping of waste until the treatment facilities were finished, clean up the bay, pay compensation for fishing losses, and make solatium payments to Minamata disease patients. (The weak, misguided Minamata Fishing Cooperative had not requested compensation for Minamata disease.) They demanded that the government quickly discover the cause of the disease, pass a strict water-pollution law, and apply the law to the Shiranui Sea.[43] The Minamata Fishing Cooperative took no part in any of these activities. Its August 30 agreement with the company prohibited asking for further compensation for damages to fishing from 1954 until the date of the agreement. Its members did not even attend the meeting on October 17 to observe or to describe their experience to the prefectural alliance. Had they attended, they might have been less isolated over the following years.

Shortly after noon, the alliance sent a delegation led by alliance president Murakami Ushita to the factory to request negotiations, but company officials refused to meet with it. The 1,500 fishermen pushed through the gate and attacked the factory security office, breaking 50 windowpanes and injuring seven guards. Murakami was finally allowed to hand the alliance's resolution to factory manager Nishida, who promised to respond "directly to the headquarters of the prefectural fishing co-op alliance on the twenty-fourth." In contrast to leaders of the Minamata Fishing Cooperative, who had traveled to Kumamoto to petition the prefectural government during their negotiations with the company, a delegation headed by prefectural fishing co-op alliance leader Murakami left that evening for Tokyo to petition the central government.

In Tokyo on October 20, the delegation met with the minister of labor and with officials at the Ministry of Health and Welfare and the Fisheries Agency.[44] The Fisheries Agency put an official on a train for Kumamoto that very day to investigate the situation. The delegation then visited Shin Nitchitsu's head office to meet company president Yoshioka Kiichi. Since Yoshioka, they were told, was out, they met a managing director named Chihara, to whom they presented the demands from the October 17 meeting and explained their difficult straits. He repeated Nishida's promise of a reply on October 24, saying: "Since our standpoints are different, I cannot promise the results you hope for, but we will show sincerity in the negotiations. In my personal opinion, we should consider the cause separately from compensation for living costs, and I do not think wastewater is the cause." Murakami replied: "I believe the wastewater is the cause. I'd like the factory to show me scientific evidence that there are no dangerous substances in the wastewater."

The next day the delegation met with the Committee on Agriculture, Forestry, and Fisheries of the House of Representatives and showed them slides and Itō Hasuo's eight-millimeter movies.[45] On October 22 the committee spent two hours questioning officials from the Ministry of Health and Welfare, the Ministry of Agriculture and Forestry, the Fisheries Agency, MITI, and the EPA:

Representative Fukunaga Kazutomi (LDP, Kumamoto): "The common understanding is that the cause is the wastewater of Shin Nitchitsu's Minamata factory. What steps are being taken by the Ministry of Health and Welfare?"

Jitsukawa Wataru, Assistant Section Chief, Food Hygiene Section, Ministry of Health and Welfare: "Overall, it has been reported that research of various types suggests organic mercury as the cause. However, the process by which it becomes poisonous is not sufficiently clear. . . ."

. . . .

Fukunaga: "The slow investigation means slowness in taking appropriate measures. I want you to solve the problem quickly."

Ōno Ichirō, Vice Minister for Political Affairs, Ministry of Agriculture and Forestry: "Investigating the cause is the key. We've been asking the Ministry of Health and Welfare to hurry."

Fukunaga: "This 'we'll think about what to do after the cause has been proved' attitude is not acceptable. As the agency overseeing Shin Nitchitsu, what has MITI been doing for the past six years?"

Fujioka Taishin, Section Chief, Industrial Water Section, MITI: "We have been looking at newspaper and magazine reports and reports from the field, keeping in touch with the Ministry of Health and Welfare, and cooperating in the investigation of the cause."

Fukunaga: "What do you mean by 'cooperating'?"

Fujioka: "Cooperating in the Ministry of Health and Welfare's research."

Fukunaga: "Specifically how?"

(no clear answer)

. . . .

Fukunaga: "Are there laws to regulate factory wastewater?"

Fujioka: "There are the Water Quality Conservation Law and the Factory Effluents Control Law, but they take at least a year [to apply]."[46]

Yoshizawa Nagamori, Section Chief, Water Quality Protection Section, EPA: "The Water Quality Protection Commission considers requests from the various ministries concerned and then selects water areas to be investigated. For 1959 these have already been decided, and we have not been contacted concerning Minamata."

Representative Kawamura Tsugiyoshi (JSP, Kumamoto): "The fishers' anger is serious. The government authorities have made a grave error in failing to take this large problem seriously. Why has the interim report of the Kumamoto University research not been made public?"

Jitsukawa: "The standing members of the Food Hygiene Investigation Committee have some doubts; so we are not at the stage where we could make it public. If mercury is the cause, evidence is lacking to show it is present in (1) the factory effluent, (2) sea water, (3) fish and shellfish, and (4) patients and cats. It could also be from a mercury mine or agricultural chemicals."

Kawamura: "What factories use mercury?"

Fujioka: "Nationwide, there are 21 factories using it in the production of acetaldehyde and vinyl chloride."[47]

The committee decided that a special law to deal with Minamata disease was needed and made plans to send a delegation to Minamata to investigate.

On October 26 the Kumamoto prefectural assembly's Minamata Disease Countermeasures Committee announced its proposed draft for a law to be passed by the Diet.[48] The law would establish three special commissions: one to investigate the cause of the disease, one to designate unsafe fishing areas and compensate fishers, and one to certify patients, whose treatment was to be provided by the Ministry of Health and Welfare. All costs under this law would be paid by the national government. The draft did not mention Shin Nitchitsu and said nothing about what was to be done once the cause of the disease had been determined. Nevertheless, it proposed far more than was ever done. The only part of this draft that was ever implemented in a meaningful way was the certification committee.

Had such activity in the prefectural and national legislatures continued, the Minamata issue might have rapidly developed into a major scandal. It is easy to see why both Shin Nitchitsu and the government, particularly MITI, were anxious to make the issue go away. For a few more weeks, the situation got worse rather than better for them, but by the beginning of the new year they seemed to have put the problem behind them.

On October 23, factory manager Nishida replied in writing to the fishermen's demands:

1. We cannot comply with the request that we shut down factory operations. However, we wish to inform you that we are now constructing facilities to enable us to end the dumping of wastewater in the Hachiman area by the last day of this month.

2. As for the other requests, at a stage in which the cause of the strange disease is still not determined, we are unable to comply with any of them.[49]

The Diet group was scheduled to arrive in Kumamoto on November 1 and be in Minamata November 2 and 3. The fishermen put their hopes in the Diet members' visit. MITI and Shin Nitchitsu were concerned about the visit as well. On October 30, the newspapers reported the final roster for the delegation and also announced that MITI had "suggested" Shin Nitchitsu take more rapid steps to deal with its waste. On October 21, the chief of MITI's Light Industry Bureau, Akiyama Takeo, had verbally suggested to the company's Tokyo head office that it stop dumping waste at Hachiman at the mouth of the Minamata River and return to using Hyakken Harbor (hence Nishida's promise to the prefectural fishing co-op alliance that he would do so). Also, Akiyama asked the company to advance the completion date of the waste-treatment facilities then under construction from March 1960 to the end of December 1959. A source in the Light Industry Bureau's Light Industry Section told the *Kumamoto nichinichi shinbun*: "This suggestion does not have the force of law; it is administrative guidance taken because the company has recently caused a social problem by dumping its effluent at the mouth of the Minamata River. We also suggested that the waste-treatment facilities be completed within the year."[50]

This treatment of Shin Nitchitsu was remarkably different from that of Honshū Paper Company's factory on the Edogawa River the previous year, when MITI's Akiyama had shut down the factory after fishermen's protests. Akiyama explained the different treatment as being due to the fact that acetaldehyde was much more important than pulp and that it was essential to attempt to meet domestic demand without resorting to imports. Akiyama was in charge of MITI's guidance of chemical factories in their shift to petrochemicals, and Shin Nitchitsu had submitted its plan to MITI in July 1959.[51]

In what was something of a rehearsal for the Diet members' visit, Kumamoto Governor Teramoto made his first visit to investigate the Minamata situation on October 31.[52] After visiting Tanoura, Ashikita, Yunoura, and Tsunagi in Ashikita *gun* (county) to the north, his group arrived in Minamata and consulted with officials at city hall. After meeting with secretary Nakamura of the Minamata Fishing Cooperative, they visited Minamata disease patients at the municipal hospital and then met with company executives at the factory. Their questions to the executives showed that the leaders of the prefectural government were losing patience with the company. Hadn't the payments to the Minamata fishing cooperative helped put public opinion on the side of the Kumamoto University theory? Surely the public was not convinced by the company's countertheories? What was the status of the new purification facilities? The company officials replied (falsely, but in line with the misleading newspaper headlines of the previous day) that all discharge of waste into the sea had ended after October 29 when pumps were brought on line at Hachiman to pump the wastewater from the settlement pools there back to the factory and to Hyakken. They said they hoped to complete the purification facilities earlier than the original target date of March, but there were limits to what they could do. After a tour of the new pumping facilities at Hachiman, Governor Teramoto visited residents of the hamlet of Yudō, including some disease victims.

Although no concrete changes resulted from Teramoto's visit, it raised hopes (and fears) that government attitudes were changing. The prefectural fishing co-op alliance was more optimistic that the Diet members' visit would help it win restitution from Shin Nitchitsu. The company, hoping perhaps to discourage the fishermen from becoming brasher in their negotiations, filed charges on October 31 with the Minamata police against the fishermen involved in the violence of October 17.[53] The police had been interviewing witnesses since the day of the incident, and had a great deal of evidence already prepared in support of the company's charges. This increased the fishermen's anger at the company, anger that was to boil over two days later.

The Diet delegation was led by Matsuda Tetsuzō (LDP, Hokkaidō).[54] It consisted of members of the Lower House from the Committee on Agriculture, Forestry, and Fisheries, the Committee on Society and Labor, and the Committee on Commerce, two representatives chosen by the LDP (one of whom was Fukunaga Kazutomi) and one from the JSP (Kawamura Tsugiyoshi). There were also representatives from the Ministry of Health and Welfare, MITI (Fujioka Taishin), the Fisheries Agency, and the EPA (Yoshizawa Nagamori). The group arrived in Kumamoto on November 1 and held a public hearing that afternoon in the prefectural legislature building.[55] Those present included Governor Teramoto and other prefectural officials, the prefectural legislature's Minamata Disease Countermeasures Committee, Mayor Nakamura of Minamata, and representatives of Kumamoto University and the prefectural fishing alliance.

The hearing became a harsh indictment of Shin Nitchitsu and the local authorities. The political system seemed to be functioning as it should, responding to demands from citizens and working for their benefit. After hearing a description of the company's dumping of mercury, Diet member Matsuda remarked: "Have the prefectural government and legislature done nothing yet? . . . To my knowledge, there is no more unreasonable factory in the whole country. This is shocking." Another representative commented: "The governor has done none of the things he should."[56] When the representatives suggested that the university had been slow to analyze the sludge and water of Minamata Bay, one of the researchers explained the financial constraints. Since 1956 the university had been given ¥400,000 ($1,110) per year in Ministry of Education scientific research assistance funds, and in both 1958 and 1959 it had also received ¥1 million ($2,780) to do research on behalf of the Ministry of Health and Welfare's Minamata Food Poisoning Subcommittee (which was soon to be disbanded). Pounding the desk, he explained that taking even one sludge sample involved travel expenses, but the science department was allotted only ¥20,000 ($56) in research funds. The shocked Diet members mumbled "only ¥1 million?" Reports of the hearing in the next day's newspapers not only raised the hopes of the demonstrators planning to petition the Diet delegation in Minamata but also angered and emboldened them.

The visitors from Tokyo were met by 4,000 demonstrators in front of the Minamata Municipal Hospital the next day. Ishimure Michiko ran from her home to observe the curious mix of obsequiousness and anger, more reminiscent of peasant protests in the Tokugawa period rather than what one might expect in Japan under its democratic constitution:

Suddenly, a cry of joy arose from the group of fishermen sitting on the pavement. . . . The hitherto silent men suddenly became animated. Their faces lit up with genuine happiness . . . .

"Hey, the Diet members have arrived." . . .

Looking back now, what struck me most was the profound respect the members of the [Minamata Disease Patients Families Mutual Aid] Society showed. . . .

Thoroughly absorbed in what was going on, several thousand members of the Yatsushiro, Ashikita, and Amakusa fishermen's unions crowded around the representatives of the Mutual Help Society, the 16 Diet members, members of the Kumamoto Prefectural Assembly, the Minamata City Assembly and other officials. . . .

Watanabe Eizō, president of the Mutual Help Society, stepped forward, visibly tense. His sunken eyes and emaciated face betrayed his great fatigue. With great deference, he took off the twisted towel tied around his head. . . . Following his example, other members of the society, standing behind him, removed their headbands, that distinctive mark of fishermen in public demonstrations. Then they folded their banners and placed them on the ground at their feet.

The Yatsushiro, Ashikita and Amakusa fishermen . . . also removed their headbands and laid down their straw flags.

The air was filled with solemn, respectful silence. People seemed to be holding their breath. . . . Another member of the Mutual Help Society, Nakaoka Satsuki, a smallish, middle aged woman, came forward and read out the fishermen's petition in a trembling voice and with frequent breaks, eloquently expressing their physical and mental torment. . . .

"We have always regarded you as fathers and mothers of the nation. . . .

"Our children are dying of Minamata Disease. . . . Our husbands are suffering from the same terrible illness and so are no longer able to sail out to catch fish. Those who can still handle their nets face poverty and hardship, because no one will buy their catches. Restrained by conscience, we cannot make a living by stealing. . . . Now we have reached the limit of our endurance. We can no longer trust anyone.

"We take your visit to Minamata to be a token of your good will and compassion toward us. You are our only hope. Please help us!"

Repeatedly nodding to the speaker's words, the older fishermen wiped their tears with the towel headbands they had just removed. The supplicating look on the faces of all the participants, their rough, dark hands resting on their knees or clasping the poles of their banners, every fold in their garments showed both despair and the fearless determination of the people sentenced to death.

The 16 members of the Diet's investigation committee listened with bowed heads in respectful silence. . . . Trying to conceal their emotion, they thanked the fishermen for impressing on the central government the gravity of the crisis . . . in such a peaceful and dignified manner and solemnly promised they would do their best. . . .

Unfolding their banners and raising them high, the fishermen thanked the Diet members for their attention and shouted "Banzai!" in unison, hurrahs of hope for a central government program that would alleviate their plight.[57]

Komori Takeshi wrote: "Can I be the only one who feels as if he were looking at a scene from a legend of *gimin* [the martyrs in Tokugawa peasant rebellions] and finds it utterly impossible to believe this is a present-day occurrence?"[58] Both Ishimure and Komori quite intentionally present the story as one of honest, determined, humble supplicants in the tradition of peasants and their martyrs. It is the pain of the still-necessary humility and obsequiousness toward authorities who have done nothing to help them, added to the suffering caused by the pollution, that makes the protesters heroes.

The delegates then entered the hospital, where they assembled in a conference room and were told by city authorities about "the weight carried by the Shin Nitchitsu Minamata factory in the city of Minamata, and by the Minamata Disease Patients Families Mutual Aid Society (Watanabe Eizō, chairman) about their distressed living situation."[59] After visiting hospitalized patients, the delegation left the hospital for Yudō, where they visited the home of ten-year-old Matsuda Tomiji, who had been blinded by Minamata disease. Finally they toured Minamata Bay by boat. They were scheduled to visit the factory the next day.

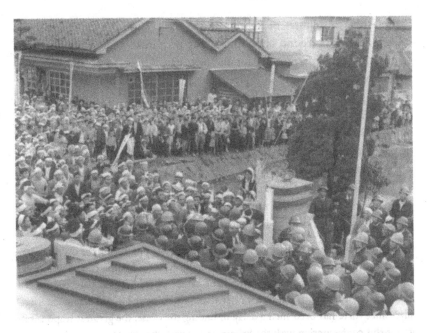

Fig. 11 Members of fishing cooperatives from the Shiranui Sea invade the factory on November 2, 1959. © *Kumamoto nichinichi shinbun.*

In the meantime, 2,000 members of the prefectural alliance of fishing cooperatives had already been to the factory. They had planned to march from the hospital to the station, send representatives to the company to demand negotiations, hold a general meeting, and finally say a respectful farewell to the Diet members from their boats on Minamata Bay before returning to their homes.[60] Instead, when the company refused to negotiate, they canceled their meeting, marched on the factory gates, and twice forced their way in and rioted.[61] At 1:50 P.M., Shinohara Tamotsu, a leader of the fishermen from Tsunagi (who developed Minamata disease a week later and died before the month ended), climbed over the factory gate and opened it from the inside.[62] A thousand fishermen rushed in and attacked the guardhouse, main offices, a laboratory, and the power station, throwing typewriters, adding machines, and teletype machines out the windows. Riot police entered from another gate, and the fishermen broke the windshield of one of their jeeps. After 40 minutes of fighting, the fishermen withdrew outside the main gate. At 6:15, however, they began throwing stones and rushed through the gate again. After 50 minutes of fighting in the dark (since the lights had been broken in the first round of fighting), they withdrew again. They dispersed at 9 P.M., planning a meeting for the next day. About 30 or 40 fishermen were reported to have been injured, along with three company employees (including factory manager Nishida) and 64 policemen, including the chief of police and the assistant chief. The company estimated its damages at ¥8 million ($22,200). Members of the Minamata Fishing Cooperative had participated in the demonstration in front of the hospital but observed the riots at the factory from a distance.

The Diet members visited the factory the next morning, November 3, and gave its executives the same sort of tongue lashing they had given the prefectural authorities two days earlier.[63] Matsuda told them:

Shin Nitchitsu's research has been only for the purpose of refuting the organic mercury theory announced by Kumamoto University. Why didn't the company cooperate with Kumamoto University to find the cause? Shouldn't you have cooperated and provided them with samples, rather than criticizing them and acting emotionally? Since there has been such a delay in finding the cause, the greatest responsibility for this confrontation with the fishermen lies with the company executives.

Representative Fukunaga continued: "The purification facilities are belated countermeasures. If you had wanted to, you could have done this sooner." Nishida could only respond that he had provided samples to Kumamoto University and would cooperate more fully in the future. That afternoon the delegation left for Tokyo. Later that month, when he was interviewed for an NHK television documentary, Shin Nitchutsu president Yoshioka commented after the recording stopped that the company itself was a "victim" of government pressure.[64]

The violence by the fishermen had two effects. On the one hand, it sparked the formation of what Ui Jun calls a "united front" to defend the company and thereby the city from violence and ruin.[65] At the same time, however, the publicity it garnered and the fears it engendered forced the company and the prefectural government to deal with the Shiranuikai fishermen.

On November 3 the factory gates were guarded by helmeted riot police.[66] Fifty investigators from both Minamata and the prefectural police headquarters swarmed over the factory collecting evidence against the fishermen. Rumors circulated in the city that there would be another invasion of the factory or that the fishermen would block the factory's drainage ditch and flood the streets with poisonous wastewater. The factory raised its damage estimate to ¥10 million ($27,800), and the police raised the count of their injured to 80.[67] The prefectural police chief announced that most of the fishermen had been drunk, and that "all the bad elements" would be arrested.[68]

On November 4, officials of the Shin Nitchitsu workers' union held an emergency meeting.[69] Their fears had been voiced during the riot by a worker's wife who was seen by Ishimure running with a child on her back and holding another by the hand, half-crazed by the sound of breaking factory windows, screaming: "Oh no, daddy's bonus will be cut. His bonus will be cut! Stop it, please!"[70] The union leaders stressed the need to find the cause of Minamata disease (although some of them may well have known the results of Hosokawa's experiments) and help the suffering fishing families. Like the Diet members, they said some responsibility for the fishermen's attack on the property with which the workers made their living lay with the factory executives and called for both sides to reconsider their actions. In the afternoon they distributed handbills advertising a "general meeting of workers" to be held that evening: "We reject violence!! Defend the factory from violence. . . . We request the attendance of workers and as many citizens as possible."[71] Two of the three employees listed on the handbill as calling for the meeting, Onitsuka Yoshisada and Gotō Haruo, were also Socialist party city council members.[72] The word "citizens" used in the call for the meeting is significant. From the time Minamata disease first became an issue, up to the present, in such contexts it has meant not all residents of the city but only those who are not directly involved. In other words, it excludes Minamata disease victims, fishing families, and company employees.

The meeting was attended by about 1,500 people.[73] One worker gave a speech entitled "An Appeal from a Victim," and Gotō titled his speech "Minamata Disease Cannot Be Solved by Violence." The meeting passed a resolution to be delivered as a petition to the prefectural fishing co-ops, factory manager Nishida, and Governor Teramoto. It asked the fishing co-ops to refrain from violence and the company to cooperate in finding the cause of the disease, to install the purification equipment quickly, and to negotiate with the fishermen "with sincerity." The governor was asked to deal firmly with those who had perpetrated the violence and take steps to prevent factory property, with which workers made their living, from being damaged again. Nothing was said about helping Minamata disease victims. The goal of this "united front" was to protect the factory in order to protect the workers and the city.

The factory was threatened by the actions of the prefectural assembly as well as by fishermen. Its Special Committee on Minamata Disease Countermeasures met November 5 and 6 and decided to call for an urgent special session of the assembly.[74] The purpose of the special session would be to pass a law halting all dumping of waste by Shin Nitchitsu, which would have meant a virtual shutdown of the factory. The committee also called on Governor Teramoto to mediate and resolve the dispute between the fishing co-ops and the company. These decisions were made over the strong objections of committee vice chairman Nagano Harutoshi, who was a Shin Nitchitsu employee and an official in its union. There was much confusion over whether the prefecture could pass a law that overlapped with the national Water Quality Conservation Law and the Factory Effluents Control Law, both of which had taken effect on April 1 that year but had not yet been enforced.[75] Tokyo, Kanagawa, and Fukuoka had their own regulations controlling pollution from factories, but these had all been established before April 1. Nagano, as well as Governor Teramoto, argued that the prefecture could not regulate Shin Nitchitsu's waste, but most of the committee, and most of the prefectural officials it heard from, believed it could be done as long as the prefectural regulations were carefully crafted so as not to duplicate the national laws.

On November 5, 1959, the Minamata city council met and decided to petition the company, the fishing alliance, and the prefecture.[76] The content of the petition was much the same as that of the resolution passed in the workers' and citizens' rally the night before. Since, after six years, the cause of the disease had still not been determined, Shin Nitchitsu should cooperate with scientists from the whole nation to find it. The fishers were suffering, but this was no excuse for violence. Future negotiations should be peaceful. Since stopping factory operations would bring serious social unrest, the prefecture should urge the factory to install pollution-control equipment quickly to make this unnecessary. The city council petition added a topic not covered in the resolution from the rally the night before: since the Welfare Protection Law did not provide sufficient aid for fishing families and patients, further steps should be taken. What these measures were, though, and who should carry them out and pay for them, was not specified. The petition was not presented until November 16, and by then events had already begun to move in the direction the city council hoped they would.

On November 6, the Standing Committee of the Kumamoto prefectural assembly called Governor Teramoto to discuss the request for a special session of the legislature.[77] Teramoto argued forcefully against a special session and against halting Shin Nitchitsu's waste output, which would mean shutting down the company. He said that Shin Nitchitsu had spent ¥60 million ($167,000) for the purification equipment that would be installed by the end of December, ¥5 million ($13,900) for three settlement pools at Hyakken, and ¥3 million ($8,330) for the new pumps at Hachiman. Therefore, "once the company announces that the toxicity of its wastewater has been reduced, the prefecture ought to back it up by publicizing the safety of the fish." About twenty delegates from the Kumamoto Prefectural Alliance of Fishing Cooperatives, waiting in a side room, agreed to a deal: the governor would begin the next day to mediate, "with sincerity," the issues of waste-water treatment, compensation for fishing losses, and aid to fishing families. The opening of a special legislative session would be "studied" while events on the national level were observed.

Also on November 6, the 3,400-member union at Shin Nitchitsu passed a resolution directed toward the prefecture, company management, and the prefectural fishing co-ops.[78] It asked the prefecture not to shut down the factory, because doing so would harm "not only its workers and their families but also the small and medium enterprises on which the factory depends and citizens in general." It also asked the prefecture to discover the cause of the disease quickly and to aid patients and fishers. The company was asked to install the purification equipment quickly, to conduct peaceful negotiations with the fishing co-ops, and "not merely insist on its own views, but cooperate with the various authorities concerned" to discover the cause of the disease. Finally, although the union sympathized with the suffering of the fishermen, they should "reconsider" their "extremely regrettable" violence.

It was not only the factory union that supported the factory against its victims. The next day, November 7, a similar statement was issued by the 5,800-member Minamata Regional Association of Labor Unions (Minamata chiku rōdō kumiai kyōgikai; usually abbreviated Chikurō).[79] This association was dominated by the Shin Nitchitsu union but included unions from small manufacturing companies, taxi companies, and JNR, as well as teach-

ers and city employees. The JNR and teachers' unions generally took relatively radical leftist stands. That they backed a statement that repeated the
resolution passed by the Shin Nitchitsu union, and even strengthened its
condemnation of the fishermen (it called their violence "morally impermissible"), is evidence of how strongly nearly all residents of Minamata identified
the company with the city.

The same day, a 50-member "all Minamata" delegation representing 28
organizations traveled to Kumamoto and petitioned Governor Teramoto
not to suspend operations at the factory.[80] The group was led by Mayor
Nakamura and included the speaker of the city council, the head of the
chamber of commerce, and the head of the Minamata Regional Association
of Labor Unions. They pleaded that "immediately halting the Shin
Nitchitsu Minamata factory's waste output is a life-and-death issue for all
citizens of Minamata." They told the governor that the city depended on the
factory for half of its ¥180 million ($500,000) tax income and that a factory
shutdown would affect all 50,000 residents in one way or another. Teramoto's reply continued the distancing from the company evident during his
factory visit a week earlier: "Both the factory and fishing are industries in this
prefecture. I want to approach the problem from this standpoint. From
what I have seen, the factory's waste treatment is all right now, but in the
past it was a bit sloppy. I would like you citizens to consider this and cooperate so that the problem can be solved in a reasonable manner."

Some members of the delegation went on to Tokyo, where they lobbied
the Fisheries Agency and other government offices. Their fears could only
have been increased by the fact that the local press was beginning to publish
more articles taking the side of the fishers. An opinion piece in the *Kumamoto nichinichi shinbun* criticized the delegation for sending 50 people to "push
their way into" (an expression comparing their actions to those of the fishermen at the factory) the prefectural capital building to lobby the governor.[81]
It went on to deplore the way the fishing families had become "isolated" and
"discouraged." "The fishers have already 'suspended operations' for a long
time. The life-and-death situation is not an 'issue' for them; it is a fact." And
it included a reminder that "the fishers are citizens too." Even before the riots at the factory, the *Minamata taimusu* noted that sardines that hatched in
Minamata and Tsunagi migrated as far north as Yatsushiro and as far south
as Nagashima.[82] Hence, over 7,000 people from over 5,000 families were
fishing in waters polluted by the factory, which had only 3,000 [sic] employ-

ees. The headline suggested a possible solution: "The Closing of the Nitchitsu Factory?"

With pressures from both sides intensifying, Teramoto went to Tokyo on November 11 and told the Ministry of Health and Welfare that the company had agreed to mediation. Pressure began building on the national level. On November 11, the JSP's Special Committee on Minamata Disease held a meeting in Tokyo with representatives from the Kumamoto prefectural legislature and the Minamata city council.[83] The upcoming meeting of the party's Policy Committee was expected to push for a special law to aid disease victims and fishers. The LDP, also planning to clarify its policy on Minamata, set up a Special Committee on Minamata Disease on November 20.[84] Back in Kumamoto, the prefectural legislature was considering holding a special session on November 14 to pass an ordinance to restrict Shin Nitchitsu's waste output.[85] The Minamata police reported rumors that Shiranuikai fishermen planned to attack the factory with dynamite on November 15.[86]

The prefectural fishing cooperatives had asked the governor to mediate on November 10.[87] Governor Teramoto met with Shin Nitchitsu president Yoshioka in Tokyo on November 12 and 13 to persuade him to accept mediation. On the thirteenth, with Yoshioka still refusing, three members of the Lower House from Kumamoto urged him to accept. He gave his verbal agreement to Teramoto later that day, deciding not to wait to draw up a formal written statement but rather to act immediately in order to head off the special session of the Kumamoto prefectural assembly scheduled for the next day. The company's official written request to the governor, dated November 16, asked that he mediate under the terms of the Water Quality Conservation Law, since this would guarantee the participation of MITI, which had criticized the company for acting on its own in the August negotiations with the Minamata Fishing Cooperative.[88] The governor preferred not to be supervised by MITI, but he did agree to enlarge the mediation committee to include one person from MITI who would have been a candidate for membership under the Water Quality Conservation Law. The other members would represent the prefectural government and legislature, the media, industry, fishing, and the local community.

The governor announced a smaller than expected committee on November 24.[89] It consisted of only five members: Governor Teramoto himself, Mayor Nakamura Todomu of Minamata, speaker of the prefectural assem-

bly Iwao Yutaka, head of the prefectural association of town and village
mayors Kawazu Toratake, and *Kumamoto nichinichi shinbun* president Izu
Tomihito. Teramoto had asked the head of MITI's Fukuoka office, a
Mr. Kase, to serve on the committee. Kase consulted with his superiors in
Tokyo, who decided a MITI representative on the committee would be seen
as favoring Shin Nitchitsu. Teramoto therefore decided that the industry
and fishing representatives—Kase of MITI and a Mr. Oka, a director of the
National Alliance of Fishing Cooperatives (Zengyoren), would serve as ob-
servers.

The committee held its first meeting at the governor's official residence
on November 26.[90] The first order of business was to decide what disputes
they were mediating, if any, in addition to that between the Kumamoto
Prefectural Alliance of Fishing Cooperatives and Shin Nitchitsu. They
agreed to leave out the Minamata Fishing Cooperative, since it had already
reached a settlement with the company in August. They could not decide
whether to accept the request of the Minamata Disease Patients Families
Mutual Aid Society that they also mediate a settlement for disease victims.

The second official meeting of the mediation committee took place on
December 2.[91] In the morning, the members heard from representatives of
the fishing cooperatives, who said their losses amounted to ¥2.5 billion ($6.9
million). Total losses since 1953, when it was then believed Minamata disease
first broke out, were ¥3.1 billion ($8.6 billion). Of this, ¥500 million was due
to a natural decline in coastal fish resources, and ¥100 million was the loss
suffered by the Minamata co-op, which had already negotiated compensation (of only ¥35 million). The remainder, ¥2.5 billion, represented the
amount of the damages now being discussed. The prefectural alliance asked
that compensation to patients be decided separately from compensation to
fishing co-ops, and that, as in the company's agreement with the Minamata
co-op, the compensation agreement cover past damages but not future. They
added two more demands: the factory should be shut down temporarily, and
the sludge in the bay should be removed. Finally, they made a threat: "If no
agreement is signed by December 10, we fear that unfortunate incidents
might occur again." The alliance may have feared the company's strategy
would be to weaken it by drawing out the negotiations.

In the afternoon the committee met separately with company executives,
including Shin Nitchitsu president Yoshioka, managing director Chihara,
and factory manager Nishida, who explained the steps the factory had taken

concerning its wastewater. They were reported to have responded to the fishermen's demands with a reply offering "nearly zero."[92] Their position was strengthened by an article by Kiyoura Raisaku of the Tokyo Institute of Technology that appeared in the *Mainichi shinbun* on the same day the newspapers reported the results of the December 2 meetings.[93] Kiyoura repeated the argument of his pamphlet distributed by MITI on November 11, saying that pollution levels in Minamata Bay were not high and that the disease may have been caused by poisonous plankton.

Teramoto left for Tokyo on December 7 to attend a conference on the development of Kyūshū and a governor's conference.[94] Before he left, he persuaded the fishing co-ops to recalculate their losses, subtracting the losses caused by factories elsewhere in the Shiranui Sea, and to agree that the next meeting could not be held until after his return to Kumamoto on December 12 or 13. In Tokyo Teramoto met with Yoshioka, and on his return to Kumamoto on December 12 he announced that he would present a concrete proposal at the third mediation committee meeting, to be held before the prefectural legislative session began on December 18.[95]

Teramoto and the other committee members spent the next few days meeting with the two sides.[96] The fishing coops had lowered their demand from ¥2.5 billion to ¥980 million ($2.7 million). The company seemed willing to pay no more than ¥40–50 million ($111,000–139,000), and Teramoto felt he needed to get them up to at least ¥100 million ($278,000) to get an agreement. He met repeatedly with managing director Chihara. What finally forced the company to agree was a story scheduled to be printed in the *Kumamoto nichinichi shinbun* the morning of December 16.[97] The article was written by a reporter who visited Kumamoto University and spoke with Dean Sera of the Medical School, who was also head of the research group studying Minamata disease. Sera told the reporter that the scientists had extracted organic mercury from shellfish in Minamata Bay. They had fed this to rats, all of whom developed Minamata disease, and were now conducting the same experiments on cats. The important news, however, was that according to Sera the researchers were on the verge of proving how inorganic mercury could become organic in the bodies of fish. Experiments with rats seemed to have explained the mechanism, and a final conclusion would be announced by March 1960. As it turned out, Sera and his colleagues were still far from explaining the process. Whether he was misunderstood, merely overly optimistic, or intentionally trying to affect the negotiations is not clear. In any case, the information had a dramatic impact on the mediation process. Since the president of the newspaper was on the mediation committee, Teramoto learned of the story in advance and decided that the committee had to present a draft agreement to the two sides before they read the article, which he feared would spark more violence.[98]

The committee began discussions in the evening on December 15 and presented its plan to the two sides at 3 A.M. the next morning.[99] The terms of the proposed agreement were:

1. The company must complete its installation of purification equipment within one week. (It was already scheduled to be completed December 20, and the newspaper reported it would mean "water as clean as river water" would flow from the waste outlet into Hyakken Harbor.)

2. The company must pay the prefectural fishing cooperative alliance ¥35 million ($97,200) to compensate its members for their losses.

3. The alliance must return ¥10 million ($27,800) of this ¥35 million to the company to cover the damage caused in the November 2 riots.

4. The company must set up a ¥65 million ($181,000) fund to help the fishing industry recover.

5. The alliance and the company will monitor the recovery of fishing and agree on conditions for return of the principal and interest of the ¥65 million.

6. The alliance will never demand further compensation, even if the waste dumped in the past by the factory is proven to be the cause of the disease, as long as the volume and toxicity of the factory's waste do not increase.

The two sides were to reply to the proposal by the next day, December 17.

The committee also proposed compensation for disease victims and presented its plan to the company. Nakamura explained it to the Minamata Disease Patients Families Mutual Aid Society when he returned to Minamata. Under this plan, the company would pay a total of ¥24 million ($66,700) to the 78 recognized patients immediately and an estimated total of ¥50 million ($139,000) in annual payments over the rest of their lives.

The company and the fishing co-op alliance held meetings to decide whether they would accept the proposal. Three of the 43 member-coops in the alliance, including those of Tsunagi and Tanoura, voted against the proposed agreement, but the leaders decided to sign.[100] Like the mediation committee in August, Teramoto said he would wash his hands of the whole affair if either side refused the agreement, and he made it clear he felt ¥100 million ($278,000) was all a company capitalized at ¥2.7 billion ($7.5 million) could possibly pay. The company, with its new pollution-control equipment coming on line soon, hoped the agreement, and the one that seemed likely to follow soon with the patients, would put the problem behind it once and for all. The fishing families, with the end of the year approaching, felt they could not sustain another round of protests and could not risk refusing.

Just before midnight on December 17, the two sides formally accepted the committee's proposal, with three amendments proposed by the company and accepted by the alliance.[101]

1. The ¥65 million fishing recovery fund, the first of its kind, was being established only because Minamata was a special case. (Shin Nitchitsu did not want to be blamed by other companies or the government for setting a precedent.)

2. No limits were to be placed on the volume of wastewater output after the treatment facilities were completed.

3. The committee would mediate solutions to any problems that might arise in the future concerning the agreement.

After the co-op alliance accepted these amendments, the company representatives suddenly announced that Shin Nitchitsu was under criticism from other companies because of the ¥65 million fishing recovery fund. They requested a break of 40 minutes to formulate a strategy to deal with this. According to a pamphlet written by the Kumamoto Prefectural Committee of the JCP, what the company actually did during this break was to get the approval of Akiyama Takeo, head of MITI's Light Industry Bureau, before signing the agreement. It was Akiyama who two months earlier had "asked" the company to switch its waste outlet back to Hyakken from the Minamata River and to advance the completion date of the pollution-control equipment.[102]

One might have expected the prefectural fishing co-op alliance to get a better settlement than that obtained by the Minamata Fishing Cooperative. The members of the prefectural alliance were not restrained by employment or other ties to the company and did not live in the city Shin Nitchitsu dominated. Their protests were more violent, garnered more media attention, and coincided with increased pressure from the Diet and the prefectural legislature. However, they never considered using the increased media attention provoked by their violence to rally support outside their own membership. Instead, their strategy evoked a strong response from the Minamata community in defense of the company, and their vastly larger numbers made it difficult for them to get as much per person as the Minamata co-op. Unlike the Minamata co-op, they lowered their initial demand drastically. In the end, they actually received a direct payment of only ¥25 million ($69,400) (after subtracting the ¥10 million for damages to the factory in the riot), which was around ¥5,000 ($13.90) per family—far less than the Minamata coop's one-time payment of ¥20 million ($55,600), which was on average over ¥67,000 ($186) per member-family. The prefectural co-ops' agreement with the company also prohibited them from demanding future compensation as long as the factory's waste did not worsen, a qualification not included in the Minamata agreement. There was more disagreement over goals and leadership in the large, loose, prefectural alliance. Perhaps most important, all sides seemed to have absolute faith that the new pollution-control equipment would actually end the discharge of dangerous waste. This prospect, the coming end of the year, and the governor's threat to abandon them made the Kumamoto Prefectural Alliance of Fishing Cooperatives decide they had to accept what they could get and not risk holding out for more.

The Victims' Struggle for Compensation

Compensating the victims of the disease, which one might have expected to be the most important issue, appears as a mere afterthought in the events of 1959 in Minamata, a brief footnote to the First Minamata Fishing Dispute, which ended on August 29, and the larger Shiranuikai Fishing Dispute, which ended on December 17. Part of the reason is that the Minamata Disease Patients Families Mutual Aid Society, founded in August 1957, was smaller, weaker, and more divided than the Minamata Fishing Cooperative or the Kumamoto Prefectural Alliance of Fishing Cooperatives.[103]

The Mutual Aid Society did have one thing these other groups lacked: a colorful, imaginative leader who could situate himself and his group in a broad context and who was not cowed by those who supposed themselves his superiors. Watanabe Eizō (1898–1986) had been a peddler before settling down to a life of fishing in Yudō.[104] His travels and life on his own had exposed him to ideas and life-styles different from those of Yudō and gave him an independent and even egotistical streak. He headed the plaintiffs' group in the 1969–73 trial, giving speeches at the University of Tokyo and elsewhere. He drew pornographic pictures in the Edo period *shunga* style.[105] During the trial he had a torrid affair with a widow who was a fellow plaintiff and Minamata disease victim. Late in his life, Watanabe built a monument to himself in his own back yard and spoke about winning the Nobel Peace Prize, and in his eighties he regularly visited a girlfriend in Uto, near Kumamoto.

Even with a leader such as Watanabe, the Mutual Aid Society in 1959 was pathetically weak and without outside support. With the "united front" supporting the company, almost the only organized group that seemed sympathetic to the disease victims was the JCP's Minamata cell, formerly headed by Tanigawa Gan. The pamphlet it issued in the name of the prefectural party committee around December 23 was, despite its jargon, the most perceptive account of the situation up to then.[106] Had its recommendations (much higher compensation payments to fishers and patients, investigation of Shin Nitchitsu for murder, cleanup of the pollution, adequate welfare payments by the prefecture to patients and their families) been implemented, the victims' lot would have been greatly improved. These measures could only have been implemented as a result of much greater public support, however, and the last section of the pamphlet hinted that the actions of the Minamata JCP cell would reduce rather than increase its support. Instead of a rallying cry for progressive groups to come to the aid of the victims, the pamphlet ends with an emphasis on the coming struggle against the renewal of the U.S.-Japan Security Treaty (usually known by its Japanese abbreviation "Anpo"). The call was not so much for groups in the Anpo struggle to come to the aid of the fishers as for fishers to be brought into the Anpo struggle. Ishimure Michiko has described what happened in September 1959 during a demonstration by the "Minamata Joint Struggle Committee of the People's Council for Preventing Revision of the Japan-U.S. Security Treaty":

No sooner had the anti–Security Treaty demonstration set itself in motion than another, much smaller group of protesters coming from the opposite direction appeared some distance away down the street. It was a forlorn, solitary body of about 300 fishermen [who had just failed in an attempt to meet factory managers]. The anxious expression on their faces, their vacant, unsteady look and the way they dragged their feet betrayed despair and weariness. The two processions advanced toward one another until their respective front ranks faced each other in close proximity. The fishermen were holding colorful flags bearing the names of their boats in large characters: "Happiness," "Clown," "Promotion." . . .

The organizers of the anti–Security Treaty demonstration completely missed the intent of the fishermen's procession. A man who seemed to be a leader stepped forward and shouted in a raspy, energetic voice: "Comrades, the fishermen are going to join forces with us. Their courageous decision was certainly motivated by a desire to be one with the will of the people, and may be seen as a direct result of our concerted propaganda work. Let us receive our new comrades-in-arms with a general clapping of hands, let us give them a hearty welcome to our movement!" . . .

Still under the shock of the unexpected welcome extended to them by the participants in the anti–Security Treaty demonstration, the fishermen were swept along across the Minamata River to the First Elementary School, where the closing meeting was to take place. They looked dazed, as if they had come along only because that was what the organizers of the demonstration expected them to do. Strangely enough, no one had hit on the idea of calling on the mass of demonstrators to support the fishermen's struggle. No one had shouted: "Comrades, let us join in the fishermen's demonstration!" The patriotic, politically-conscious residents of Minamata had missed yet another opportunity to join forces with the victimized fishermen. . . . In spite of stirring visions of "the solidarity between peasants and laborers," of "the glorious alliance with farmers and fishermen," of "a movement firmly rooted in the reality of our regional society," the citizens made no attempt to take the side of the fishermen. . . .

Thus the historical moment when the foundation for mutual understanding and a real merging of interests between the anti–Security Treaty movement representing a large portion of the Minamata citizens and the fishermen could have been laid, was irretrievably missed by both sides. . . . Like two processions of ants carrying bits of food to different destinations, the fishermen and the participants in the apparently more momentous political demonstration met briefly, walked side by side for a while, placidly and without signs of recognition, then parted again without looking back.[107]

The party was tightening its focus on the top and center, and those who were too independent in thought and action, including Tanigawa Gan and Ishimure Michiko, resigned or were expelled. Tanigawa, who had left Minamata in 1958 for the coal fields of Chikuhō and then went to the Miike mines during the historic strike there, was expelled in June 1960, along with members of his Circle Village (Sākuru mura) group, which published a journal of the same name. Ishimure Michiko left the party and issued a "declaration of independence":

Because Tanigawa Gan was away . . ., the Japan Communist Party's attacks on the *Circle Village* in Minamata were directed mainly at me. I was even disparaged as "a mere woman." For belonging to the Circle Village group, which was openly critical of the party, and for contributing manuscripts to the journal for the benefit of the well-intentioned masses, I was accused of Trotskyite deviation and of aiding and abetting the enemy by confusing the masses. . . .

"You refuse to recognize the decision of communist parties the world over that Soviet and Chinese nuclear experiments are preferable to those conducted by American imperialists, believing that you alone are correct. Criticizing the local party authorities and defying the communist parties of the world, you assert the correctness of Tanigawa Gan's political and literary thought. You must consider yourself very grand. Through its official organs and its current drive to double membership, the party is giving its all to the attempt to succor the masses. We should like to hear the scheme with which you intend to achieve that end, working on your own outside the party."

Never having publicly declared my party affiliation, I did not bother to report this ludicrous incident to the editorial staff of *Circle Village*. A few months later, humiliated and feeling like a stray dog, I left the party.[108]

Even before they demanded restitution from Shin Nitchitsu, the Minamata disease patients, most of whom were fishers in families that had immigrated to the city, were objects of discrimination. For many Japanese, fishing hamlets represented a rural life-style considered to be poor and dirty, and in 1959 most of Japan's city dwellers were not far enough removed from the countryside—in most cases they were only a generation or two away—to feel nostalgia for it. The fishing life-style in particular, with its suggestions of rootlessness, marginality, and individualism, lacked the cultural weight of rice-growing.[109] *Nōhonshugi* thought (agriculturalism, a stress on farmers as the soul of Japan) had dignified the role of farmers from the Meiji period into early Shōwa, and in wartime and the postwar period the government has subsidized rice farmers by purchasing their rice for a price higher than that at which it is sold to consumers. Fishers lacked comparable sources of social approval, self-respect, and financial support.

When such a community is threatened and looked down upon, it is natural for it to turn on some its own members. Those who were afflicted with Minamata disease or who demanded compensation for fishing losses were seen to be harming the whole community by making it impossible to sell fish and by attracting the animosity of the company and the city. This combined with a traditional abhorrence of uncleanness and disease and the feeling that

the community could not afford to antagonize the company to create discrimination against patients and those active in demanding restitution. A
sense that the community was threatened by economic disaster intensified
this. Being ostracized by the community in such a way was understandably
more fearful than disease or financial distress for many people.[110]

The phenomenon happened everywhere the disease occurred and persisted long beyond the early days of the Minamata disease incident. Irokawa
Daikichi once asked an old woman in Yunokuchi hamlet on the island of
Shishijima to tell her story.[111] She had been examined by Dr. Harada Masazumi some time between 1965 and 1974. Her symptoms were severe, and the
doctor urged her to apply for certification; she did so and began receiving
compensation. The villagers accused her of doing this for the money and
said that because of her they would no longer be able to sell their fish. She
was shunned. No one would speak to her, and she soon refused to leave her
house. Her daughter-in-law then became the focus of the hamlet's anger,
and with no one on whom to turn her anger but her mother-in-law, she
stopped serving meals to the old woman. The grandmother told Irokawa she
wished she had never been examined by Harada and had never applied for
certification. She said it would have been better just to die of the "strange
disease."

As of November 1959 there was still no compensation for disease patients.
Their increasing numbers, their worsening financial situation, and the examples of the Minamata and prefectural fishing cooperatives finally over-
came the problems of disunity and reluctance and impelled them to demand
restitution. Like the fishing cooperatives, they began with petitions and
switched to other tactics when these got them nowhere. Mutual Aid Society
leader Watanabe Eizō had prepared a petition to Shin Nitchitsu on September 17, using a word for "petition" (*tangansho*) reminiscent of Edo-period
petitions by peasants to their lords and of prewar labor disputes, but he
never delivered it. On November 16, when the governor was beginning to
form his mediation committee, some 50 members of the Mutual Aid Society, led by Watanabe, met with Mayor Nakamura Todomu, city council
speaker (and fishing co-op head) Fuchigami Sueki, and Hirota Sunao, a
member of the city council's Minamata Disease Countermeasures Committee.[112] They complained that the city's leaders, including Nakamura, appeared to be petitioning the central authorities on the company's behalf, and

asked, "How long will those of us who have been sacrificed have to cry our-
selves to sleep?" They requested that the plant be shut down. Fuchigami
promised them ¥30,000 ($83) for the society's operating expenses, and
Nakamura promised to do what he could to satisfy them. Five days later
Mayor Nakamura accompanied 50 Mutual Aid Society members by bus to
Kumamoto, where they met with Vice Governor Mizugami Nagayoshi and
other officials and presented a petition.[113] Watanabe told Mizugami: "I have
the feeling that because the fishermen made a fuss, the focus in the Minamata disease issue has moved from the patients to fishing problems."
Mizugami replied: "You are not being forgotten by the prefecture," but he
made no specific promises. On their way out, the delegation met the governor in the hall, and he promised to do what he could for them.

Like the fishing coops when their petitions had no effect, the Mutual Aid
Society finally approached the factory directly.[114] Six representatives of the
58-family association met with Kawamura Kazuo, chief of the General Affairs Section, on November 25 and handed him the following demand:
"From 1953 to the present, the total number of patients of Minamata disease,
caused by the factory's wastewater, is 78. As compensation money for this
damage, pay ¥234 million (¥3 million per person) [$650,000 ($8,300 per person)]." They requested a written reply by November 30. Kawamura responded that since the Ministry of Health and Welfare had not concluded
that the factory's waste caused the disease, the company would be unable to
reply promptly. The association insisted that "the mercury theory is absolute
fact," and Kawamura finally agreed to reply by the thirtieth.

On the day the Mutual Aid Society met with Kawamura, there was new
evidence of the spread of the disease in the Shiranui Sea. A 61-year-old fisherman named Ogata Fukumatsu was examined by doctors at the Minamata
Municipal Hospital.[115] They announced that because he was unconscious, it
was impossible to make a firm diagnosis, but from their examination and the
information provided by his family, it seemed almost certain that he had
Minamata disease. Ogata was from the isolated fishing hamlet of Meshima
in the town of Yunoura, 20 kilometers north of Minamata, and was the first
in his area to come down with the disease.

The *Nishinippon shinbun* reported on November 27 that Watanabe believed the company was certain to offer the Minamata Disease Patients
Families Mutual Aid Society nothing.[116] The prefectural and central governments had taken up the fishing issue only because of the two major inci-

dents of violence, Watanabe said, and the patients were now hidden in the shadow of the fishermen's struggle and being forgotten. To make their demands heard, the Mutual Aid Society might have to do something dramatic as well, without waiting for the company's reply. He suggested they might march all the way to Tokyo to petition the central government. Such marches had been attempted in 1897, 1898, and 1900 by farmers suffering from flooding and pollution caused by the Ashio copper mine in Japan's first serious modern pollution incident. The march would have taken more money and strength than the Minamata patients had, however, and was never carried out. In the Ashio incident, the farmers were supported by a militant Diet representative, Tanaka Shōzō, but the Minamata victims had no such political support.[117]

Watanabe hinted at violence, but the tactics he suggested, and the ones the Mutual Aid Society actually adopted, were nonviolent. Their numbers were far too small to invade and ransack the factory. Instead, 50 of them (including Hamamoto Fumiyo and her brother Tsuginori, when he was not at work at the company) began a sit-in in front of the factory gate on the afternoon of November 28.[118] News of the deaths of two victims from north of the city made their pleas more urgent. Ogata Fukumatsu of Meshima had died the previous day, and Shinohara Tamotsu of Tsunagi, who had climbed over and opened the factory gate during the November 2 riots, had died early that morning.[119] Late in the afternoon of November 28, representatives of the Mutual Aid Society met with assistant factory manager Ishino, who gave them a written reply repeating what Kawamura had said three days earlier: since no connection had yet been established between factory waste and Minamata disease, the factory, although it sympathized with their plight, could not accede to their demand.[120] The delegates left and decided to ask a factory security officer to return the company's reply along with their written request for another answer. Finding no one to do this, they left the company's reply at the guardhouse inside the gate, and all but the women and oldest men continued their sit-in overnight.

For the sit-in, the Mutual Aid Society used a tent borrowed from the union, but the union soon demanded it back on the excuse that the protesters' fire was dirtying it. The story of the women of the Mutual Aid Society washing the tent in the cold water of the Minamata River before returning it became one of the most oft-told tales of Minamata, symbolizing the isola-

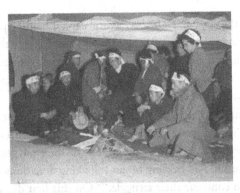

Fig. 12 The patients' Mutual Aid Society's sit-in at the factory gate, November 1959. © *Kuwamoto nichi-nichi shibun.*

tion and privation forced on the victims when they were abandoned by the cold-hearted citizens of the city.[121]

On November 29, members of the Mutual Aid Society marched through the city carrying placards asking for support.[122] They attempted to meet with Nishida, Kawamura, and Ishino at their homes in Jinnai, but all were out. The next day seven angry Mutual Aid Society members met with Mayor Nakamura and city council speaker Fuchigami, fuming that the city authorities had done nothing and had "not shown a bit of sincerity."[123] When the city authorities did not offer to take any action, the delegates stormed out. City officials then met with the city council and agreed that representatives from the city would travel with Mutual Aid Society members to Kumamoto the next day to petition Governor Teramoto to include compensation for patients in his mediation. On the afternoon of November 30, Mutual Aid Society representatives met with factory manager Nishida and asked him to request company president Yoshioka to allow the mediation to include compensation of patients, but Nishida refused. That same day, Minamata disease patients with relatively lighter symptoms had demanded to be allowed to leave the municipal hospital to join the sit-in, hoping their presence would garner some sympathy from factory executives, but the doctors refused to allow them to leave.[124] When the victims did make sure that more visibly affected patients joined their activities beginning in 1968, they made good use of the publicity to draw public sympathy.

On December 1, 51 members of the Mutual Aid Society traveled with city officials to Kumamoto to petition the governor.[125] They marched the three kilometers from the station to the prefectural capital holding placards in one hand and blankets in the other, prepared for a sit-in to force the governor to meet them. Fuchigami and prefectural legislators from Minamata persuaded Teramoto to see them, however, and he promised to ask Shin Nitchitsu to include compensation of patients in the mediation.

The sit-in seemed to be having some effect. Sitting in front of the factory gate, the disease victims were visible to passers-by, to workers entering and leaving the factory, and to people coming out of the train station. On December 4, the Mutual Aid Society began collecting donations on street corners to help them continue their struggle.[126] On this first day they collected ¥9,620 ($27), and the next day brought them about ¥26,000 ($72), including one large donation of ¥11,200 ($31) from the singer Shimakura Chiyoko, in town for sold-out concerts, ¥2,500 ($7) from her band, and ¥10,000 ($28) from factory manager Nishida's wife, Shinako. On December 12, the 2,400 families in the factory's consumers' cooperative, Suikōsha, donated ¥35,000 ($97) and 200 items of clothing.[127]

The patients then went farther afield, sending nine people each to Yatsushiro and Kumamoto to collect donations.[128] It was the year-end bonus and shopping season, and in Kumamoto they solicited money in the Shimotōri shopping district. They also handed out flyers reading: "It has been six years since Minamata disease began. Over 30 people have already died. This is a terrible disease. The Shin Nitchitsu factory will not compensate the patients, who are the direct victims. We ask that you try to save the victims with your impartial public opinion." These handbills represent the patients' first organized attempt to mobilize public opinion on their behalf. They were well aware of the advantages of doing this in Kumamoto, outside of Minamata and close to the governor, his mediation committee, and the media. Had they been able to continue with their sit-in and appeals to public opinion for several months, they might have gone further toward breaking out of their isolation. However, the mediation committee was moving quickly, and the protesters, unwell to begin with, were suffering from the increasingly cold weather.

When Teramoto's committee announced its proposed solution to Shin Nitchitsu and the Kumamoto Prefectural Alliance of Fishing Cooperatives on December 16, it also announced its proposal for "solatium" payments to the 78 recognized victims of Minamata disease.[129] Company acceptance had been confirmed on December 7, when Yoshioka, informed that the committee would suggest a total of ¥74 million ($206,000) for disease patients, replied to Teramoto: "That's not very different from what I was thinking."[130] Since no Mutual Aid Society representatives had been invited to the meetings with the mediation committee in Kumamoto, Mayor Nakamura returned to Minamata and explained the proposed agreement.

The Ministry of Health and Welfare would establish a certification committee to determine who would receive payments. The company would pay adult patients ¥100,000 ($278) per year, and children (including those now adults who had contracted the disease as children) would receive ¥10,000 ($28) per year. The family would receive ¥300,000 ($833), plus ¥20,000 ($56) for funeral expenses, for each patient who died. Payments covering the time since each patient had contracted the disease would be made as soon as the agreement was signed, and would total ¥24 million ($66,700). The balance of ¥50 million ($139,000) was the estimated total of future annual payments and was based on the assumptions that no new patients would appear and that patients would live to an average age of 60. The total of nearly ¥950,000 ($2,640) per person was far less than the ¥3 million ($8,330) demanded. Yet the offer of nearly a third of the patients' original demand was relatively better than the settlement accepted by the Prefectural Alliance of Fishing Cooperatives, which was 4 percent of their original demand and 10 percent of the last amount they had asked for.

Watanabe Eizō announced on December 17 that the plan was unacceptable and that the sit-in would continue.[131] The Mutual Aid Society had agreed that the total of ¥74 million was acceptable, but wanted the entire amount paid immediately, or if necessary over a period of three years, with every patient getting an equal amount.[132] Families with child victims were particularly unhappy with the amount offered to children. Governor Teramoto sent the prefecture's Mining and Industry Section chief Yokota to Minamata to work with Nakamura to persuade the Mutual Aid Society to accept the proposal as presented.[133] The city council's Minamata Disease Countermeasures Committee decided on December 21 to urge the society to accept and offered to assist with the mediation if necessary. The mediation committee reminded the patients unnecessarily that Minamata disease was incurable and said it feared that if all the money was paid at once, the patients would use it up quickly (true enough, considering how low the payments were); because of this, annual payments were "the kindest payment method."[134] These arguments were repeated on December 22 when the mayor accompanied the Mutual Aid Society's leaders to a meeting with the governor, where they were also told that when the cause of the disease was confirmed, they could go to court to get compensation.[135]

Families with children who had the disease continued to oppose the proposal, but they made up only a small proportion of the Mutual Aid Society's members. (Although many congenital Minamata disease victims had been born, none was diagnosed as such because the congenital form of the disease was not yet recognized.) The society's resolution was also weakening as the cold weather began to take its toll, and the ranks of those sitting in at the factory gate began to thin around December 20.[136]

On December 25, the day the official signing ceremony was held concluding the agreement between Shin Nitchitsu and the fishing co-ops, the Ministry of Health and Welfare established the Minamata Disease Patient Examination Commission (Minamatabyō kanja shinsa kyōgikai) in preparation for the expected agreement between Shin Nitchitsu and the patients. The members were Hosokawa Hajime, Itō Hasuo, two Kumamoto University Medical School professors, the director of the Minamata Municipal Hospital, the vice president of the Minamata doctors' association, and the head of the Kumamoto prefectural Hygiene Department. Only those certified by this board as Minamata disease patients would receive payments from the company. From this time to the present, diagnosis and certification of Minamata disease patients have been as much political and financial issues as medical questions.

On December 25, Teramoto and the mediation committee agreed to raise the annual payment to child victims from ¥10,000 to ¥30,000 ($83).[137] That evening the Mutual Aid Society voted by a margin of just one vote not to accept the new proposal, although Watanabe Eizō and most of the group's other leaders were in favor of it. On the morning of December 27, Nakamura and city council speaker Fuchigami met with four of the society's leaders, who agreed to try once again to persuade the members to accept. They failed to break the deadlock, and that afternoon Watanabe, negotiating committee chairman Nakatsu, secretary Ogami Mitsuyoshi, and two other negotiating committee members announced their resignations. This shocked the members of the society into meeting and voting again at 8:00 P.M. This time they accepted, and the resignations were withdrawn. The next day the sit-in ended, a month after it began.

On December 29, the two sides assembled in Mayor Nakamura's office to give their formal acceptance.[138] At the last minute, when Mayor Nakamura asked if either side had any further comments, the company asked that an extra clause be added: "If in the future it is determined that the cause of Minamata disease is not the factory's wastewater, [the company] shall end the payment of solatium money after that month." This would precede the clause reading: "Even if in the future it is determined that the cause of Minamata disease is the factory's wastewater, [the patients] will make absolutely no further demands for compensation money."[139] The Mutual Aid Society's negotiators met privately and agreed to accept the new clause, but when the two sides met again the issue of adjusting the payments for inflation came up.[140] Discussion continued until 1:00 A.M., when they agreed to attach the following "note" to the "memorandum of understanding," which, along with a "protocol," would be attached to the "contract": "If in the future there are significant changes in prices, the amount of the yearly payments may be adjusted on the basis of joint discussions requested by either [the company or the patients]."

The signing ceremony was held in the mayor's office at 12:15 that afternoon, December 30, 1959, and less than two hours later the Minamata Disease Patients Families Mutual Aid Society received ¥23.5 million ($65,300) from Shin Nitchitsu for 79 patients. This was an average of ¥297,468 ($830, or 2.1 times Japan's per capita annual GNP in 1959) per person. The largest amount received by a single family was ¥1,205,000 ($3,350) (for two people who had died and one living patient); the smallest was ¥15,000 ($42) (for a child). Although the press continued to refer to the payments as "compensation" (*hoshō*), the agreement specified that they were "solatium money" (*mimaikin*). At the time they received this solatium money, 13 of 58 families in the Mutual Aid Society (and a total of 64 fishing families in the city as a whole) were receiving welfare payments.[141]

The statements made by Nishida and Watanabe borrowed from those made by the company and the Minamata Fishing Cooperative when they announced their agreement on August 29. Nishida said: "We are pleased that with the efforts of the mediators agreement has been achieved. For the factory, the amounts of money and other points are unsatisfactory, but in order to relieve social anxieties and to honor your [the mediation committee's] efforts, we have accepted it." Watanabe's statement began: "I would like to thank the members for swallowing their tears and accepting the contract and protocol, and to express my heartfelt gratitude to Mayor Nakamura and the other mediators for their efforts." He continued with a conciliatory remark reassuring the townspeople that the patients did not mean to threaten the company's dominance in Minamata: "I have not changed my belief that Minamata owes everything to Shin Nitchitsu, and hope that we can continue to get along well with each other."

"As Clean as River Water": The Third Leg of the "Solution"

With the conclusion of agreements with the fishing cooperatives of Minamata and of Kumamoto prefecture and with the patients, the first "full and final" solution to the Minamata disease issue was almost complete. If new patients appeared, the mechanisms were in place to certify and pay them. If other fishing cooperatives (from Kagoshima prefecture to the south) demanded compensation, they could be dealt with in the same way as those from Kumamoto prefecture.

The agreements with the fishing cooperatives and the patients were two legs of the solution. The third promised to make it stable. This was the pollution-control equipment the company had rushed to install. If the factory's waste were clean, it would not matter what had caused the disease, since existing patients were already provided for and no new ones would appear. For this strategy to work, it was necessary only to make people believe the waste had been made safe. Amazingly, the company succeeded rapidly in this, although the facilities about which it boasted did not remove any mercury from its waste.

Shin Nitchitsu had been expanding its sedimentation pools at Hachiman for some time. Wastewater was allowed to sit in these until solids settled out. On October 30, 1959—just in time for the Diet members' visit—a pumping system was completed so that the surface water could be pumped back into the factory and reused. This was presented by the company as a total recycling system, eliminating the dumping of waste into the sea. In fact, the ground under the pools was permeable, and a great deal of the wastewater, with its dissolved mercury, seeped out into the river and the sea. And although the company did not announce this to the public, MITI knew that after January 1961, when the factory discovered that the recycled water was not clean enough to be used safely, the pumps were rarely turned on.[142]

An even more highly publicized system consisted of a "Cyclator" and "Sedifloater" designed by the Ebara Infilco company. It was completed on December 19, 1959, and began full operations on January 20, 1960. At the completion ceremony on December 24, Yoshioka drank a glass of water from the Cyclator in front of the assembled dignitaries, including Governor Teramoto.[143] None of the guests was told that the wastewater from the acetaldehyde plant was not being put through the Cyclator. Neither did they know of Dr. Hosokawa's cat #400, which had developed Minamata disease in October after being fed wastewater from the acetaldehyde plant.

The Cyclator was planned before Kumamoto University announced its organic mercury theory (although not before the factory knew it was dumping organic mercury) and was designed to remove carbide tailings from the wastewater. The lawyer Gotō Takanori later confirmed directly with an Ebara Infilco engineer that it was never intended to remove substances such as organic mercury that dissolve in water.[144] The failure of Shin Nitchitsu to run the acetaldehyde waste through the Cyclator for Yoshioka to drink suggests strongly that they knew it would not remove the mercury. The most damning evidence came out in 1970 in the first Niigata Minamata disease trial, when managing director Andō Nobuo of Shōwa denkō, which caused the Niigata Minamata disease, testified: "At that time we contacted Chisso [Shin Nitchitsu], and Chisso replied [that their] 'purification tank was built as a measure to solve social problems, and it has no effect in removing mercury.'"[145]

In December 1959, though, none of this was known outside the company. The Cyclator and Sedifloater were marvelous public relations tools, well worth their cost to the company. In early 1960, Shin Nitchitsu sent Kumamoto University Professor Irukayama samples of what it said were "original wastewater" and "wastewater after treatment." He announced that the former contained 20 ppm of mercury and the latter none; thereafter he stated in a number of reports and publications that there was no more mercury in factory waste. MITI, knowing that most of the acetaldehyde waste was being sent to the Hachiman Pools and seeping from there into the river and the Shiranui Sea, nevertheless sampled mercury concentrations only in Minamata Bay, where they declined.[146] For years afterward it was assumed

by most people, including doctors, that there could be no new Minamata
disease patients because no more mercury was being dumped into the sea.

The three-part "solution" of 1959 was a clear-cut victory for the company
and for the government, especially for MITI. All sides were locked into a
narrow view of Minamata disease. It was believed that the disease had begun
in 1953 and almost completely ended by 1960. Only the most acute form of
the disease was recognized, as described in 1956 and 1957. Since the Cyclator
and Sedifloater were supposedly making the factory waste safe, there was no
need to search for patients, as had been done in 1956. The dispute over the
cause was merely an academic issue if the victims had been compensated.
Even if the factory waste was the cause, the "Solatium Contract" prohibited
the patients from demanding further compensation. The fact that fishers
and patients were now being paid directly by Shin Nitchitsu meant that
they no longer made their livings independently but were utterly dependent
on the very company that had poisoned them.

Production and pollution continued. The company was able to avoid
admitting its responsibility for the disease, and the local and national governments were not held to account for allowing the disease to occur and to
continue. The issue was handled in an extra-legal manner, through mediation in which traditional authorities retained control, rather than through
the courts or the ballot box. Neither the opposition parties nor the media
made the victims' cause their own or used it to challenge the existing power
structure. Minamata's tragedy did not become a national issue, and civil society did not serve as a link between the victims and the state.

All three groups demanding compensation from Shin Nitchitsu—the
Minamata Fishing Cooperative, the Kumamoto Prefectural Alliance of
Fishing Cooperatives, and the Minamata Disease Patients Families Mutual
Aid Society—followed similar courses. All three began by presenting their
grievances directly to the company, city, and prefecture through institutional
channels. When these petitions brought no results, there was no serious discussion of suing the company. Instead, they resorted to the extra-
institutional methods of violence or sit-ins. Belated attention from the media
combined with the involvement of the police (except in the case of the Mutual Aid Society) and the possibility of action by the prefectural or national
legislature to bring about mediation. The mediation was carried out at the
lowest possible levels, by prefectural and municipal rather than national

authorities. Nor did members of the mediation committees content themselves with merely facilitating the negotiations. Instead, committees whose members were better aware of the importance of the company to the city and prefecture than of the suffering and loss caused by its pollution dictated settlements. These settlements were based more on the company's ability to pay than on any calculation of actual losses by the victims. These agreements left the victims dependent on the company and contained built-in barriers to further demands.

All parties involved learned important lessons from the events of 1956 through 1959. Shin Nitchitsu and the government, at all levels, were able to put these lessons into practice with little opposition. It was not until 1968, however, that the victims could begin to apply the lessons they learned at such cost.

Both the government and the company discovered that they could successfully suppress information and manipulate opinions about the disease and its cause, playing center against periphery. Much of the responsibility for this lies with the media.[147] In this first round of responses to Minamata disease, the media failed to inform the nation adequately of this local incident or to recognize its national implications. Reports on Minamata disease appeared in the Kyūshū editions of the *Asahi* in 1956, but not in Tokyo. Tokyo readers of the *Asahi* first heard of Minamata through a small article in April 1957 announcing that the Ministry of Health and Welfare would be studying the "strange disease." The first article they saw on Minamata disease that originated in the newspaper's Kumamoto bureau was a small article in August 1957, reporting (falsely) that fishing in Minamata Bay would be banned. The *Asahi* scoop of July 1959, reporting the Kumamoto University mercury theory, did not run in Tokyo. It was not until November 1959 that the Tokyo edition of the *Asahi* ran a major story on Minamata, reporting the fishermen's riot at the factory. Even this did not appear on the front page, but at the top of the "society" section.

This weakness of the media in reporting local stories combined with another weakness, its attempt to be "neutral," to help the company and government confuse the issue of the cause of the disease and delay full acceptance of the mercury theory. Announcements by Kumamoto University were far less likely to be reported than those made in Tokyo by Shin Nitchitsu's head office, by MITI, by the Japan Chemical Industry Association, or by professors at Tokyo universities. And the media's concern with

maintaining a neutral stance led it to give equal credence to all theories of the
cause, rather than to question the objectivity of Shin Nitchitsu, MITI, the
industry association, and the scientists whose research they supported.

After 1959, Shin Nitchitsu knew that the fishing cooperatives could continue to be bought off with money and land (and soon, with jobs) at a cost
the company could bear. This pattern of relations between the fishing cooperatives and the company continued for decades. The company learned that
prefectural and national legislators could pressure it uncomfortably, but that
the mayor and governor would mediate settlements that would not kill the
company, provided it was willing to compromise. The more local the level to
which the dispute was confined, the greater the relative weight of the company. Government officials learned that the more the incident was confined
to the local level, the easier it was to control. Handled in this way, it need
have no significant effect on Japan's political system.

The victims were never quiescent or cowed. They learned that violence
brought results but undermined public support. Soon, they were to learn
that it brought punishment as well. They experimented with or considered
tactics that, while difficult to sustain, offered promise: sit-ins, the participation of visibly affected patients in public actions, and the soliciting of funds
and distribution of handbills, especially in Kumamoto city. They became accustomed to the vocabulary that has surrounded the Minamata disease incident ever since—"sincerity," "swallowing tears," "a full solution"—but in
these early years they rarely used the terms "rights" or "public opinion."

What are we to make of Watanabe Eizō's comment after the signing of
the solatium agreement, seemingly accepting the fact that the city put the
company first? Did he and the members of the Mutual Aid Society think of
Minamata in terms of a Confucian hierarchy despite the postwar constitution's guarantee of democratic equality and rights? Why did the fishing cooperatives and the Mutual Aid Society not attempt to obtain redress
through the courts? Were their actions no different from those of peasants
who rebelled in the Tokugawa period, or the farmers arrested at Kawamata
in 1900 while protesting pollution from the Ashio copper mine?

It is partly true that the victims acted according to old values and patterns. In 1959, those who had been educated under the old imperial system
were still the vast majority. Patterns of thought and action are not changed
overnight by the adoption of a new constitution, and even today there are
some who say their main motivation for seeking redress is that they "want to

be recognized by [their] superiors" (*okami ni mitomete moraitai*) as human beings who have suffered through no fault of their own and whose complaint is just. It takes time to adjust to the change from subject to citizen.

It is also true, as Komori Shigeto noted, that some of the events of 1959 resemble peasant rebellions (*ikki*). Compare them with Herbert Bix's description of the typical stages of an *ikki*:

> These included an initial short, preparatory stage, noted by the designation "unrest" (*fuon*) or even "disturbance" (*sōdō*). In the process, some villagers might seek redress of grievances through legal appeal or petition (*shūso*); others might take flight (*chō-san*). Simultaneously, instances of illegal appeal to higher levels of authority (*osso*), sometimes outside the fief itself, would appear once the situation burst into a full-fledged forceful appeal (*gōso*), that is, an ikki involving the entire fief, often accompanied by "house-smashing" (*uchikowashi*).

Bix notes an increase over the Tokugawa period, as the economy developed, in "house-smashing," "a traditional sanction in the form of total or partial property destruction levied on individuals considered guilty of intolerable social abuses."[148]

It is tempting to describe the events in Minamata as an *ikki*, nearly a hundred years after the end of the Tokugawa period. Minamata saw all these stages, including the "escape" by many people to urban areas to the north and east in search of work. The damage inflicted on factory offices in 1959 is certainly reminiscent of house-smashing. It is easy to find parallels between peasant martyrs (*gimin*) and the Minamata disease victims who participated in protests and later died of the disease or were convicted for their violent acts, especially since Minamata was often referred to as a "castle town" and Shin Nitchitsu as its "feudal lord." Furthermore, as in many *ikki*, in Minamata the victims gained some small alleviation of their misery—and, they hoped, encouraged those in power to end the cause of that misery—without challenging the existing power structure or system of political morality.

There are some key differences between the events of 1959 and Tokugawa *ikki*, however. The most important is that the protesters of 1959 were not risking their lives or livelihoods by protesting. Appeal to higher authorities was not illegal in 1959. The difference in the terminology used to describe events with surface similarities reveals the more important fact that the participants' views of their political worlds were very different. Except for *sōdō* (disturbance), I have not found any of the terms from Bix's description of *ikki* used in contemporary accounts of the 1959 events. The struggles of 1959 were *funsō*—"disputes" or "strife." The petitions were *seigan* or *chinjō*. The destruction of factory property was not "house-smashing" but simply "violence" (*bōryoku*).

The disputes in Minamata were not merely a question of legal rights. The victims knew they had the legal right to sue the company. Some would argue that cultural restraints inhibited them, and it remained true even in the 1990s that those who sued the company were sometimes criticized by their neighbors for their supposed selfishness and for making trouble.[149] The real crux of the matter, however, was an imbalance of power. Suing the company would have meant challenging the privileged position of the company in the city and, by extension, the political economy of the nation as a whole. In 1959, the victims lacked the political, social, and economic power necessary to do this; instead they did what was practical and possible. Later, thanks to changes in Minamata and the nation and to the roles played by a few creative leaders, they would find ways to gather such powers in their support.

Frank Upham uses Minamata as an example of how Japan's elite rulers—in the LDP, in business, and in the bureaucracy—maintained their power by controlling processes of dispute resolution and keeping them informal.[150] He sees "a common pattern of conflict" in Tokugawa peasant uprisings, the Ashio copper mine case, and Minamata: "appeals to government benevolence followed by collective, often violent, protest, and eventually resulting in effective government action. The overriding legal characteristic of such conflict, however, is informality."[151] The solatium agreement is for him the perfect example of how the elite handled disputes so well, keeping them out of the courts and under control:

The agreement reestablished social harmony in the Minamata area and bought several years of quiescence for Chisso and its government supporters. Had not events elsewhere dramatically altered the balance of power in Minamata, redirected the attention of the national media to pollution, and brought the victims new political allies, the 1959 negotiations might have come to represent one more instance of successful Japanese informal dispute resolution.[152]

In fact, "social harmony" did not increase in Minamata after December 30, 1959, but it is certainly true that those in power had successfully controlled and limited the dispute with the patients by keeping it informal. The same may be said for the company's disputes with the fishing cooperatives. The relative ease with which this was accomplished is striking, as is the fact that most of the work was done by the governor, mayor, and factory managers. *Local* elites—not as seamlessly woven into a nationwide fabric of elites at all levels as Upham implies—were able to handle the disputes themselves, with only occasional assistance and direction from central bureaucrats and politicians, corporate headquarters, and corporate alliances.

The victims were not passive in 1959, but they were unable to find the support needed to tip the balance of power in their favor. When victims and their supporters brought the struggle to Tokyo over a decade later, they changed the rules of the game, and changed them more permanently than Upham suggests. But that is a later chapter in the Minamata story. If citizenship is defined by behavior and consciousness and not just by results, then many of the Minamata victims were already acting and thinking much like democratic citizens in 1959, well before the explosion of local citizens' groups in the 1960s.[153] Had these patterns of thought and action not already been partly developed, the victims could not have been so effectively integrated into the new national network of support that brought better results for them a decade later.

Before the Minamata settlement in 1959, Minister of International Trade and Industry Ikeda Hayato had begun putting together his plan for doubling GNP and individual income within a decade. The idea was first presented to the cabinet in December 1959—the month after he had warned the cabinet against deciding that Shin Nitchitsu's mercury caused Minamata disease.[154] A year later, after Ikeda had replaced Kishi Nobusuke as premier in the wake of mass protests against the U.S.-Japan Security Treaty, the cabinet approved the plan to double income by making Japan a mass consumption society through bureaucratic guidance. With the settlement in Minamata, the decks had been cleared of what could have become an obstacle to this continuation and acceleration of Japan's high-cost high growth. A political "solution" had turned Minamata into a problem merely of compensation, and the question of responsibility was ignored. With few exceptions, this has been the government's policy ever since.

PART III
"Years of Silence"?

Maintaining the Solution

"Year after year withered and fell off neatly, like dead leaves or the brain cells of the victims of mercury poisoning."

—Ishimure Michiko

The years between December 30, 1959, and June 14, 1969—from the solatium agreement between patients and Shin Nitchitsu to the filing of a suit against the company by 112 patients and family members—are often referred to as the "ten years of silence" or the "ten years of isolation."[1] In fact, the patients were by no means silent, but so little attention was paid to them that they might as well have been. The patients were so isolated and ignored that it seemed the company and government authorities at the local level could maintain the 1959 settlement indefinitely. During these years, however, important changes in Minamata and Japan slowly undermined the 1959 settlement and brought the questions of compensation and responsibility for Minamata disease before the nationwide forum of civil society. The end of this period of isolation and "silence" is properly placed not ten years after the first "solution" was constructed at the end of 1959 but eight years later, when the Citizens' Council for Minamata Disease Countermeasures (Minamatabyō taisaku shimin kaigi) was established on January 12, 1968. For those involved in the Minamata disease incident, this organization signaled the beginning of a period of experimentation with new forms of social citizenship and a sea-change in citizen-corporation-state relationships.

The Fishers

In the eight years after 1959, each of the three parts of the settlement—compensation to fishers, consolation payments to recognized patients, and waste-treatment facilities—was expanded, but overall the nature of the settlement was not changed. From the 1920s to the present, the company has preferred to deal with fishing cooperatives more as if they were other companies rather than organizations of citizens or victims. The cooperatives, especially the one in Minamata, have usually accepted this pattern of negotiation and agreement. Nominally, the settlement trades fishing rights for money and reclaimed land. But, whether or not this is made explicit in the agreement, both sides have always understood the money and land to be compensation for losses caused by factory waste. Violence has been relatively rare.

In 1959, the cooperatives overstepped these bounds, with the August violence by the Minamata co-op and the more serious November 2 riots by the prefectural co-ops. Prosecution and conviction of participants in the November riots served as a warning to the fishers and showed that they could not yet use the law and the courts to their advantage. On December 19, two days after Shin Nitchitsu and the prefectural alliance of cooperatives reached an agreement, 205 prefectural police officers searched 26 locations, including fishing cooperative offices and private homes, for evidence in connection with the riots. The chief of the prefectural police commented: "I am well aware of the fishers' desperate situation, but in a nation ruled by law violence is absolutely impermissible."[2] Ui Jun suggests that the start of the investigation was carefully timed. Had it begun before the compensation agreement was reached, it might have provoked further violence. It also was carried out just eight days after the Miike mine in Ōmuta, near the northern border of Kumamoto prefecture, announced the layoff of over 1,200 miners, and Ui believes the prosecution of those involved in the Minamata riots was intended to warn against similar violence there.[3]

On January 12, 1960, the prefectural police set up an investigation headquarters in the Minamata police station and proceeded in ways calculated to strengthen the message implied by their actions. At 7:30 that morning, they arrested five fishermen and called in fifteen others for questioning. Two more were arrested later that day.[4] Beginning at 7:00 A.M., January 16, six more were arrested, and ten people were called in for questioning.[5] The pattern continued until January 26, when another round of arrests included a number of leaders of the various co-ops and brought the total number of people arrested to 25.

Governor Teramoto commented that he thought the police investigation "too severe" and worried that "this may worsen relations between the police and the people of the prefecture."[6] Police sources applied pressure on those both in and out of jail by letting the media know that the eleven co-op leaders under arrest had not yet admitted to planning the violence in advance and that more arrests were likely if they did not confess.[7] The governor and prefectural police chief criticized each other in comments to the press for several days. Since governors have little actual control over Japan's centralized police system (in which prefectural police chiefs are paid by the central government), Teramoto, safely free of direct responsibility, may have been making his mildly critical comments in an attempt to appear moderate and sympathetic to the fishermen.

The Kumamoto district public prosecutor indicted 55 fishermen on April 30, 1960, and all were found guilty on January 31, 1961. The judge decided that the evidence of premeditated forcible entry was clear. The alleged ringleaders, the heads of three fishing cooperatives, were given suspended sentences, with the judge noting the suffering of the fishing families and the fact that the co-ops had already paid the factory ¥10 million ($27,800) in compensation for damages. The 52 others were fined between ¥15,000 ($42) and ¥25,000 ($69) each. Lacking money, support, and experience, the fishermen did not appeal and did not turn this first (and often forgotten) trial in the Minamata disease incident into a judgment on the company's negligence.[8]

Irokawa Daikichi compares the results of this trial unfavorably with the trial of the farmers convicted in the Kawamata incident of 1900. In that trial, a lower court convicted the farmers whose land had been flooded and poisoned by runoff from the Ashio copper mines and who had fought with police while attempting to march to Tokyo of rioting, but they appealed their case and a higher court dismissed the case against them. It may have helped that they had a very vocal advocate in Diet representative Tanaka Shōzō, who continually brought their plight to the attention of the media and the Diet and even attempted to appeal directly to the emperor. Irokawa also found that by 1980, of the 55 fishermen convicted in the Minamata incident, three had committed suicide, thirteen had been certified as Minamata disease victims, seventeen more had applied for certification, and nineteen had died.[9]

When Minamata disease began appearing over the prefectural border in Kagoshima, fishing cooperatives in Kagoshima prefecture decided to demand compensation like that given the fishing cooperatives in Minamata and elsewhere along the Shiranui Sea in Kumamoto. The governor of Kagoshima met with Shin Nitchitsu officials on December 19, 1959, and gained their agreement that Kagoshima fishers would be compensated at the same level as those in Kumamoto. City officials, including the mayor, in Izumi in Kagoshima joined the Izumi fishing cooperative's negotiations with Shin Nitchitsu. Unlike Minamata, Izumi was not politically or economically dependent on the company. With the mayor joining the fishers in their negotiations, progress was relatively smooth.

The Izumi negotiators asked the company for ¥82 million ($228,000) in compensation on January 23, 1960, but Shin Nitchitsu offered only ¥9 million ($25,000). At the end of January, the fishers asked Kagoshima Governor Terasono Katsushi to mediate, but he refused.[10] The fishers lowered their demand to ¥30 million ($83,300). The company raised its offer to ¥12 million ($33,300) in March and then sent Managing Director Chihara to negotiate with the Izumi fishers at the Izumi city hall on May 20. Governor Terasono now consented to mediate, and a final agreement was hammered out and signed in his office on May 23. The compensation for fishing losses was set at ¥15 million ($41,700), and the company promised to give priority in hiring to young fishers from the Izumi area. The five fishing cooperatives in the Izumi area agreed never to ask for more compensation as long as the factory's waste did not worsen, even if it was determined to be the cause of Minamata disease.[11]

In the meantime, the Minamata Fishing Cooperative had decided to seek further compensation from the company. Minamata disease and the decline in fish stocks, not to mention the low prices and low demand for the few fish they caught, continued to worsen. Over 300 households had fished in 1957, but by 1961 the number who still fished had been cut approximately in half.[12] In January 1960, the prefectural fish sellers' association voted not to sell fish from the Minamata Bay area. In February, Kumamoto University announced the results of surveys of mercury levels in hair. Some Minamata disease patients were found to have 700 parts per million (ppm) just after developing the disease and 300 ppm three months later. Samples taken from residents of Kumamoto City averaged 2–3 ppm, but some "healthy" residents of Minamata's coastal areas had 100 to 150 ppm.[13] To put this in perspective, although it is impossible to specify an exact level at which Minamata disease is triggered, doctors consider a hair mercury concentration of 50 ppm dangerous, and the normal level for Japanese ranges up to about 10 ppm.[14]

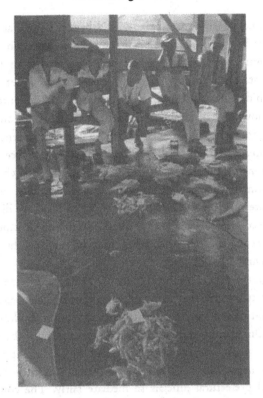

Fig. 13 Fishermen with little to sell and no customers, in the Marushima fish market, Minamata, 1960.
© Kuwabara Shisei.

The Minamata city government sent a delegation to Tokyo with petitions asking that surveys of the pollution be expedited and that fishing be
banned in dangerous areas in order to restore consumer confidence. They
made their case to the special Minamata disease committees of the LDP and
JSP, as well as to officials of the Ministries of Health and Welfare, Agriculture and Forestry, Transport, and MITI and the EPA. They were told
that the EPA's survey of the bay would take a year to complete and that, like
the prefecture, the central government remained unwilling to impose a ban
that would require compensation of those prohibited from fishing. They
also met with executives at Shin Nitchitsu's head office and asked them to
hire unemployed fishers. After raising the issue at an executive conference,
Managing Director Chihara promised municipal officials that the company
would do its best to help.[15]

The Minamata Fishing Cooperative had begun a sit-in at the factory's main gate on February 15, 1960, demanding compensation for damages due to Minamata disease, which had been excluded from their August 1959 agreement. On February 23 co-op representatives met with factory manager Nishida Eiichi to explain their demands and presented him a detailed chart showing their total estimated losses from 1955 through 1961 to be ¥283,151,000 ($787,000).[16] Shin Nitchitsu suggested Governor Teramoto should mediate. The municipal delegation made its unsuccessful pleas in Tokyo beginning on February 27. On March 21, the co-op, whose membership had declined from 297 the previous summer to 214, held a formal meeting to vote on tactics. The majority chose to press for direct negotiations with the company rather than mediation. They also decided to resume their sit-in that night. They held several peaceful marches through the city over the following days.[17]

On April 7, the new co-op head Matsuda Ichijirō and some 30 members traveled to Tokyo, where they met company officials. They began a sit-in on April 9 in front of company headquarters in the Tokyo Building, near Tokyo Station. On April 13, they petitioned a joint session of the special committees on Minamata disease in both houses of the Diet to intervene in their compensation negotiations.[18] Matsuda explained that they did not trust municipal and prefectural officials to mediate fairly. The committees decided to require mediation under Article 21 of the Water Quality Conservation Law. The formal mediation committee system provided for by this law had never been put into practice, but the EPA, which was the relevant authority, promised to notify Governor Teramoto that he must set up a committee according to the law. The governor never assented, and the law was not applied.[19] Following the more typical and probably expected pattern, the mediation that eventually took place was informal and was not carried out under the Water Quality Conservation Law.

On April 14, ten of the protesters, wearing their usual towel headbands and work clothes, met Kiyoura Raisaku, the Tokyo Institute of Technology professor who two days earlier had explained his arguments against the mercury theory to the EPA-directed study committee. His intentional "leak" to the press that his amine theory was undermining the mercury theory in the committee's discussions helped weaken the Minamata fishers' case.[20] They angrily refused to accept his explanation that fish and shellfish from Minamata Bay did not cause Minamata disease in experiments, and promised to send him fresh samples to prove their case.[21]

The protesters were beginning to be noticed in Tokyo. Passers-by and employees at the nearby Tokyo Central Post Office began to donate money and supplies. A restaurant in the vicinity provided food. The Minamata municipal government, with the situation slipping out of its control, hurriedly sent a delegation headed by the vice mayor to persuade the fishermen to accept mediation and come home. Governor Teramoto, also in Tokyo, told municipal officials he would consider mediating only if asked by both sides to do so. The municipal officials visited Diet members from the prefecture, but the latter insisted that since the dispute did not involve matters of national policy, it should be solved at the prefectural and local level.[22]

A meeting was held in a Diet office building on April 20, attended by Shin Nitchitsu's Managing Director Chihara, the head of the factory's General Affairs Section, fishing co-op head Matsuda, the fishing co-op's secretary, four members of the House of Representatives and two from the House of Councilors, Minamata's vice mayor Ishihara Waketake and City Council speaker Fuchigami Sueki, two members of the City Council's committee on Minamata disease, two other City Council members, and two officials from Kumamoto prefecture's Tokyo office. The understandably cowed co-op head Matsuda, with no other choice as long as the company refused to conduct direct negotiations, agreed that the co-op would accept mediation by the governor. He saved a bit of face by insisting on vague conditions guaranteeing an impartial mediation committee and by explaining that the fishermen were likely to get sick from exposure if they continued their protest. They boarded the train for home that night. Thus, the first sit-in at Shin Nitchitsu's headquarters, and the first "Tokyo negotiations" in the Minamata disease incident, ended in failure. There had been no negotiations, and the co-op was forced to accept the mediation it had tried to refuse.[23]

Governor Teramoto formally agreed on May 13 that he would mediate. He named a seven-member committee composed of himself, the head of the prefectural government's Commerce Section, Minamata Mayor Nakamura, the speaker of the City Council, the head of the City Council's Minamata disease committee, and two other City Council members. Reflecting a condition insisted upon in Tokyo by the fishing co-op, this time no committee member was a Shin Nitchitsu employee.[24] The co-op staged a sit-in demonstration in front of the prefectural capitol building in Kumamoto on June 2 to urge quick action by the committee, which held its first meeting June 7, but the company maintained its hard line. President Yoshioka Kiichi announced: "As compensation for factory waste in general, excluding Minamata disease, we paid ¥35 million ($97,200) last summer, and we are paying ¥2 million ($5,600) per year for development of the fishing industry; so now, with the cause of Minamata disease yet to be confirmed, we can pay no more. Instead, we will have our subsidiaries hire some fishers who wish to work."[25] Fishing co-op officials responded that it was unfair for the regional alliance of fishing cooperatives to get compensation for Minamata disease while the Minamata co-op, the most directly affected, received nothing.

The company's refusal to offer monetary compensation and a growing split within the co-op over whether to accept jobs with Shin Nitchitsu stalled the mediation process. The company offered to hire about 100 of the coop's 200 members and to contribute to a fishing-promotion company if one were established, but the co-op held to its demand for ¥283,151,000 and refused to submit a list of applicants for jobs.[26] The governor had asked the five Minamata members of the committee to work out a solution, but they concluded this was impossible. On August 13, Teramoto called co-op head Matsuda and Managing Director Chihara to the governor's office and informed them that the committee had given up mediation.[27] Henceforth the two sides would have to negotiate on their own. The company and co-op were back where they had started six months earlier, when the fishers first demanded compensation for Minamata disease.

Chihara told reporters: "There is absolutely no basis for the demand for ¥280 million. And it is clear from the results of last August's compensation that even if we paid some money, it would not support the fishers. For this reason the company thought of long-term measures such as hiring, and it is a shame that the co-op leaders refused to consider these. If the co-op does not change its stance, negotiations will be meaningless."[28]

The co-op, ¥4 million ($11,000) in debt and now without prospects of help in the near future for its members and their families, who totaled 1,000 people, issued a statement the next day:

1. The hiring the company proposed would involve 80 or so people being hired by Shin Nitchitsu and other companies, and no compensation would be paid to the remaining 150 or 160 people, who make up two-thirds of the cooperative member-

ship. This would be no different from abandoning them to their deaths. We requested that the compensation issue be resolved first, and then those fishers who are hired could return their compensation, but the company refused to consider this.

2. Concerning the establishment of a fishing-promotion company—The fishers of Minamata have no experience with fishing in distant or nearby deep waters, and even if we fish in coastal waters, we cannot sell the fish we catch. Therefore the company would be certain to fail within a year.

3. The company had said it would compensate the Minamata Fishing Cooperative along the lines of the compensation it has paid to the Shiranui Sea coastal fishing cooperatives and the Izumi fishing cooperatives, but at the last minute it changed its position and said it would not pay compensation. That is why we and the company are in opposition.[29]

There was a great deal of grumbling within the cooperative over the leaders' policy of refusing to accept the company's offer of jobs until the compensation issue was decided. The leader of the opposition was Satō Takeharu of Modō, who had participated in the April sit-in in Tokyo.[30] Like many members of the fishing co-op, he had worked at other jobs besides fishing. Satō had started work at Nitchitsu after graduating from junior high school, but after the war worked for Japan National Railways. Laid off during a rationalization, he joined his father in full-time fishing. Later he again worked for the railway, and there he met Kawamoto Teruo of Tsukinoura, who had a temporary job maintaining tracks. In late June 1960, Satō visited Kawamoto to enlist his help in persuading co-op leaders to accept Shin Nitchitsu's offer of jobs. Satō was by this time a member of the co-op, but Kawamoto was not, since for each family only one person, the family head, could be a member. Teruo's father, Katōta, was the member for the Kawamoto family, although he was ill with what Teruo assumed must be Minamata disease.

Kawamoto Teruo's story is important not only because his is an example of a family afflicted with Minamata disease but also because he was to become one of the central figures in the Minamata disease incident a decade later. Teruo's father had moved with his wife, Kana, from Ushibuka in the Amakusa islands to work at the Nitchitsu factory. He had always fished in his free time, and when he retired from the factory in 1946 he became a full-time fisherman, pole fishing from a rowboat. The illiterate Kana cleared some land and grew mandarin oranges and vegetables.

Teruo, born in 1931, was the eighth of eleven children, five of whom worked for the company. He was a good student, but his family could not afford to send him away to a decent school. In April 1945, while attending the Minamata Agricultural and Technical School (which later became Minamata High School), he and his classmates were mobilized and sent to the factory. There they loaded equipment onto trucks for transport to the mountains, where it would be safe from the air raids that factory manager Hashimoto Hikoshichi knew would destroy most of the factory. On August 9, from outside his school, Kawamoto saw a flash far beyond the Amakusa islands, saw a gourd-shaped cloud begin to grow, and then heard a distant explosion. A few days later a soldier passing the Kawamotos' house on his way to Kagoshima stopped to ask for a drink of water and told them Nagasaki had been destroyed.

In August 1947, since his elder brother Shigeru could no longer pay Teruo's school fees, Teruo dropped out and worked at a series of day jobs with construction companies doing repair and maintenance work at the factory. Among other work, he roofed most of the factory's buildings and repaired the pipeline carrying carbide tailings to the settlement pool at Hachiman. His mother died in 1958; since all his brothers and sisters had moved out, Teruo and his wife, Miyako, remained with his father. Miyako had married Teruo in 1957, even though he had begun to feel a tingling in his hands and feet and assumed it was Minamata disease. Teruo fished with his father when not doing day labor, which was getting harder to find, and they began to eat more fish. A son was born in 1958, and it was difficult to live on Teruo's unemployment insurance of ¥700 ($1.95) per week. He pawned his only suit to buy rice. He noticed that his father put rubber bands on his toes to try to force the nerves to feel something. Teruo himself was losing feeling in his left foot and took to wearing rubber boots since other types of footwear tended to fall off without his noticing.

In June 1960, the desperate Kawamoto agreed to help Satō Takeharu in the campaign against the co-op leaders' refusal to accept the company's offer of jobs. This campaign was in fact funded by Shin Nitchitsu, through Yamataka Matanori of its General Affairs Section, who paid Kawamoto, Satō, and others hoping to work for the company ¥500 ($1.39) per day, 25 percent more than the going rate for day labor. They rode in a three-wheeled truck and used megaphones to publicize their demands that the co-op leaders compromise, that those who took jobs with the company not be punished, and that the co-op leadership be changed and "democratized."

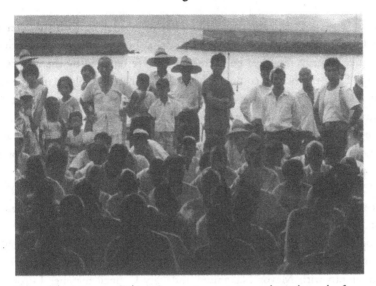

Fig. 14 The Minamata Fishing Cooperative meets to expel members who favor accepting the factory's offer of jobs, 1960. © Kuwabara Shisei.

Co-op head Matsuda made the rounds of members' homes on August 15, two days after the committee had suspended its mediation, to win support. Matsuda called an emergency general meeting for the next morning.[31] Satō, Kawamoto, and the other rebels criticized the leaders strongly at this meeting, arguing that they were acting in an arbitrary fashion and had misjudged the situation ever since the sit-in in Tokyo, that this had lost the co-op all sympathy it might have had from the citizens of Minamata, and that the leaders should therefore resign. Instead, Satō Takeharu and six others were expelled from the co-op. One of those expelled was Kawamoto Katōta, as punishment for his son's activities. At the same time, seven other fishermen and four *amimoto* were warned that they might be expelled. Matsuda commented: "It's too bad they didn't accept my arguments. Now that mediation has been cut off, I will have a meeting of representatives from each district on the seventeenth to work out a clear strategy: whether we will conduct direct negotiations with Shin Nitchitsu, request a resumption of mediation, have Diet members mediate, or take the dispute to court."[32]

Matsuda's authority and the co-op's ability to stand up to pressure from the company and the local authorities declined as its unity crumbled in the face of the challenge from the younger members expelled for wanting to accept work with the company. The offer of jobs, along with the offer to fund a fishing-promotion company, was a highly effective divide-and-conquer strategy. Younger co-op members were tempted by the chance to escape from the fishing co-op, which was dominated by older, more traditional leaders who had not won enough compensation money to support the fishers and their families. And *amiko* (who worked for net owners, the *amimoto*), in addition to hoping to escape financial difficulties, may have welcomed the chance to work as regular employees of a fishing-promotion company on an equal footing with other workers.[33]

On August 18, Matsuda and co-op secretary Nakamura, accompanied by Vice Mayor Ishihara, pleaded with Governor Teramoto to reopen mediation. Teramoto refused on the grounds that nothing had changed, and the co-op criticized him for not following the example of the reopening of negotiations at Mitsui's Miike coal mine.[34] Five days later Matsuda returned to Kumamoto with Mayor Nakamura and City Council member Hirota to meet with the head of the prefectural Commerce and Fisheries Department, Morinaga Ryūzō. Matsuda told Morinaga he would be willing to reduce the demand for ¥280 million, so long as the compensation was comparable to that paid to the Izumi and Shiranui Sea co-ops. Morinaga countered that the committee might be willing to resume mediation if the co-op agreed to binding arbitration on compensation, hiring, and the fishing-promotion company. Matsuda refused, saying he would accept a hiring plan if compensation were paid, but that the fishing-promotion company plan was unrealistic and unacceptable.[35]

On August 26, however, the co-op informed the local members of the mediation committee that it would in fact submit to full binding arbitration on all three issues—only ten days after expelling members for disagreeing with its decision not to change or reduce its demands.[36] The decision to give in was not made at a general meeting but by the co-op leaders alone. Matsuda announced: "The company has violated our rights, and we want compensation. I believe public opinion supports us."[37] The company had yet to accept binding arbitration, however, and the co-op leaders' arbitrary actions worsened the split in the co-op.

Shin Nitchitsu found, as usual, that delay worked to its advantage, and it took a hard line under its new factory manager Kitagawa Kinsai. The local members of the mediation committee asked the company on August 27 to accept binding arbitration, and Kitagawa promised to reply on August 30.

On that day, however, Kitagawa asked the committee to wait until Managing Director Chihara's visit to Minamata on September 3. He also suggested that the company doubted the legitimacy of the co-op's decision to accept binding arbitration. City Council speaker Fuchigami reassured him, incorrectly, that the decision had been made by vote of the co-op members.[38] In Shin Nitchitsu's official reply to the committee on September 3, the company refused binding arbitration or the legitimacy of the co-op's decision to accept binding arbitration and continued to insist on a solution composed of hiring and a fishing-promotion company, with no financial compensation.[39]

At this time, a new controversy arose over the resumption of fishing by co-op members. They were, of course, desperate for both food and income. Elections for members of the prefectural committee that allocated fishing areas to cooperatives were upcoming, and prefectural law stipulated that only those who had engaged in commercial fishing 90 or more days during the year preceding September 15 could vote. Members of the Minamata co-op had done almost no fishing since the city's fish sellers had stopped buying their fish over a year earlier. The co-op promised that its members would now fish only for their own consumption, would not market the fish they caught, and would fish 300 to 500 meters from shore and not in the Hyakken and Hachiman areas. The prefecture advised the fishers not to sell or even eat fish from dangerous areas but remained unwilling to ban fishing because of the compensation such a step would require. City residents were justifiably frightened, since some fish from the Minamata area undoubtedly made their way into the shops. On September 10, the fish sellers renewed their pledge not to buy any fish from the Minamata fish market, even those caught in distant waters.[40] They had asked the company to compensate them for their losses, but it, of course, refused, arguing that there was no proven connection between the factory and the disease and declining fish catches. Finally, in August 1961 an arrangement was worked out whereby the fish sellers' association would borrow ¥1 million ($2,800) from the Higo Bank and the company would repay the loan. The share of each association member came to ¥7,575 ($21).[41]

On September 15, 1960, members of the mediation committee met at company headquarters with executives including Shin Nitchitsu President Yoshioka and Managing Director Chihara, but to no effect. The company continued to refuse to pay compensation, but when Mayor Nakamura returned to Minamata, he reported that he thought the company might in fact pay something. He also announced he had visited a prawn farm in Kisarazu, Chiba prefecture, which might serve as a model for the fishing-promotion company being discussed in Minamata.[42]

On September 20 the internal rebellion in the Minamata Fishing Cooperative flared again when thirteen current and former members opposed to the "dictatorial" leadership's strategy issued the following call in a newspaper insert addressed "To All Members of the Fishing Cooperative":

We are confident that if new leaders negotiate with Shin Nitchitsu, we can reach a compromise better than we could through binding arbitration. . . .
Our requests:
1. The holding of a special general meeting. The prompt holding of an election to replace the current leaders.
2. Concerning Hiring
Consult with the company to have it hire as many fishers as possible.
3. Concerning the fishing-promotion company, consult with municipal authorities in order to rapidly realize its establishment and to enable all members to participate in it.
4. We want to negotiate the financing of a recovery fund for those to whom points 2 and 3 do not apply.
5. Investigate current rumors about impropriety by officers.
6. Let us build a democratic fishing cooperative.

The co-op leaders promised but put off a general meeting.[43]

The company was finally forced to take action by pressure from groups other than the pollution victims. In the fall of 1959, it had been spurred to act by moves in the Diet and prefectural legislature. Now, a year later, there was for the first time pressure on the company and the municipal government from opinion leaders in Minamata. This pressure was partly due to the fears fanned among residents by the co-op's resumption of fishing. An official of the Minamata Chamber of Commerce wrote to the editor of the *Kumamoto nichinichi shinbun*:

The truth of this frightful disease is known throughout the world through reports on the miserable situation of the patients, but no concrete measures have been taken to eliminate the cause. . . . The fishers, utterly dependent on compensation from Nitchitsu, have no rice for today, much less tomorrow. If bad sludge still remains, why have the authorities and Nitchitsu made no serious attempts to remove it? At this stage one action is more important than 10,000 words denying responsibility.[44]

The publisher of the *Minamata taimusu* aimed his criticism at the committee:

More than three months have passed [since mediation was begun], but [the committee] has not been able to achieve a compromise. It has gone along with Nitchitsu's delaying tactics and set aside its purpose of aiding the fishers, who are in the depths of poverty. Criticisms have begun to be raised, saying a committee so incapable of mediating ought to resign promptly to make way for qualified people. . . . Dangling jobs in front of the cooperative in order to split it has been effective to some extent, and what aids this tactic of the company is the indecisive attitude of all the members of the mediation committee.[45]

The company sent Chihara to Minamata on October 4. On October 11, undoubtedly after preliminary discussions, Shin Nitchitsu told prefectural Commerce and Fisheries Department head Morinaga Ryūzō (a member of the mediation committee): "Because we want a full solution to the situation that has come to an impasse, we will not necessarily continue to hold fast to the same way of thinking."[46] The committee met immediately and presented its proposal the next day. The proposed agreement consisted of four points, plus an attached memorandum. First, the company was to pay the co-op ¥7.5 million ($20,800) as a recovery fund. Second, Shin Nitchitsu would hire 30 to 50 fishers, a subsidiary would hire 20, and related companies would hire a few more. In addition, children of co-op members who were not hired were to be given preference in admission to the company's technical school. Third, the company would invest ¥5 million ($13,900) in the fishing-promotion company being planned by the city to provide jobs raising prawns for former full-time fishers. The fourth point was a familiar qualification: "Even if it is learned in the future that factory waste is the cause of Minamata disease, the cooperative shall make absolutely no requests for further compensation." Finally, the memorandum stipulated that to promote "the development of Minamata city," the company would reclaim 330,000 square meters of land in the Hachiman area and pay the co-op ¥10 million ($27,800) in compensation for the loss of fishing rights.[47]

The co-op's original demand of over ¥280 million would have meant ¥1.3 million ($3,600) for each of its 216 members. The proposed agreement would pay the co-op a total of ¥17.5 million ($48,600), including the ¥10 million for the reclaimed land, which was only ¥81,000 ($225) per member, or 6 percent of the original demand. Because of this, and because of the scandalously low price for the reclaimed land, the *Nishinippon shinbun* wrote that the fishing co-op, "isolated and lacking support," was "totally defeated." The ¥10 million for the reclaimed land was only ¥100 ($0.28) per *tsubo* (3.3

square meters). A former leader of the co-op recalled that ¥200 per *tsubo* had been paid for the right to reclaim land in the area in 1934, when prices were hundreds of times lower, and he called the proposed agreement "a suicidal act." As the *Nishinippon shinbun* concluded, the company was killing "two birds with one stone" by gaining valuable land that it urgently needed for waste disposal, while resolving the compensation problem. The co-op's leaders perhaps feared further splintering of the co-op if they delayed and may have decided that with a ¥4 million deficit they had to take what they could while they could get it.[48]

They did ask for some changes. Both sides were to give formal responses to the proposal October 17, and it was to be signed October 20. The company agreed on the seventeenth to accept it without modification, but the co-op asked for three changes. It wanted the company to be required to hire "50 or more" fishers rather than "30 to 50." Second, the proposal specified that the recovery money of ¥7.5 million would be paid to the 216 members of the co-op as of May 2, but the co-op leaders did not want to share the money with members who had been expelled since then. No changes were made in the text in response to these requests, but the committee agreed informally that the co-op would be responsible for distributing the money on its own. Finally, the co-op asked that the area of reclaimed land be reduced.[49]

Shin Nitchitsu at first refused to accept a smaller area, and the signing was postponed. Emperor Hirohito, well known for his interest in marine biology, visited Kumamoto to attend the National Athletic Meet held there in 1960, and on October 21 he asked Governor Teramoto about the situation in Minamata.

According to Governor Teramoto, His Majesty, appearing particularly concerned about Minamata disease, asked: "What is the situation now regarding Minamata disease?" When the governor replied: "The academic theories have not yet been confirmed, but facilities to prevent Minamata disease have recently been installed, and it appears that the compensation issue has been mostly resolved," he appeared satisfied.[50]

An emperor's (or more properly, his handlers') expression of concern with current affairs is never taken lightly, and this may have been what brought the company back to the bargaining table. Negotiations resumed at Minamata City Hall the evening of October 24 and continued through the night. When the company agreed at 4:49 the next morning to reduce the area to be reclaimed from 330,000 to 298,320 square meters and to give 27,921 square

meters of it to the fishing cooperative, the agreement was signed.[51] Once
again, the agreement was portrayed as putting the Minamata disease problem in the past. The committee member who had taken the leading role in
the negotiations, prefectural Commerce and Fisheries Department head
Morinaga, announced: "From now on, we want to continue to make efforts
to help Minamata's fishers recover and to prevent a second occurrence of
Minamata disease." The *Kumamoto nichinichi shinbun* concluded: "The focus
in the Minamata disease problem will be reduced from now on to clarifying
the cause and preventing and treating the disease."[52]

The well-justified criticism of co-op head Matsuda made the split in the
co-op abundantly clear. One fisher commented: "It's co-op head Matsuda's
fault. Going from the demand for ¥300 million right back to binding arbitration, doing things any way he pleases, that's why we've come to this sort
of split."[53] Never again would the Minamata Fishing Cooperative play a
leading role in the Minamata disease incident. The *Minamata taimusu* was
still nearly alone in its scathing public criticism of the mediation committee,
but the attitude of its publisher helps explain why some patients never again
accepted mediation. Three days before the agreement was signed, the newspaper editorialized:

> If you're a big capitalist, it seems you need have no shame even if you discharge bad
> water and cause the Minamata disease that kills 30 people, condemns 15 infants to a
> dark future due to "infantile paralysis," and results in many sick people with no hope
> of recovery. You are supported by the government and the city. . . . The problems
> requiring mediation have not been solved, and impartial mediation cannot be ex-
> pected; so the mediation committee members should resign their positions at once.
> In a situation like this, warriors of past times would slit their bellies to take respon-
> sibility, but the convenient world of the postwar present knows no shame, and they
> can retain their posts.[54]

Ui Jun attributes the defeat of the fishing co-op not only to the power of
Shin Nitchitsu and the poverty of the fishers but also in particular to the co-
op's lack of the sort of structure and leadership needed to make it an effective pressure group. Watanabe Eizō, the leader of the patients' Mutual Aid
Society, could never have been elected to head the fishing co-op, says Ui.
The co-op was run by an elected head, a secretary, one or two staff members, and district representatives. "Class" differences based on scale and type
of fishing operations—pole fishing, several kinds of net fishing, octopus
pots; boat and net owners (*amimoto*) and the *amiko* they hired—meant the

co-op could not easily act as a unit. Furthermore, the co-op and its members had little experience acting independently of "local bosses" such as City Council members. Finally, the leaders were chosen because of their prominence in this patriarchal system of "bosses." Able leaders with the flexibility and creativity necessary to deal with this situation were unlikely to emerge. The traditional leaders, says Ui, were unable to go outside the network of the "boss" system to forge links with other groups.[55] Matsuda's actions exemplify these limitations, as well as the difficulties of democratic practice in local contexts where traditional patterns persisted long after Japan's "democratic constitution" took effect in 1947.

It would seem that the fishing cooperative's leaders were often chosen precisely because they were *not* primarily fishermen but because they were politicians with the connections and power necessary to promote the co-op's interests. Prewar and wartime co-op head Fukami Yoshitake was mayor from 1936 to 1946, and Fuchigami Sueki, who led the co-op through the 1950s, was vice mayor (1946–50) and a city councilman (serving as speaker in 1959–63 and 1975–79).[56] Ironically, this power was also a weakness, since it confined them to the established network and social hierarchy of political power.

Yet the Mutual Aid Society was not significantly more successful than the co-op in gaining compensation. Certainly its sit-in and its experiments with appeals for money and support in cities other than Minamata were more effective, and more similar to the successful tactics used in the second round of responses to Minamata disease, than those of the co-op. Yet the Mutual Aid Society, like the co-op, was forced to give up these tactics without significant gains. This suggests that the balance of power in Minamata and the difficulty of gaining national public or governmental support were as much to blame as the structure and tactics of the Mutual Aid Society and the fishing cooperative for the paltry settlements they won.

The city's plans to provide jobs for fishers by establishing a "fishing-promotion company," to which the October 1960 agreement committed Shin Nitchitsu to invest ¥5 million, were never realized. A specialist from the Chiba prawn farm Mayor Nakamura had visited in September 1960 was invited to investigate conditions in Minamata in March 1961. His report concluded that no "seed prawns" could be found nearby, and that they would have to be brought in from far to the south in Kagoshima prefecture. Getting permission to take them, since fishing rights belonged to local fishing co-ops, would be difficult, and transporting them would be expensive, with significant losses along the way. Since conditions and food in the waters around Minamata were not appropriate, tanks would have to be built to raise the prawns, at a cost of ¥30 million ($83,300) or more.[57]

Nevertheless, Yamaguchi Yoshito (LDP), chair of the City Council's committee on Minamata disease, announced on July 14, 1961, that the company would be established, capitalized at ¥10 million ($27,800), and would begin operations in November. The total start-up cost would be at least ¥20 million to ¥25 million ($55,600 to $69,400). The amount not covered by Shin Nitchitsu and the city would be borrowed. Water would be piped from "clean" areas far offshore to some 200 tanks built in the Marushima area, the "seed prawns" would be caught in the Shiranui Sea by the Minamata Fishing Cooperative, and technical guidance would be provided by the prawn company in Chiba. An ice-making company capitalized at ¥20 million to ¥30 million ($55,600 to $83,300) would also be established, and the prawns would be sold in major cities such as Tokyo, Osaka, and Fukuoka for ¥4,000 to ¥5,000 ($11 to $14) per *kan* (3.75 kg).[58]

Yamaguchi's plan was impractical, could not be funded, and was never put into practice. No "fishing-promotion company" was ever established. Yamaguchi went on to attempt an equally impractical project on his own, raising turkeys—when most Japanese had never tasted turkey—on land in Yunoko rented from fellow City Council member and ideological opponent Hiyoshi Fumiko (JSP). The neighbors (including an elementary school) complained of the noise and smell, and after fights that spread to the City Council floor, Hiyoshi evicted Yamaguchi.[59] Earlier, the city had tried to help fishing co-op members attempt deep-water fishing around the island of Tsushima, between Kyūshū and Korea, but this venture also failed.

Since the fishing-promotion company never materialized, the jobs promised by Shin Nitchitsu were the only jobs provided under the October 25, 1960, compensation agreement. The co-op collected 53 job applications from its members by the October 31 deadline.[60] Shin Nitchitsu hired 35 to work at the factory; nine more were hired by its subsidiary Senkō un'yu (Senkō Transport). Those hired included Satō Takeharu (whose share of the settlement with Shin Nitchitsu had come to ¥160,000, or $444) and all the others expelled from the co-op except for Kawamoto Katōta, who, in addition to being too ill to work, was ineligible because he had already reached the mandatory retirement age and retired from the company.[61] Shin Nitchitsu, although it had used Kawamoto Teruo against the fishing co-op leaders, did not hire him because he had not been a member of the co-op. Both sides had abandoned him.[62]

Kawamoto found work in a small factory, and both he and his father got sicker. Teruo's wife, Miyako, quit her job to care for Katōta, who finally had to be hospitalized in the fall of 1961. Teruo insisted his father had Minamata disease, but the doctors, expecting no new patients because of Shin Nitchitsu's new Cyclator and believing Teruo was only trying to get compensation money, disagreed. After two months Teruo's elder brothers could no longer pay the hospital costs, and Katōta was brought home. The lower half of his body was paralyzed, and he attempted to hang himself. In January 1962, Miyako gave birth to a daughter, and soon afterward Shin Nitchitsu finally gave Teruo a job. He worked near open vessels of hot calcium carbide and on occasion burned his feet, but he rarely noticed this due to the loss of sensation caused by his mercury poisoning.[63]

The Patients

Certified Minamata disease patients received payments from Shin Nitchitsu under the December 1959 solatium agreement, but the money was far from enough to support those who had no other income. Receiving the solatium money made them ineligible for welfare payments, but by March 1960 five families had already spent all their solatium money and gone back on the welfare rolls.[64]

At the same time, evidence continued to mount that the disease was spreading, despite the persistent but mistaken belief that it could not do so because people had stopped eating local fish and because Shin Nitchitsu's Cyclator made the factory's effluent safe, and that in any case only those who ate fish from Minamata Bay could get the disease. The results of tests of mercury levels in hair, carried out from late 1960 to early 1961 by Kumamoto and Kagoshima prefectures, document not the reduction in mercury levels that would have been expected if the factory waste was safe, but a frightening spread of mercury (see Tables 4 and 5).

The findings were shocking—one woman in Goshonoura in the Amakusa islands was found to have a concentration of 920 ppm—but what is more shocking is that the subjects were never informed of the results of the

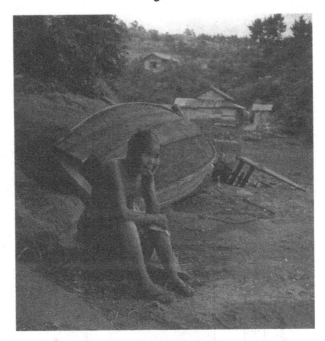

Fig. 15 An old woman in the fishing hamlet of Tsubodan, 1960.
© Kuwabara Shisei.

tests. A decade later, researchers from Kumamoto University attempted to find some of these people and discovered that many of them had died of "unknown causes."[65] Had the subjects known the results, they, their neighbors, and their customers might have stopped eating the fish they caught. This would have saved lives, even though it would have put many people out of work. It would have given the potential patients a chance to demand certification and compensation. It would have further undermined the myth that Minamata disease was confined and over with, and it might have brought the issue to a head again much sooner.

Instead, no government action was taken in response to the surveys. In March 1960 the Kumamoto prefectural assembly dissolved its special committee on Minamata disease. The certification committee, the municipal hospital, and doctors throughout the area were well aware that certification of more patients meant increased costs for Chisso and troubles for the city. They tended to diagnose and certify only those patients with the classic Hunter-Russell symptoms. For most of the bureaucrats, doctors, and

Table 4

Mercury Concentrations in Hair, Minamata Area and Kumamoto City, 1960–1961

Area	Number of persons / % of total			Total number of persons tested	Highest ppm
	0–10 ppm	10–50 ppm	> 50 ppm		
Minamata City	38 (19%)	100 (50%)	61 (31%)	199	172
Tsunagi Village	12 (12%)	61 (60%)	29 (28%)	102	191
Yunoura Town	0	14 (58%)	10 (42%)	24	139.4
Ashikita Town	1 (3%)	19 (48%)	20 (50%)	40	192
Tanoura Town	6 (18%)	15 (45%)	12 (36%)	33	200
Kamegatake Town	24 (28%)	57 (66%)	6 (7%)	87	167
Goshonoura Town	59 (12%)	334 (69%)	89 (18%)	482	920
Kumamoto City	22 (71%)	9 (29%)	0	31	42.5

NOTE: Due to rounding, percentages may not total exactly 100.
SOURCE: Kumamoto-ken eisei kenkyūjo and Kumamoto-ken Minamata hokenjo, "Minamatabyō ni kan suru mōhatsu chū no suigin ryō no chōsa (dai ippō)," May 1961, MBJSS, 2: 1504.

Table 5

Mercury Concentrations in Hair, Kagoshima Prefecture Areas near Minamata, 1960–1961

Area	Number of persons / % of total			Total number of persons tested	Highest ppm
	0–10 ppm	10–50 ppm	> 50 ppm		
Komenotsu area,					
Izumi City	185 (42%)	117 (26%)	148 (33%)	445	642
Akune City	26 (79%)	4 (12%)	3 (9%)	33	338
Takaono Town	2 (20%)	3 (30%)	5 (50%)	10	89.9
Higashi Town	18 (24%)	32 (43%)	25 (33%)	75	142

NOTE: Due to rounding, percentages may not total exactly 100.
SOURCE: Kumamoto-ken eisei kenkyūjo, "Mōhatsu suigin ryō no chōsa," 1962, MBJSS, 2: 1519–20. The original document is marked "not to be made public."

researchers involved, the nearly universal assumption that the factory's waste-treatment facilities had solved the problem of Minamata disease must have made it easier both to justify their failure to break the taboos surrounding the issue and to directly or indirectly acquiesce in a cover-up.

Of course, people were still contracting the disease. The most obvious evidence was the fact that cats continued to get sick, "go crazy," and die. According to Ui Jun, there was a concerted effort to conceal this fact by the fishing hamlets and by Itō Hasuo, head of the city's Public Health Office.[66] When a city hall worker's cat developed Minamata disease, however, it could not be kept secret, and the authorities, the fishing co-op, and the fish sellers struggled to contain the damage. The *Asahi shinbun* reported on May 16, 1961, that a cat belonging to Hamasu Yoshitaka, who lived in the Hyakken area and worked in the agriculture section at city hall, had been sent to the Kumamoto University Medical School and confirmed to have Minamata disease. The city, the newspaper said, was in "shock" to find that what had erroneously been reported to be a fishing family's cat actually belonged to an "average" family.

The family reported that they had fed the cat the guts of some fish they had bought in late April, and that the cat had gone crazy four or five days later, bumping into pillars. Since Hamasu had never fished in the ocean, residents feared that the fish bought in the markets could cause Minamata disease. The prefectural authorities tested the family's hair for mercury, and the city tried to determine where the fish had come from. The family lived only 300 meters from a site where the co-op dried fish it caught in the bay for the city to provide to Kumamoto University for experimental use, and it was suggested that the cat might have eaten poison fish there. The fishing co-op said it had been patrolling the dangerous area of the bay since February to prevent fishing there and was certain the fish in the markets were safe.[67]

The fish retailers' association met on May 19 to reaffirm its August 1959 resolution not to buy Minamata fish and ask the city to take steps to prevent "average citizens" from fishing along the shores of the bay. On May 20, the *Kumamoto nichinichi shinbun* reported a different explanation from Hamasu of how his cat got sick. He said that on April 28 he had caught two fish 500 meters southwest of Koiji Island, and fed them to his pig and cat the same day. The next day the cat began dancing about crazily, and he controlled its symptoms with Jintan, a popular cure-all remedy. It acted sick again on

May 4 and was later confirmed by Kumamoto University to have Minamata disease.[68]

If this story were true and the fish Hamasu caught had caused the disease, then there was a good chance fish in the markets were dangerous, since he had apparently caught them near the border of the no-fishing zone the fishing co-op was trying to police. However, the prefectural public health laboratory announced that the results of its tests of the Hamasu family's hair showed only normal levels of mercury. This meant, said the *Kumamoto nichi-nichi shinbun* in an article contradicting its earlier story, that "what gave the cat Minamata disease was not the fish Hamasu bought, but probably fish it ate at the site where poison fish were dried for experimental use by Kumamoto University."[69]

The most heartrending development during these "years of silence" was the confirmation that the many children born with "cerebral palsy" and other problems in fact had a congenital form of Minamata disease. It had long been realized that there were extremely high rates of miscarriages, stillbirths, birth defects, cerebral palsy, and mental retardation in the areas where Minamata disease was most concentrated, and it was logical to suspect links with the disease.[70] But if the affected fetuses and children had not consumed poison fish, how could they have gotten Minamata disease? In many cases the mothers did not appear to be ill. Medical schools the world over taught that natural barriers protected two vital areas in the body from poison: the brain and, in pregnant women, the fetus. It was not yet known that although this is true for most poisons, including to some extent even inorganic mercury, the exact opposite is true for organic mercury. It passes through these supposed barriers and actually concentrates in the brain and fetus.

Professor Harada Takayoshi of the Kumamoto University Medical School reported to a regional meeting of the Japan Pediatric Association on June 11, 1961, that since 1959 he had been studying seventeen children from Modō and Tsukinoura, born from 1955 to 1958 and diagnosed with cerebral palsy. He found that sixteen of them had concentrations of 50 to 100 ppm of mercury in their hair; in comparison healthy children in Kumamoto City had none. He also found mercury in their mothers' milk and in their umbilical cords.[71] (The custom of saving umbilical cords has helped a great deal in research on Minamata disease, and a high concentration of mercury was later found in an umbilical cord from 1932, the year the factory began producing acetaldehyde using mercury.) In the areas and period he studied, 7.46 percent of the children had been born with cerebral palsy, whereas the normal rate of occurrence was estimated to be 0.2–0.6 percent.[72]

One of Harada's subjects, Iwasaka Yoshiko, died in March 1961. Her father had died of Minamata disease, and an autopsy at Kumamoto University confirmed that her brain cells had been attacked in the manner typical of organic mercury, and she, too, had had the disease.[73] The parents of the other children, along with most of the researchers from Kumamoto University, urged that the other sixteen be certified as well. The certification committee met on August 7 and agreed that Iwasaka had died of Minamata disease but disagreed over whether to certify the others. Hosokawa Hajime argued against doing so, since he believed at least two of the children definitely had cerebral palsy and not Minamata disease. The committee decided that "at present, without autopsies we cannot confirm [whether they have the disease]."[74]

The families were forced to wait for another child to die. Six-year-old Iwasaka Mari died on September 15, 1962, and once again an autopsy by Professors Takeuchi Tadao and Matsumoto Hideyo proved she had Minamata disease. Like Iwasaka Yoshiko's, her brain was roughly half the normal weight. It was certain that she, too, would be certified. The question was whether the surviving children would again be rejected, but two things had changed since the previous summer. First, a new certification committee had been formed, this time not including Hosokawa, who had resigned his job with Shin Nitchitsu. Moreover, the company and the city were now in the midst of a bitter, divisive strike (see Chapter 6).

Takeuchi and Matsumoto decided to announce to the Kumamoto Medical Association, on November 25, their discovery of the existence of congenital Minamata disease. This would make it likely that the committee would certify all the children at its November 29 meeting. Harada Masazumi, then a lecturer and still working on his degree, remembers arguing with Professor Tatetsu Seijun, who insisted that it would be unfair to Shin Nitchitsu to harm it during the strike by making such an announcement. Despite Tatetsu's reservations, Matsumoto and Takeuchi made the announcement. On the twenty-ninth, the committee (of which Takeuchi was a member; Harada attended as an observer) debated for seven hours before finally certifying Iwasaka Mari and the surviving fifteen children, who ranged in age from four to seven years and included Mari's younger sister Sueko.

Former president of the patients' Mutual Aid Society Watanabe Eizō, whose four-year-old grandson Masaaki was one of those certified, made a telling remark: "I'm grateful that they rose above politics and made a purely medical decision." Iwasaka Masaki, father of Mari and Sueko, told the press: "I now want to discuss compensation as calmly as possible."[75]

The factory manager immediately promised to compensate the newly certified patients according to the 1959 solatium agreement. The center of gravity in the Mutual Aid Society was now shifting further toward families with children who had the disease. These families were particularly dissatisfied with the low payments for children, and they pushed the society to request that the solatium payments be renegotiated. They put their request to Shin Nitchitsu, in November 1962, but the company asked them to wait until its labor troubles were solved. The strike ended in January 1963, but when the Mutual Aid Society approached the company again in March, it was asked to wait a little longer, until the company had finished putting things in order again after the strike. Actual discussions did not begin until the end of 1963.

In September 1963, Shin Nitchitsu's General Affairs Section chief Misawa explained to the *Nishinippon shinbun* what the company thought the solatium payments meant: "When poor neighbors get sick, the people who have money give them some. That's all that's happening here." Patients told the newspaper: "We've lived by taking fish in waters recognized by the government as public. We haven't done anything wrong. . . . If we make too much of a fuss, the townspeople don't like it. They tell us that without Shin Nitchitsu the town will be ruined."[76]

The negotiations that began in late 1963 were conducted directly, without publicity and without a mediation committee. The Mutual Aid Society wanted to avoid the defeat imposed on it by the mediation committee in 1959, but it had no new cards to play in these negotiations. Agreeing to a delay of over a year so the company could settle its labor troubles had weakened its position. It did nothing to gain publicity that could bring it support. There were no newspaper reports on the negotiations and only a short article in the *Kumamoto nichinichi shinbun* on the final agreement. When there seemed to be no way to resolve disagreements over how much to raise the payments to compensate for inflation, one Mutual Aid Society member remarked that perhaps they should take their complaints to court and let the court decide which side was right. General Affairs Section chief Misawa retorted: "Go ahead and try, if you can. The Ministry of Health and Welfare and the EPA haven't issued any conclusions [about the cause of the disease]. All we have to do is wave our hand and nobody will believe you—not lawyers, and not prosecutors or judges either. And I wonder if you've got enough money to take us to court."[77]

The agreement signed on April 17 gained little for the patients.[78] Adult patients were now to be classified by the certification committee into those with light and those with severe symptoms. This added even more political and financial implications to the supposedly medical decisions by the committee. The annual payments to members of the first group increased only 5 percent, from ¥100,000 to ¥105,000 (from $278 to $292). Those with more severe symptoms would receive ¥115,000 ($319). The 1959 contract had paid those who contracted the disease as children only ¥30,000 ($83) per year, even after they became adults. Under the new agreement, they received ¥50,000 ($139) up to age 25 and ¥80,000 ($222) thereafter. (This was a curious age to choose, since the age of majority in Japan is 20; 25 had been the minimum voting age under the "universal" [for men only] suffrage from 1925 to 1945.) Payments for deaths—¥300,000 ($833), plus ¥20,000 ($56) for funeral expenses—were not increased. As of April 1964, then, Shin Nitchitsu could still be quite confident of maintaining the 1959 settlement with only minor adjustments, avoiding court disputes and minimizing uncomfortable publicity.

What little support and encouragement the patients did receive did not yet seem to portend any great change. Hokusei gakuen, a private girl's high school in Sapporo, Hokkaidō (nearly as far from Minamata as one can get in Japan), sent ¥80,000 ($222) in donations to researchers at Kumamoto University from 1956 to 1960. In 1961 students at the school began sending handicrafts, *origami* cranes, and money to Minamata disease patients in the Minamata Municipal Hospital. As the *Kumamoto nichinichi shinbun* put it, "These girls are still continuing their relay of love for Minamata disease patients, passing it on as they graduate to the students who follow them." The money was used to buy a television, and according to a nurse other donations began to trickle in from around the country in 1962 and 1963.[79]

The city, and Mayor Hashimoto Hikoshichi (elected again in February 1962; he served a total of four terms from 1950 to 1958 and 1962 to 1970), put the brightest possible shine on the March 22, 1963, visit to Minamata of a teacher, a graduate, and a student from Hokusei gakuen. Hashimoto and the visiting teacher traded praises for each other's cities, with Hashimoto expressing envy and amazement at the growth of Sapporo's population to 650,000 from the 50,000 it had been when he was a junior high school student there. The visitors toured the municipal hospital and cried when they were introduced to Minamata disease patient Matsunaga Kumiko, who had been in her bed in the hospital, unable to see or hear, for six years. They then met the less severely handicapped patients and played a tape they had brought of their schoolmates singing hymns. The final stop was the young people's club in Yudō, where they met and spoke with some 30 patients before leaving for home.[80]

After the delegation returned to Hokkaidō, the school sent the municipal hospital a donation of ¥13,800 ($38). In June, they sent lilies of the valley by air to Minamata to thank the city for inviting them and to the researchers at Kumamoto University. When Hokusei gakuen was damaged by a fire late in 1963, Minamata disease patients collected ¥11,000 ($31) and sent it to Sapporo.[81]

SIX

Change Undermines the Solution

Changes in Minamata

In the mid-1960s, it by no means seemed that pressures underneath the surface in Minamata were building toward an explosion. Patients and fishers were being compensated, following the patterns established in 1959. Two new hospitals, one for "rehabilitation" and one for patients too ill to live at home, were under construction in Yunoko, a seaside hot spring area to the north (and out of sight) of the city center and the factory. Outsiders concerned about disease patients, such as the Sapporo schoolgirls, were no threat to the established order. Yet changes were taking place in Minamata and Japan that would inaugurate a second round of responses to Minamata disease in 1968.

INDIVIDUALS AND SOCIETY

In 1959, almost no "average citizens" of Minamata (those not affected by the disease and not employed by Shin Nitchitsu) showed, or acted on, any feelings of sympathy for the disease victims. During the next several years, a few residents took the side of the patients, and a few outsiders did the same. A historical determinist would argue that if these particular individuals had not acted as and when they did, circumstances would have brought others to take their places, but I believe this is at most only partly true. Without these key creative individuals, the course and timing of the second round of responses could not have been the same.

The first of these people, and the one about and by whom the least has been written, was Akasaki Satoru, a city government employee.[1] Akasaki, like Ishimure Michiko, was a member of the literary group led by Tanigawa Gan. Working at the Public Health Office, Akasaki served as liaison between patients and the city government, driving patients to the hospital and bringing university doctors to the patients' homes. In 1958 he secretly showed Ishimure the 1956 report by the Kumamoto University research group, and he took her with him on many of his visits to patients, alone and with researchers. His own daughter had been stricken with infantile paralysis at the age of two, and he resolved to do what he could for the patients to try to make up for what he thought was the city government's callous treatment. Akasaki was a quiet, gentle man, known for his drinking, and the fishers eventually accepted him.

Akasaki was once assigned to guide a television crew from Tokyo that came to film a report on Minamata disease. Shin Nitchitsu's general affairs manager called the Public Health Office with a warning that Akasaki should not show them anything embarrassing. Akasaki went ahead and brought them to the home of a severely affected, bedridden patient. Later he was transferred to a job as a radio operator at a distant, inland branch office of the city government. He was eventually transferred back to city hall, and when the Association to Indict [Those Responsible for] Minamata Disease (Minamatabyō o kokuhatsu suru kai) was established in Kumamoto in 1969 and began publishing a monthly newsletter, Akasaki wrote a regular column on the lives of the patients.

Ishimure Michiko has been by far the most important person in the movement on behalf of Minamata disease patients.[2] Born in 1927 in Amakusa, she has lived in Minamata since her infancy. Tanigawa Gan and the Circle Village group helped her develop a distinctive writing style, using the local dialect and marked by a strong sense of place and a reverence for a way of life and connection to nature being destroyed by "modern civilization." Like Tanigawa, she attempts to be a "facilitator," distilling and presenting the experiences of common people.[3] She has published over a dozen books and won numerous awards. Her best-known book, *Kugai jōdo: waga Minamatabyō*, published in January 1969, describes events in Minamata through 1968 and is the first part of a trilogy.[4] A compelling mix of journalistic and poetic styles, the book describes actual events but changes some names. The central text in the dominant narrative of Minamata, it presents the Minamata story as a condensed version of the tragic story of "modernity" (*kindai*) in Japan, exemplifying capitalism's destruction of a rather romanticized pre-industrial way of life.[5] It has been through many printings, inspired plays, been analyzed in books and dissertations, and is even used in high school classes.

Ishimure Michiko began working as a substitute teacher before the end of the war and married Ishimure Hiroshi in 1947. He soon left his job in construction to work as a teacher. She sold makeup door to door and traveled inland by train with their baby son strapped to her back, trading fish for black market rice that she hid between her baby and her back. In 1954 she met Tanigawa Gan, who influenced her writing and her politics through his radical literary group.

When Ishimure's son Michio was in the Minamata municipal hospital with tuberculosis, his room was near those for Minamata disease patients. She decided to visit one of them, Sakagami Yuki, in May 1959 and, on her way to Sakagami's room, was struck by the sight of another patient, Kama Tsurumatsu.

Up to the time of my first visit to the hospital I'd been an inconspicuous, self-effacing housewife. . . . I had a preference for old songs and ballads, and occasionally dabbled in poetry. I was, of course, incurably in love with the calm expanse of the Shiranui Sea and with the smooth, endless tideland it exposed when it ebbed into the distance. Judging by the average life expectancy of Kyūshū women, it seemed to me that I could live to be over 70. However, I contemplated without enthusiasm the remainder of my life, thinking that it would continue to unroll itself in the same drab, uneventful way as the life I was leading then.

On the day I saw Tsurumatsu, above all else, I despised myself unbearably for being a part of the despicable human race. From that day forward, the image of his pathetic, blind body lying there like a piece of deadwood, and his restless, unforgiving spirit took up residence somewhere deep inside me.[6]

The "restless spirits" of the Minamata disease victims are one of the most pervasive images in Ishimure's work, and reflect her conviction that it is her fate not to rest as long as they are unable to do so. Her parents and husband criticized her for neglecting her family, but she felt "I simply had to be present where I was needed."[7] Her husband eventually came to be involved in the movement himself through the teachers' union, especially after he began teaching at Fukuro Middle School, which is attended by children from Detsuki, Tsukinoura, Yudō, and Modō—some of the worst affected areas.

Ishimure Michiko was moved by her visits to patients, at their homes and in the hospital, to begin writing their stories. The first part of what became *Kugai jōdo: waga Minamatabyō* was published in 1960 in *Sākuru mura* (Circle village), a journal founded by Tanigawa Gan and others. Another chapter appeared in *Nihon zankoku monogatari* the same year. Ishimure and friends established the journal *Gendai no kiroku* in 1963, intending that the remaining installments of what would clearly become a book would appear in it, but the journal folded after one issue. More of the book was serialized under the title *Umi to sora no aida ni* (Between sea and sky) in the journal *Kumamoto fudoki* in 1965 and 1966. The journal's founder and editor, Watanabe Kyōji, was later one of the founding members of the Association to Indict [Those Responsible for] Minamata Disease. Ishimure's book finally appeared in 1969.

During these years Ishimure continued visiting patients, writing letters, and working with people in Minamata and from outside. One of these outsiders was the photographer Kuwabara Shisei, who first visited Minamata to photograph patients and fishing hamlets in 1960. He exhibited his photographs in Tokyo in the fall of 1962 and published them in book form in 1965.[8] Ishimure wanted the people of Minamata to see Kuwabara's work.

Toward the end of 1963 I pleaded with Hashimoto Hikoshichi, the Mayor of Minamata, to organize an exhibition in town with Kuwabara's . . . shattering photographs of Minamata Disease patients and their families. We had the following conversation. [Hashimoto was the former Shin Nitchitsu engineer and plant manager who had invented the acetaldehyde production process that used mercury as a catalyst.]

"Your occupation?"

"I beg your pardon? Er . . . I am a housewife. I am writing a book on Minamata Disease. I've only written one or two chapters. There's plenty to do at home, you know. Besides, we raise pigs, so I haven't much time."

"I see. Do you know Araki Seishi?"

"Yes, I do."

"I mean, does he know you personally?"

"Yes, he does."

"If so, what's his opinion of you? Where does he place you among the younger generation of writers in Kumamoto?"

"Pardon me? Er, I'm afraid I'm not exactly what you would call a writer. I've never had the honor. . . ."

Without letting me finish, the mayor summarily refused to answer my request. Araki Seishi was the patriarch, the uncontested authority in the literary world of Kumamoto. I wrote a letter containing the same request to the director of *Kumamoto nichinichi*, the most influential local newspaper. This time also the answer was a polite, but firm, refusal.[9]

Ishimure was finally able to organize an exhibition of Kuwabara's photographs at the Tsuruya Department Store in Kumamoto with help from the teachers' union. She also visited Hosokawa Hajime, the former director of the factory hospital who had discovered the disease and proved with his "cat no. 400" that the acetaldehyde waste caused it, who had retired to the island of Shikoku.[10]

In Minamata, Ishimure's efforts were helped by the work of Hiyoshi Fumiko. Hiyoshi was an elementary school teacher and administrator, an active member of the JSP, and a City Council member from 1963. Like Ishimure, she was inspired by a hospital encounter with Minamata disease patients. She was greatly moved by the patients she saw when she accompanied the delegation from Hokusei gakuen in Sapporo on their hospital visit. She was particularly concerned that the public schools provide for the needs of children with Minamata disease. It was to address these needs, as well as other concerns she had as an activist member of the teachers' union, that she ran for the City Council.[11] According to Ishimure, Hiyoshi donated her City Council salary to Minamata disease patients at the municipal hospital.[12] This small, determined woman, a tenacious debater and questioner, was nicknamed "Fireball" by Eugene and Aileen Smith.[13] In 1968, Hiyoshi helped found the Citizens' Council for Minamata Disease Countermeasures (Minamatabyō taisaku shimin kaigi) and served as its first president.

At the same time as the photographer Kuwabara Shisei became active in Minamata, another "outsider" whose work and publications would play important roles in the Minamata disease incident was closely observing the lives of patients. This was Harada Masazumi of the Kumamoto University Medical School. Other doctors usually conducted examinations by asking city officials to assemble patients at the municipal hospital or in meeting halls, and Harada did this himself at first. One of the most heartbreaking pictures in the Minamata disease story was taken by Harada when he assembled sixteen children diagnosed with cerebral palsy at the municipal hospital—children who, of course, actually had congenital Minamata disease.

Before long Harada began to spend a great deal of time walking around the seriously afflicted areas and getting to know the residents. His initial motivations were to avoid inconveniencing them and having to pay their transportation costs, but he soon realized the main benefit of visiting them at home was that he learned much more about them and their disease. Perhaps because doctors were unable to cure the disease, many patients and their families felt they were being used as research subjects and mistrusted

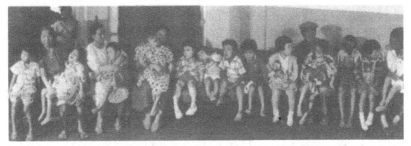

Fig. 16 Congenital Minamata disease patients assembled by
Dr. Harada Masazumi, 1962. © Harada Masazumi.

doctors. On one of his early visits to Minamata, he encountered a sign at one home reading: "Newspaper reporters stay away! Kumamoto University doctors get out!"[14] With patience, sympathy, and an interest in their life-styles and psychological stresses as well as their physical symptoms, he gradually gained their trust. Because of this he made the most important contribution in the uncovering of congenital Minamata disease.

In August 1961, after leaving the home of a bedridden patient in the Myō-jin area, he encountered two young brothers playing.

"Where's your mommy?"
After a long, long time, the elder brother finally answered "Ocean."
"And your daddy."
Again, after a long time, he answered "Dead."
In fact, their father had died of Minamata disease in May 1960. The child spoke with great difficulty, and it was hard to understand him; he obviously had a speech defect. The younger brother was unable to speak or hold his head steady, and as is characteristic of children with this type of handicap, his body jerked and his legs kicked out. And yet he had a broad grin.

Soon . . . their mother came up [from the shore] with a plate of sliced fish. I asked "What do these children have?" . . . She replied "The older one has Minamata disease. The younger one doesn't have Minamata disease, but cerebral palsy." . . . When we called the patients to Minamata Municipal Hospital for examinations, the elder one had come, but the younger brother was left alone at home, unseen by us. . . .

I asked her to let me examine him, but she said it was unnecessary. She had lost faith in doctors, and given up. . . . The mother said "There are a lot of other children like this one among those born that same year. My cousin has one too." Pointing across the bay toward Yudō, she said "You know, they say there are six or seven in that hamlet.[15] And in Modō, all the children born that year have the same thing." ... When I asked "Why isn't it Minamata disease?" the mother laughed for the first time. She simply said, "Shouldn't you doctors know? It's because they didn't eat fish; they were born with it."[16]

Harada Masazumi later came to know Ishimure Michiko, whom he had often seen sitting in a corner while he examined patients. He continued his close relationship with the patients and their communities. He was a member of the Minamatabyō kenkyūkai, the research group formed in 1969 that assisted the plaintiffs and lawyers in the first suit by writing a report proving the company's negligence. Harada's work with victims of carbon monoxide poisoning from the November 9, 1963, explosion at the Miike mines in Ōmuta convinced him even more of the need for doctors to understand their patients' lives and communities and to consider their psychological as well as physical wounds. It also gave him experience working with union members, something he did as part of the Minamatabyō kenkyūkai.[17]

Harada has written a dozen or more books on Minamata disease, including a children's book, and testified frequently in Minamata disease court cases. He has received an award from the United Nations and has been sent by the Japanese government to help Brazil investigate mercury poisoning in the Amazon. Harada is probably Kumamoto University's most famous professor since Natsume Sōseki, Japan's first great modern novelist. And yet, because the academic establishment frowns on "commitment" to a "cause," he was still not a full professor when he retired in 1999.[18]

Ui Jun is another outsider whose commitment harmed his career in academia.[19] He graduated from the University of Tokyo in applied chemical engineering in 1956 and remembers that Shin Nitchitsu still had a high reputation among his fellow students. Only the best students could even take its employment examinations.[20] He took a job at Nihon zeon, where he helped set up a waste-water system that, like Shin Nitchitsu's, discharged mercury. Shocked at what he heard about Minamata, he quit his job, returned to the University of Tokyo to enter graduate school, and began studying the situation in Minamata. He first visited Minamata in 1960 and in 1962 went with the photographer Kuwabara Shisei to speak with Dr. Kojima Akikazu at Shin Nitchitsu's hospital. Probably intentionally, Kojima excused himself from the room for a few minutes, leaving on his desk an internal memo reporting the results of Dr. Hosokawa's cat experiments.

Kuwabara photographed the document.[21] Ui then traveled to Shikoku to visit Hosokawa, who confirmed the authenticity of the memo.[22] (Hosokawa had resigned in March 1962 after submitting a report on his final experiments, which had proved the existence of organic mercury in the acetaldehyde plant's waste and shown that it caused Minamata disease in cats.)[23] But Hosokawa cautioned Ui against taking the story to the news media, saying the company could easily mobilize enough support to crush any allegations from a young university assistant.[24]

At Hosokawa's suggestion, Ui told Ishimure Michiko of the discovery. She and Akasaki Satoru helped Ui collect and organize a huge volume of materials on Minamata disease, including newspaper reports, company pamphlets, and journal articles. He published an annotated collection of these documents in serial form, using the pen name Tomita Hachirō, in *Gijutsu shi kenkyū* beginning in 1963; and the series continued in the chemical industry union journal *Gōka* in 1964. An abbreviated version was published in book form in July 1968 as *Kōgai no seijigaku: Minamatabyō o otte* (The political science of pollution: on the trail of Minamata disease). The book criticized not only the Chisso corporation but also government at all levels and the capitalist system in general. Together with Ishimure's *Kugai jōdo*, published six months later, it brought the disease to the attention of many readers and inspired some to get involved. The original journal articles were privately printed by the Association to Indict in 1969 and are an invaluable collection of documents for the period up to the mid-1960s.[25]

Ui Jun became an assistant at the University of Tokyo in 1965 and had still not been made a professor, despite the many books he published, when he left to become a professor at Okinawa University in 1986. The previous year, 1985, had seen the end of his Jishu kōza, an evening lecture series on pollution that he had begun in 1970 as an open school to counter the elite, closed nature of Japan's most prestigious university.[26] In 1991 he was given a Global 500 award by the United Nations Environment Program. Ui provided important links in the Minamata movement—between activists and scientists, activists and academia, Minamata and Tokyo, Minamata and Niigata, and activists in Japan and throughout the world. Most important, in his 1968 book and in his role in the movement, he pioneered linkages between the science and politics of pollution.

Along with Akasaki, Ishimure, Kuwabara, Hiyoshi, and Harada, by the mid-1960s Ui had shown that citizens, from Minamata or from far away, could be active on behalf of Minamata disease victims. His book of July 1968 and Ishimure's of January 1969 were widely read and inspired others to follow.

COMPANY AND ECONOMY

In the early and mid-1960s, the weakening of Shin Nitchitsu and the bitter splits within both the union and much of the city removed some of the constraints on those in Minamata who might wish to join Ishimure and Akasaki in activism. The company reached its postwar high point around 1960. Shin Nitchitsu's market share for octanol was 64 percent in 1961, and it held 26 percent of the market for acetic acid, 25 percent for ethyl acetate, and 9 percent for vinyl chloride. The city, whose fortunes always reflected those of the company, had a budget surplus that year for the fifth year in a row.[27]

But the company's postwar success was built on a rapidly aging foundation. Nitchitsu had been a pioneer in what John Dower calls Japan's "second industrial revolution" before and during the war.[28] By the beginning of the 1960s, however, Shin Nitchitsu was already being left behind by Japan's third industrial transformation, the move to petrochemicals, automobiles, and electronics. Shin Nitchitsu had been downsizing and rationalizing its Minamata factory since the early 1950s. The plant had nearly 5,000 employees in 1950, under 4,000 in 1960, and under 2,000 in 1970.[29] The company moved into petrochemicals (which MITI had suggested back in 1955) later than some of its competitors, and never again was it at the forefront of technological development in the chemical industry. When it did build a petrochemical plant, it did so at Goi in Chiba prefecture, near Tokyo, where it began producing polypropylene in 1963 and acetaldehyde in 1964. In September 1964 the new plant produced acetaldehyde at a cost of ¥43,365 per ton; the comparable cost in Minamata was ¥48,987.[30] Workers and other Minamata residents feared the company was at least partly abandoning the city.

The Goi plant was run by a separate company, Chisso sekiyu kagaku (Chisso petrochemical), which was established in order to improve labor relations in the new factory. A 1965 company publication about the building of the Goi factory contains a remarkable explanation:

In reflecting on our operations in light of the Minamata disease incident, we considered it most important to reconsider our company's basic way of thinking about local society, in particular our colonialistic attitude. The Nihon chisso Minamata factory had been there over 40 years since 1907. But the colonialistic conditions had continued without the slightest change. The factory was capital with no connection to the locality. Concerning labor, too, distinctions between *shain* and *kōin* had persisted until very late. This was a relationship typical of Japan's dual structure, with local areas dependent on low-productivity agriculture, and industry requiring a high level of technology. At Goi we made it a major policy to build on such self-reflection and aim at harmony.[31]

In 1962, while the Goi plant was under construction, Shin Nitchitsu broke with its tradition of promoting engineers to top management positions by bringing in Egashira Yutaka from the Industrial Bank of Japan to serve as managing director and help the company through difficult times.[32] Egashira replaced Yoshioka Kiichi as president in December 1964, and on January 1, 1965, Shin Nihon chisso Hiryō K.K. changed its name to Chisso K.K. The renamed company sped up the reduction of the labor force at the Minamata plant, whose carbide-based processes were losing competitiveness compared with those at the Goi plant. The five-year plan announced in August 1967 called for the elimination of 1,500 jobs in Minamata, leaving only 1,200. From 1968 to 1971 the Minamata plant ceased production of acetaldehyde, octanol, dioctyl phthalate (a plasticizer for vinyl chloride), ammonia, acetic acid, nitric acid, and calcium carbide.[33] These circumstances made the company and its civic supporters more fearful of anything that might increase Chisso's burden in paying compensation for Minamata disease. They also made it possible for the company to play on these fears by threatening to cut its operations in Minamata even further, or pull out completely, whenever there were suggestions that it should be forced to pay more compensation.

These changes and the divisions caused by a strike and lockout from 1962 to 1963 narrowed the company's base of support in Minamata but increased the determination of its local partisans. At the same time these changes led others, including some workers, to begin to see themselves as being harmed by the company rather than benefiting from it and to sympathize with Minamata disease patients as fellow victims.

The strike was a response to management plans to reduce labor strife and financial uncertainty, and in particular to eliminate the annual "spring labor offensive," as the Minamata work force was reduced and the Goi plant came on line. Like the 1953 strike against the division of workers into *shain* and *kōin*, the 1962–63 strike in Minamata mirrored what unions had attempted elsewhere, especially at Mitsui's Miike coal mines in Ōmuta to the north.

The 313-day Miike strike and lockout that ended on November 1, 1960, is described by Andrew Gordon as "a turning point in postwar history," the decisive defeat of the attempts in the 1950s to create a more democratic, worker-dominated "workplace culture."[34] In both Miike and Minamata, the workers were responding to rationalization and downsizing in industries suffering from the shift from other resources to petroleum. In both cases, management was attempting to change the wage structure and weaken the union and had the backing of industry and government. Both unions fought hard and often violently, with significant outside support. In Miike much of this support came from the Sōhyō union federation and the anti–Security Treaty movement (the treaty was signed in Washington on July 1, 1960); the Minamata strikers were assisted by the General Council of Trade Unions of Japan (Sōhyō) and veterans of the Miike struggle. Both at Miike and at Minamata, management outlasted the strikers, formed a "second union" more willing to cooperate, and won a total victory.[35] Kawamoto Teruo had begun working at the Minamata factory in January 1962, and the very next month the union began its spring labor offensive with a demand for a pay increase of 10 percent, or an average of ¥2,375 ($6.60) per month.[36] Beginning monthly salaries would be ¥12,500 ($35) for middle school graduates, ¥15,000 ($42) for graduates of the company's technical school, ¥16,000 ($44) for high school graduates, and ¥25,000 ($69) for university graduates. Layoffs, the union demanded, should be prohibited, and transfers of union members should not be carried out without prior consultation. The union staged short strikes in March and April.

The company responded on April 17 with an offer of a "stable wage system" (*antei chingin seido*), which would guarantee wages through 1965 in return for a "peace agreement," a promise by the union to accept the company's rationalization plans and not to strike.[37] The pay level for 1962 would be ¥500 ($1.39) per month less than the average for the six major chemical companies. This would mean ¥11,000 ($31) for company technical school graduates and female high school graduates, ¥12,000 ($35) for male high

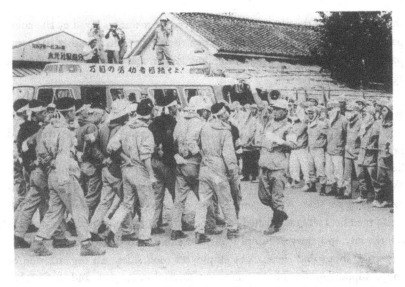

Fig. 17 The "Stable Wage Struggle" strike that split the union and the city in 1962–63. Strikers from the original union are attempting to prevent members of the new, second union from entering the factory to work. The sign on the truck reads "Workers of the world, unite!" Photograph courtesy of Chisso rōdō kumiai.

school graduates, and ¥19,000 ($53) for university graduates. Monthly pay would then be increased by ¥500 in 1963, by ¥1,000 ($2.78) in 1964, and again by ¥1,000 in 1965.

The union, unwilling to give up its only weapon against rationalization of the workforce, continued its intermittent strikes. More than the immediate question of pay for the fiscal year beginning in April 1962, the key issue for most workers was how to retain some bargaining power to protect themselves as the factory rationalized further. The company announced a total lockout on July 23, and the union declared an unlimited strike. A "new union" of about 350 workers was formed the next day.

Kawamoto Teruo fell between the cracks widening in the company and its city. He was classified as a temporary worker, not eligible for membership in or support from either union. Unable to support his family on unemployment insurance, he was paid ¥500 ($1.39) per day by the No. 1 (antimanagement) union to help with the picketing. Kawamoto approached members of the No. 2 union as they left the factory, telling them how poorly management had treated the fishers seeking compensation, but it turned out that a number of the former fishing cooperative members hired by the company had joined the No. 2 union. When the strike ended, neither the company nor the union had need of him any longer, and he found himself once again without a job.[38]

The strike lasted through the fall and most of the winter. There was a great deal of violence at the factory gates, at the tunnel connecting the factory with its private port at Umedo, and at company housing. A thousand prefectural policemen—over half of the total in Kumamoto—were mobilized, and labor organizers arrived in droves from the Miike mines. Women's groups and students, even those in elementary school, were mobilized by each side. A Minamata Farmers' Association (Nōminkai) with 2,504 members was established to support the strikers. As the strike dragged on, the city and every group in it divided along with the workers. Even the city's 672 shops and their 2,484 employees took sides. An organization of shops supporting the No. 2 union was formed in August, and in October the No. 1 union began a boycott of these shops.[39]

In the broadest sense, the struggle between the No. 1 union and management was viewed as one of labor in general versus capital in general, in the form of the Japanese Federation of Synthetic Chemistry Workers Unions (Gōka rōren) and the General Council of Trade Unions of Japan versus the Japan Chemical Industry Association and the Japan Federation of Employers' Associations (Nikkeiren). When the No. 1 union finally voted to give up on January 13, 1963, the company was victorious. Wages would be higher than the levels the company had offered in April 1962, but the company had clearly won: it had created a second union and would be able to carry out its rationalization plan.[40] The workers were called back to their jobs in stages beginning February 1, but the splits in the community never completely healed. Minamata was not a big enough town to allow anonymity. Everyone knew which side their neighbors had taken—and they never forgot.

Onitsuka Iwao, who was an active union member and used his still and eight-millimeter movie cameras to document the strike, remembers the "leaflet wars" during the strike. Flyers were put out by the company, the unions, and other groups and distributed by hand, as newspaper inserts, and even dropped from airplanes by the No. 2 union. One from the new union read: "The Minamata factory has resumed production, starting with carbide. Members of the old union, you are being deceived by Gōka rōren and Sōhyō. Don't delay, get on board the 'S.S. Stable Wages' before it's too late."[41] The new, company-supported Minamata City League for Peace (Minamata-shi heiwa dōmei) tried to drive a wedge between the organizers from Miike and the strikers: "Are you sure there are none among you willing to see the company fail? . . . As long as it is possible to damage the city of Minamata further, their work will continue. They are dogs come from outside to destroy our paradise."[42] Similar attacks on outside agitators and on domination by the General Council of Trade Unions were made by a group called the Association to Protect Minamata (Minamata o mamoru kai), backed by the city government.[43] This tarring of the No. 1 union with the brush of association with radicals from outside, bent on destroying the company and the city, seriously weakened the strikers.

The most interesting group to appear during the strike, and the most important in the long term because of the way the seeds it sowed blossomed five years later, was the Minamata Cultural Collective (Minamata bunka shūdan).[44] The group included Ishimure Michiko, Akasaki Satoru, and Matsumoto Tsutomu, a friend of Akasaki's from city hall. These three people, along with Ishimure Hiroshi and Hiyoshi Fumiko, became the founders and core of the Citizens' Council for Minamata Disease Countermeasures in January 1968. The attacks by the Cultural Collective on "Minamata nationalism" (to use Kikuchi Masanori's term), which branded supporters from the outside as enemies of the city, were often repeated in the second round of responses to Minamata disease, which saw its own "leaflet wars."

The Minamata Cultural Collective's other main contribution was to link the labor struggle with the Minamata disease issue for the first time and to suggest an alliance between the union and the patients. They asked in one flyer who was really destroying the city: "As can be readily seen from the example of Minamata disease, the company does not think twice about doing things that bring harm to the citizens and does absolutely nothing to improve the welfare of the citizens. Driving the workers hard for low wages, squeezing all that can be squeezed out of Minamata—that's how the company operates."[45] Another pamphlet, supposedly the words of "an unemployed woman," was written in heavy Minamata dialect and compared the use of the police against fishers in 1959 and against the strikers in 1962, using the word *citizens* to refer to both groups: "What have the citizens ever done wrong? The police were like that when the issue was Minamata disease, too. They only went after the fishers. They didn't investigate the company that killed 89 people. They say the fishers were violent. Who are the real violent ones? The company committed murder."[46]

The new union at Shin Nitchitsu remained smaller than the No. 1 union for longer than at many other companies. This was despite great pressure put on strikers who refused to join the new union after they went back to work. They were called back to work in eleven stages from February 1 to March 9, 1963. Of the 2,368 strikers who returned, only 594 were sent back to their own jobs. The remaining 1,774 were transferred to other work.[47] In part, this was because management used the opportunity to carry out its planned restructuring, but the fact that 75 percent of the returning workers were assigned to new jobs is also evidence that management was putting pressure on those who refused to go over to the company union.

Onitsuka Iwao went back to the factory on February 21 and soon was called to what the workers referred to as the "persuasion chamber," a tiny room where managers attempted to coerce them into joining the new union.[48] He had already been told what to expect:

They would start by asking something like "What do you think of the No. 1 union and the new union now?" Then they'd ask about your past record, your brothers and family and children, their advancement in school, your neighbors, even relatives you couldn't remember. . . .

They'd say "We have a record here of mistakes you've made. . . . If you come over to the new union, we'll make sure this record is kept here and not shown to anyone, but if you can't do that. . . ."

They'd be forceful like this, and then use the soft touch: "In the company, it wasn't like this before the strike; everyone got along well. What we're telling you now, we're doing because we're thinking of your own good. If you tough it out and stick with the old union, we don't know where you'll end up. You'll have no future, and may just end up hanging yourself. Now if you could come over to the new union instead. . . ."[49]

Some people were kept in the persuasion chamber for a whole day, but Onitsuka found a way to shorten the unpleasant experience. The second time he was called in, he refused to say a word, and was excused after just ten minutes.

When the No. 1 union agreed to end its strike, the company promised not to discriminate against its members in any way. After the strike, however, the new foremen were almost all No. 2 union members, and many vet-

erans who refused to switch to the new union were assigned to the most unpleasant and menial tasks or moved to the night shift.[50] Onitsuka, a twenty-
year employee, was made to clean ditches, pick weeds, and clean toilets,
storerooms, and windows. He resisted by working slowly, sometimes clean-
ing only two or three panes of glass in a day.[51] Another worker recalled being
ordered to move a pile of ashes removed from a boiler back and forth.[52] Such
discriminatory treatment and the suggestions made by the Minamata Cultural Collective in its flyers prompted some of the defeated strikers to begin
for the first time to sympathize with Minamata disease patients as fellow
victims.

The pressure on No. 1 union members and the thinning of their ranks
through transfers and retirements meant the new union approached the old
in membership within a year, but for some years thereafter there was little
change in their relative sizes. When the strike ended, the old union still had
2,471 members to the No. 2 union's 992, but by the end of the year the numbers were 1,655 and 1,522, respectively. Only 62 more workers switched from
the No. 1 union to the No. 2 union from 1964 through 1968, although far
more members of the old union than the new accepted "voluntary" early retirement. By 1976, only 28 percent of the 1,473 employees were No. 1 union
members, and when Onitsuka Iwao retired in 1983, twenty years after the
strike ended, 79 percent of the factory's 830 employees were members of the
No. 2 union.[53] Still, the No. 1 union had retained more members than those
of many other companies, and its losses were due not only to defections but
also to transferring of far more of its members than members of the No. 2
union away from Minamata.

Expressions of resentment against Shin Nitchitsu became more common
from around the time of the strike. Just before the strike began, the company
secretly asked leading figures in the city to make public comments in its support, but Fuke Masaki, who headed the doctors' association (and who served
four terms as mayor beginning in 1970), remarked: "It seems that Chisso
thinks of Minamata as its colony, and it is painful for the citizens to see the
way the managers swagger."[54] During and after the strike, the popularity of
the story of one man who had fought against the domination of Minamata
by Noguchi Shitagau and his company reflected this new interest in resistance to the company. The story was told and retold as a myth and morality
tale. It was written down and published in the union journal *Gōka* in 1972 by

Okamoto Tatsuaki, who for a time headed the No. 1 union. Irokawa Daikichi heard the story from several old women who served as his informants
on Minamata history.[55]

Ogata Korenori, born around 1871 and better known as "Hiranoya no
danna" (the master of the Hiranoya), was the second biggest landlord in
Minamata and boasted that he could walk on his own land all the way from
the harbor to Yunotsuru hot spring, a distance of two *ri* (7.86 km). The
story tells of his fall from the pinnacle of Minamata society, at the time Noguchi built his factory in 1908, to 1946, when he starved to death in a chicken
coop in the hills. In 1909, Ogata's income of ¥2,160 ($1,070) was the sixth
largest in Minamata. In the coming decades, he used all his strength and all
his assets in a futile fight to prevent Nitchitsu from taking economic control
of the town away from the traditional elite.

Ogata attempted to prevent the people who worked his land, many of
whom were still called *nago* (landless peasants at the bottom of the Tokugawa rural social scale who were virtually serfs), from taking jobs at the factory. He built an observation platform on a hill and called down to workers
he knew who were on their way to the factory, offering to pay them more
than Noguchi if they would work for him. He operated a movie theater, a
fancy restaurant, and several pawnshops and sponsored circus performances
and *sumō* tournaments. He established a bank that soon failed and experimented with new crops. He slowly lost his fields and woodlots and even had
a large plot near the harbor repossessed. Nitchitsu bought that piece of land
and used it for the acetaldehyde plant that caused Minamata disease.

Ogata squandered more money building homes for mistresses and paraded around town in a black-lacquered horse-drawn carriage modeled after
the emperor's. His children grew up and left, and he was cared for as he aged
by his lover, a faithful *nago* named Otoku. With Otoku he had a daughter,
who later went mad and drowned herself in the Minamata River. He and
Otoku moved to Otashiro in the hills behind the city and started making
and selling *tōfu*, but they could only take in 45 sen per day. They were unable
to pay their rent, and their landlord removed the roof to force them out.
Ogata, the story goes, sat calmly in the bathtub in the rain, holding an umbrella over his head. Around the start of the Pacific War, he moved into a
chicken coop in Yunoko on land owned, ironically, by Maeda Eiki, who had
led the successful drive to convince Noguchi to build his factory in Mina-

mata. Otoku brought him food from time to time, and then a woman named Yamanouchi Naso did the same. She found him there one rainy night in 1946, starved to death. He had outlived Noguchi Shitagau by two years.

Changes in Japan

The changes in Minamata in the years after 1959 gave more and more people reason and opportunity to support a renegotiation of the 1959 settlement. Changes that occurred in Japan as a whole over the same years suggested new patterns of organization and action and built a small but significant nationwide constituency of potential supporters. In other words, these changes made possible entirely new levels of citizen participation in Japan's democracy in the decade after 1959. To begin with, the very economic growth that caused Japan's pollution problems gave the nation the financial security and ability to pay the costs of that growth.

ECONOMIC GROWTH

Japan's per capita GNP was ¥105,000 ($292) in 1956, when Minamata disease was discovered. It reached ¥205,000 ($569) five years later, ¥385,000 ($1,069) in 1966, ¥763,000 ($2,184) in 1971, and ¥1,476,000 ($4,978) in 1976. In 1958, around 30 percent of nonfarm urban households had washing machines, 15 percent had televisions, and 5 percent had refrigerators; by 1970 each of these appliances could be found in over 90 percent of all households.[56] In the context of this kind of change, the sympathy payments to recognized victims, low enough to begin with, became scandalous. The annual payments were raised in 1968—when Japan's GNP passed West Germany's to become second largest in what was still called the "free world"—to just ¥140,000 ($389) for adults and ¥75,000 ($208) for children. Because of Japan's rapid economic growth, even after these increases, the annual payments were still far *smaller* in real terms than they had been in 1959: for adults, 27 percent of per capita annual GNP in 1968 as opposed to 70 percent in 1959, and for children, 14 percent as opposed to 20 percent.[57] It is not surprising that "we can do better" arguments began to carry more weight in a newly wealthy Japan.

Japan's "miracle growth" brought with it improvements in transportation and communication, such as faster rail travel and the spread of television, that brought Minamata closer to the rest of the country. By the mid-1960s, nearly all families in Japan had a black-and-white television. Within a few years activists learned how to use this medium, and the television networks became willing to regularly bring the disease into people's homes. Also, more people had the money and time to travel to Minamata, and the books by Ishimure Michiko, Ui Jun, and Kuwabara Shisei would soon inspire a few to do so.

As important as the increase in Japan's overall income was the equality of income distribution. By around 1970, according to Margaret McKean, Japan was at or near the top of major industrial democracies in terms of economic equality. The after-tax income of the richest 20 percent of the population was 5.19 times that of the poorest 20 percent, a slightly more equitable distribution than in Sweden and Norway and far better than the 9.53 ratio in the United States. This meant that protest by the established left had to be ideologically oriented, since distribution was not an issue.[58] The demands for compensation for Minamata disease victims were therefore less frightening than they might have been, because they were not linked to broader demands for systemic changes or class conflict over the distribution of wealth. And McKean finds that inequality peaked in the postwar period between 1959 and 1962, the period in which the first round of responses to Minamata ended, and that equality increased thereafter until 1974, just after the second, and very different, "resolution" of the Minamata issue.[59]

In some ways, however, despite Japan's increased equality of income distribution overall, high growth widened the already broad gap between Minamata and Japan's major urban centers. Patients and fishers, of course, were left behind as high growth more than doubled incomes in the 1960s, even accounting for inflation, and created a mass consumption society. By no means were they a part of the "new middle mass" described by Murakami Yasusuke, a society in which everyone was expected to consider him- or herself a part of a homogeneous middle class.[60] Chisso employees in Minamata saw their factory steadily shrink. No longer was it the hub of an international industrial empire, as it had been until 1945. Now it was on the periphery. More and more of Japan's industrial growth came from new factories such as Chisso's Goi plant, in an industrial belt along the Pacific coast from Tokyo Bay to northern Kyūshū.

Yet the widening gap between Minamata and Japan's advanced urban centers did, in time, give Minamata and more traditional lifestyles a new attraction. In the mid-1950s, fishing families were seen as poor, dirty, and backward reminders of a way of life most Japanese were anxious to escape. By the 1970s, big city–dwellers were another generation removed from their rural roots, aware of the dark side of industrial growth, and beginning to feel pangs of nostalgia for the simpler times and places of their real or imagined pasts. This new nostalgia was the occasion for the Japan National Railways' "Discover Japan" advertising campaign and led to a *furusato būmu* (old hometown boom).[61]

CITIZEN AND STATE

Another change in Japan as a whole that had decisive implications for Minamata was the rise of a new stream of leftist opposition, the citizens' movement of progressive groups and individuals who were politically active but kept the established parties at arm's length. The Left had come to prominence in the protests against the renewal of the U.S.-Japan security treaty in 1960. The huge strikes and demonstrations in May and June of that year, many of which turned violent, involved not only organized labor and the Socialists, but students, intellectuals, and literally hundreds of thousands of people who had never expressed themselves politically outside a voting booth. Prime Minister Kishi was forced to step down after the treaty was extended, and Ikeda Hayato, the minister of international trade and industry who had argued forcefully that the Minamata dispute needed to be contained, took his place. As prime minister, Ikeda instituted his famous plan to double income within a decade, hoping thereby to turn the nation's energies and attention in a less divisive direction.

But the Left did not disappear after 1960. In bringing together the Marxist and non-Marxist opposition and sparking so many people to engage in political activism for the first time, the Security Treaty protests created new possibilities for mobilization on other issues. In addition to the existing Communist and Socialist parties, two new streams developed: the New Left and the citizens' movement. The New Left and its student sects took over the struggle against the construction of the New Tokyo International Airport and alienated most Japanese with their violence and radical ideology.[62]

The other new stream on the left, the citizens' movement, had two branches. The issue around which one of these coalesced was the Vietnam

War. Left-wing intellectuals led by the writer Oda Makoto formed the League for Peace in Vietnam (Beheiren) in 1965.[63] The league made an important contribution with its focus on a single issue and its organizational philosophy. Oda and the members of the league opposed hierarchy and control and were fearful that even "democratic" organizations could be inflexible, overmanaged, and coercive. Consequently the league had no real headquarters and remained apart from established institutions of the Left. Any concerned citizens, anywhere, could form a group and call it a local branch of the League for Peace in Vietnam. They demonstrated, conducted sit-ins and teach-ins, published pamphlets and newsletters, helped deserters from U.S. bases in Japan, solicited contributions, and established a loose network of communication among groups nationwide that served as a model and provided members for other citizens' groups, including those supporting Minamata disease patients.

Another branch of the citizens' movement consisted of local groups concerned with environmental issues.[64] The best-known example is the movement by citizens in the Mishima-Numazu area, which in 1964 successfully prevented the construction of a petrochemical complex.[65] This was, however, a before-the-fact, preventive movement, whose members tended to be on higher rungs socially and economically and often already more politicized than those who were seeking compensation for pollution diseases in places such as Minamata. It was the other pollution diseases—and most particularly the Niigata Minamata disease—that did the most to spur activity in Minamata in the late 1960s.

OTHER POLLUTION CASES

Responses to other major pollution cases that appeared in postwar Japan were far more instructive to those in Minamata than the Mishima-Numazu case. The "Big Four" were the organic mercury poisoning in Minamata, air pollution in Yokkaichi city, cadmium poisoning in Toyama prefecture, and the "second Minamata disease" in Niigata prefecture north of Tokyo (see Table 6). The Minamata victims were the last to file a lawsuit. Despite the changes in Minamata and Japan during the 1960s, Minamata disease and its victims might well have remained mostly unheard and forgotten without the catalyzing effect of the Niigata outbreak.

Table 6
Japan's "Big Four" Pollution Cases

Name	Disease	Suit filed.	Court decision
Toyama Itai-Itai (ouch-ouch) disease	cadmium poisoning	Mar. 9, 1968	June 30, 1971
Niigata Minamata disease	mercury poisoning	June 12, 1967	Sept. 29, 1971
Yokkaichi air pollution	asthma	Sept. 1, 1967	July 24, 1972
Kumamoto Minamata disease	mercury poisoning	June 14, 1969	Mar. 20, 1973

A petrochemical complex was built at Yokkaichi on Ise Bay in 1959, and the sulfur oxides and other pollutants in its smoke soon began causing severe respiratory problems. Victims filed suit in September 1967 and, to the surprise of some legal experts who believed it would be impossible to prove causation and corporate negligence, won their case in July 1972. In Toyama, cadmium in waste from Mitsui's Kamioka mine on the Jinzū River caused people's bones—especially those of women—to become painfully brittle. Villagers there sued in March 1968 and won in June 1971.

Niigata Minamata disease was caused by a factory owned by Shōwa denkō at Kanose on the Agano River, which used a similar process to make acetaldehyde and discharged the same type of organic mercury as Shin Nitchitsu in Minamata.[66] The difference in Niigata was that most of those who caught and ate the fish that caused the disease lived downstream in areas that had no ties to the factory, unlike the residents of Minamata, Chisso's "castle town." A few scientists (including Ui Jun), doctors (including Hosokawa Hajime and Harada Masazumi), activists from the New Left and the citizens' movement, and lawyers associated with the JCP rushed to Niigata after the disease was discovered in June 1965, partly out of shame at having done so little for Minamata. They quickly confirmed what was happening, helping to limit the damage, and set up a support network for the victims, who sued the company in June 1967 and won in September 1971. With Ui Jun as go-between, a delegation of patients from Niigata visited Minamata in January 1968 and sparked the beginning of the second round of responses to the disease in Minamata.

PART IV

The Second Round of Responses, 1968–1973

SEVEN

Bringing the Issue to the Nation

In 1968 the Minamata victims began to find that they were no longer alone and ignored. Patients of pollution diseases elsewhere in Japan, a few fellow citizens in Minamata, and concerned people in Kumamoto and throughout the nation began to show an interest in their plight. The victims had never stopped speaking up, even in the supposed "years of silence," but beginning in 1968 they and their new network of supporters found ways to reach a new, and newly receptive, national audience. A small but critical mass of support was achieved rapidly, and the resulting reaction replaced the already substantially undermined 1959 settlement with another "solution" that was far more fair and comprehensive, although still less than complete, in 1973.[1]

1968

The moment that marked the beginning of this new and ultimately decisive round of responses to Minamata disease was the creation on January 12, 1968, of the Citizens' Council for Minamata Disease Countermeasures (often called the Shimin kaigi).[2] The immediate reason for the establishment of the Citizens' Council was the need for an organization to host the upcoming visit, facilitated by Ui Jun, by patients of Niigata Minamata disease, who had filed suit against Shōwa denkō on June 12, 1967, and some of their lawyers and supporters.[3]

The Citizen's Council did not appear as suddenly as it might seem, however. Ishimure Michiko and Akasaki Satoru had been in close contact with patients for years, and Ishimure, through her contacts with Ui Jun, was well aware of the way victims and supporters were organizing in Niigata. Matsumoto Tsutomu, who with Ishimure and Akasaki had been a member of the Minamata Cultural Collective during the strike at Chisso, had been corresponding with the victims' group and lawyers in Niigata, with lawyers in Kumamoto, and with victims in Minamata regarding possibilities for organizing and suing in Minamata.[4] Matsumoto had also asked Yamashita Yoshihiro (better known by an alternative reading of his given name, Zenkan), who worked in Chisso's laboratory and was a member and later head of the No. 1 union, to give Niigata researchers information about Minamata disease, and Yamashita had done so secretly.[5]

The core members of the new Citizens' Council were Ishimure Michiko, Matsumoto Tsutomu, Akasaki Satoru, and the chairperson, Hiyoshi Fumiko. Hiyoshi, a City Council member and former teacher, was already well known as an advocate for education and for Minamata disease patients. Ishimure and Matsumoto decided she would be the most appropriate leader for the new group.[6] In addition to being widely known in the city, she had political experience, was an able speaker, and was firmly committed to the cause. Matsumoto was chosen to be the secretary.

Interestingly, with Hiyoshi and Ishimure as two of its most important leaders, the Citizen's Council does not fit the pattern of the citizens' groups described in a study by Margaret McKean, who found no women leaders except in women-only groups.[7] The explanation for the leadership roles of women in Minamata (although not in the patients' Mutual Aid Society, whose official leaders and negotiators were always men) is not mainly that the circumstances or culture were different in Minamata. (McKean's groups were mostly prevention-oriented urban groups in the Tokyo area.) These were simply remarkable women, working with unusual men such as Akasaki and Matsumoto who were sensible enough to recognize and accept Ishimure's and Hiyoshi's abilities. But it was still the women who served tea.

Among the Citizens' Council members were several Chisso employees from the No. 1 union, including Onitsuka Iwao and Yamashita Yoshihiro. The council eventually formed subcommittees for research (to support negotiations and later the trial), support of patients, publicity, and fundraising; it also issued a newsletter.

The Citizens' Council's goals and rules were brief:

Objectives

1. To carry out activities to make the government confirm the cause of Minamata disease and to prevent a third and fourth outbreak of Minamata disease.

2. To demand relief measures for patients and their families, and to support them both materially and spiritually.

Council Regulations

1. We shall work to realize the Council's goals of protecting life and truth.

2. The membership fee shall be ¥30 [$0.08] per month, and activities shall be funded by seeking donations as necessary.

3. The management of the council, concerning violations of council rules and other matters, shall be decided democratically by the executive committee.[8]

Cooperation and trust from the patients did not come quickly or easily. One of the speakers at the founding meeting was Nakatsu Miyoshi, who chaired the patients' Mutual Aid Society and expressed their lingering bitterness and suspicion: "If you had set up your association and joined hands with us at least ten years ago, you could perhaps have saved many lives and spared us a lot of suffering."[9]

Ishimure, who was present at, and instrumental in, the creation of the most important support organizations for the patients and at virtually all the most significant and dramatic events in the entire history of the Minamata disease incident, describes her own role in the meeting: "Like a *kuroko* in a Kabuki drama [the actors' assistants, dressed in black and intended not to be noticed], I tried my best to remain invisible and inaudible."[10] This comment is an example of how the dominant groups in the Minamata disease support movement, who also became the tellers of the dominant narratives of the movement, consciously attempted to play down the roles of individual leaders, especially those who were not patients. As Ishimure's fame grew, especially with the publication of her book about Minamata the next year, she worked increasingly hard to stay out of the spotlight. She had observed the strikes at Miike and in Minamata and disliked what she considered the unions' high profile, autocratic leadership.[11]

The visitors from Niigata—six patients from the Niigata Organic Mercury Poisoning Victims' Association (Niigata yūki suigin chūdoku higaisha no kai; later the Niigata Minamata Disease Victims' Association [Niigata Minamatabyō higaisha no kai]), a documentary film crew, members of the Niigata Prefecture Council of Democratic Groups for Minamata Disease Countermeasures (Niigata-ken minshu dantai Minamatabyō taisaku kaigi; usually abbreviated Minsuitai)—arrived with Ui Jun on a snowy Sunday, January 21, 1968. The Minamata and Niigata groups had been corresponding for several months.[12] The visit was historic, as was the presence at the station to meet them of not only Minamata patients and the Citizens' Council but also a delegation and bus from the factory's No. 1 union. Looking ahead, says Ishimure, they were "conscious of our part in the prologue of a drama." Ishimure very intentionally places them in the context of past struggles and national issues as they marched from the station to the factory:

Since the mid-1950s many a public demonstration and mass rally had walked down the road we were now passing: the demonstrations for the reversion of Okinawa, the demonstration against A- and H-bombs, the demonstration against the amendment of the Police Law, the anti-Japan-U.S. Security Treaty demonstration, the demonstrations of the Minamata Fishermen's Union and the Minamata Fish Retailers' Union, the lonely, ghost-like processions of the Minamata disease patients, the large-scale demonstration of the Shiranui fishermen in November 1959, the demonstrations of the Chisso worker's union against the company's wage stabilization plan and, after the splitting of the union, the separate demonstrations of the First and Second Union.[13]

On January 24 the four groups—one patients' group and one support group from each prefecture—issued a joint statement:

We realized that the Kumamoto and Niigata incidents are one....

We demand that the government clearly recognize the scientists' conclusions [about the cause of the disease] and take responsibility for solving the issue, and that it take concrete steps with the prefectures and cities to provide living support for the victims....

As we citizens of Minamata and Niigata firmly clasped hands in our three days of exchanges, we understood that the only path to the elimination of industrial pollution is for the people of polluted areas to unite and fight together.

People of the nation, let us fight together to protect lives, health, and livelihood.[14]

A month after their Minamata visit, members of the Niigata Victims' Association visited asthma patients in the city of Yokkaichi, who had sued the companies in the neighboring petrochemical complex in September 1967. On March 9, 1968, 28 patients and relatives in Toyama prefecture sued Mitsui Mining for ¥61 million ($169,400) in compensation for the *itai-itai* disease. Among the Big Four pollution cases, only the Minamata patients had yet to sue. Thanks partly to Matsumoto Tsutomu's lobbying, there was strong support for suing among members of the Citizens' Council, but relations with the patients' Mutual Aid Society were still delicate. On March 16, the two groups jointly petitioned the prefectural assembly to exempt the solatium payments under the 1959 agreement from income limits for welfare recipients, to help patients find work, and to set up special classes for children hospitalized with Minamata disease. Ten days later the two groups joined the Victims' Association from Niigata in asking the government to issue its expected conclusions regarding the causes of Minamata disease in Minamata and Niigata simultaneously. With these petitions, in the first months of 1968, patients in Minamata were cooperating for the first time with other citizens and with pollution disease groups from another part of Japan.

The legal challenge to Shōwa denkō in Niigata was less difficult than a suit against Chisso would be. Although the Niigata case was filed first, the plaintiffs there had only to prove that the company had illegally caused a tragedy similar to one that had already happened elsewhere—in Minamata. Even so, the fight in and out of court against Shōwa denkō did not go smoothly. The company borrowed pages from Chisso's playbook, issuing pamphlets disputing the argument that organic mercury in its waste caused the disease. One of its theories was that the disease was caused by pesticides that had spilled into the river during the magnitude 7.5 earthquake in Niigata on June 16, 1964.

In May 1968, the patients' Mutual Aid Society in Minamata voted not to sue, while in Niigata a second suit was filed against Shōwa denkō in July by 21 more people in sixteen families, demanding over ¥40 million ($111,000). Chisso made its Minamata factory a subsidiary in June, with a president ranking above the factory manager, and rewarded the patients for not suing by giving them a "special solatium" of ¥3,000 ($8.33) and packages of sugar in August.

Pressure was building in many ways, however. In May a National Alliance for Pollution Countermeasures (Kōgai taisaku zenkoku renraku kyōgikai) was established, with the Niigata groups as its core members. On July 13 the Agano River Research Group (Aganogawa kenkyūkai) was formed. A week later, one of its leading members, Ui Jun, published his book on Minamata disease, *Kōgai no seijigaku: Minamatabyō o otte.* Ui's book was a harsh indictment of Chisso, the national, prefectural, and local governments, and the capitalist system that sacrificed fishing families for power, profits, and growth. Four years earlier, Shōji Hikaru and Miyamoto Ken'ichi's *Osoru beki kōgai* (Fearful pollution) had begun to awaken Japanese to the destruction of their environment in much the same way that Rachel Carson's *Silent Spring* had in the United States in 1962.[15] Now, Ui laid blame squarely on Chisso and the government, and issued a call for action.

On August 27, 1968, the All-Japan Prefectural and Municipal Workers' Union (Zen Nihon jichi dantai rōdō kumiai; commonly known as Jichirō), met in Kumamoto and voted to support the Minamata disease patients, and on September 5 the board of education for the Minamata region did the same thing. On August 30 the Kumamoto public prosecutor conducted a brief and inconclusive (but undoubtedly disturbing to Chisso) investigation of the legality of the December 30, 1959, solatium agreement. On August 29, the No. 1 union halted the company's attempt to export 100 tons of mercury-laden waste to South Korea.

On August 30, the No. 1 union made Japanese labor history by issuing its famous "declaration of shame" (*haji sengen*):

Minamata disease has killed dozens of people and disabled dozens of living people; it has disfigured dozens of innocent children at birth. It was said from the start that the cause of Minamata disease was Chisso's factory waste, and this is now common knowledge not only among the citizens but throughout Japan.

What sort of fight have we fought against this Minamata disease? We were not able to fight at all.

For some six years since the wage stabilization struggle, we have fought tenaciously against the company's attacks on workers.

That experience has taught us that the struggle is not only within the company and that it must be fought together with the workers of the whole nation and together with the citizens, as well as that at the same time the struggle is a burden we must bear on our own shoulders.

Why were we unable to fight against Minamata disease? That we, who know from our own experience what struggle means, have been unable until now to fight against Minamata disease, is truly shameful to us as human beings and as workers, and we must reflect on this from the bottom of our hearts.

The company's actions toward workers are exactly the same as its actions regarding Minamata disease, and the fight against Minamata disease is also our fight.

Even today, the company refuses to recognize that the cause of Minamata disease is the factory's waste, and it hides all its documents. We resolve to devote all our energy to making the company admit responsibility for Minamata disease, to support the victims of Minamata disease, who even today are in the depths of suffering, and to fight against Minamata disease.[16]

This declaration, like the creation of the Citizens' Council, was less sudden and unexpected than it might seem. As explained in the previous chapter, the company's treatment of No. 1 union members after the 1962–63 wage stabilization struggle had led some of them to sympathize with Minamata disease patients. A number of union members, including Onitsuka Iwao, had joined the Citizen's Council, and the No. 1 union had greeted the Niigata visitors at the station in January and provided a bus for them. Still, the declaration was dramatic and unprecedented. An equally hard blow to the company was an *Asahi shinbun* article on August 27 that revealed Hosokawa Hajime's secret experiment with "cat no. 400," which had proved in October 1959 that the factory's acetaldehyde waste caused Minamata disease.[17]

It seemed likely from early 1968 that the government would finally issue an official conclusion regarding the causes of Minamata and Niigata Minamata disease, nearly nine years after quashing the report of the Ministry of Health and Welfare research group in November 1959. It was no coincidence, but rather evidence of MITI's success in stalling, that no such announcement was made until after Chisso had stopped producing acetaldehyde in Minamata (becoming on May 18, 1968, one of the last two factories in Japan to give up the carbide-acetylene process and switch to petroleum-based acetaldehyde production). For the same reason, the Water Quality Conservation Law and the Factory Effluents Control Law (usually referred to as the "two water-quality laws"), in force since 1959, were not applied to Minamata Bay until this time.[18]

The new minister of health and welfare in the second Satō Eisaku cabinet was Sonoda Sunao, an LDP diet member from Kumamoto prefecture who was expected to push for an announcement. On January 18, as he was leaving a school for handicapped children in Kumamoto, Hiyoshi Fumiko ran up to him and with tears in her eyes presented a petition and asked him for help. He cried as well, and in front of Governor Teramoto and the media he told her that he knew Chisso's mercury caused the disease. He said the Science and Technology Agency wanted to announce the causes of both the Minamata and Niigata diseases simultaneously in May.[19] On May 15, the Citizens' Council petitioned Sonoda to exempt the solatium payments from income limits for welfare recipients and to make sure the government finding left no doubt about the cause of Minamata disease. On the same day, the *Kumamoto nichinichi shinbun* reported that he had promised again that announcements regarding Niigata and Minamata would be simultaneous.

The process was a long one, however, involving a great deal of "adjustment of opinions" between the Ministry of Health and Welfare, MITI, and the Science and Technology Agency. The agency circulated a proposed draft of an official government finding regarding Niigata in April 1968, but the Ministry of Health and Welfare asked for changes. Sonoda commented to the press on July 6 that previous research was sufficient and there need be no delay to conduct further research. The interministerial negotiations were conducted behind closed doors, but the mercury issue remained constantly in the news. In August Sonoda issued government guidelines for safe levels of mercury in factory waste, in fish, and in human hair. In September the *Kumamoto nichinichi shinbun* reported that Chisso's vinyl chloride plant was also discharging waste laden with organic mercury.[20]

There was no doubt that the government would find Chisso to be the cause of Minamata disease, and all parties concerned began to position themselves for what would happen after the announcement. Chisso said it would negotiate with the patients after the government finding, if necessary. Governor Teramoto said that Chisso Minamata President Tokue Takeshi had admitted that mercury had continued to be discharged after the Cyclator was completed in 1959, and Teramoto said he might mediate new negotiations to increase the solatium payments. The No. 1 union repeated its demand that the company admit responsibility and urged it to make the data from all of its cat experiments public.

The pro-management No. 2 union brought up an issue of concern to many civic leaders when it asked the company on September 12 to revise its five-year plan, issued in August 1967, under which 1,500 jobs were to be cut. The same request was made by the Yunoko Tourism Association on September 18, and by the Minamata Chamber of Commerce on September 19. On September 19, however, Chisso Vice President Shimada Ken'ichi announced that a smaller reduction was impossible, and the plan would be carried out unchanged. On September 25, 30 organizations including the Chamber of Commerce and the tourism association formed the Citizens' Conference for the Development of Minamata (Minamata-shi hatten shimin kyōgikai). They pledged to work for the reconstruction of the city and of the company. In the code understood by everyone in Minamata, this meant protecting the city by urging Chisso to limit its cutbacks, and protecting the company by attempting to minimize the burden of any further compensation Chisso might be forced to pay.

On September 22, when Minister of Health and Welfare Sonoda visited a hospital in Minamata, one of the most haunting incidents in the entire Minamata disease story occurred. When Sonoda passed by, a Minamata disease patient named Murano Tamano began to have convulsions, as she often did. As doctors held her down to inject her with a sedative, she suddenly shouted "Long live the emperor!" (*Tennō heika banzai*), and then began singing "Kimi ga yo" (His Majesty's reign), the de facto national anthem. As Ishimure tells the story, "Unable to bear the raw ghastliness of the scene, Sonoda and his party hastily left the room."[21] In Irokawa Daikichi's interpretation, Tamano was not "an ignorant woman who knew nothing of postwar democracy," but one who, in her suffering at the lowest levels of Japanese society, held on to the desperate hope that the person at the pinnacle of that society would save her.[22]

Whatever the explanation, Murano's outburst is a reminder of how the ghost of the emperor system floats in and out of the Minamata disease incident and indeed all of Minamata's history, from the gifts of white turtles at the beginning of the city's history through Nitchitsu's role in Japan's empire to Hirohito's visits to the factory and his questions to Governor Teramoto in 1960. The emperor has also been used, as Irokawa does in explaining the incident above, as a symbol of the political and social hierarchy of imperial Japan that persisted in the postwar period and put the Minamata disease victims at its lowest levels.

The *Asahi shinbun* had reported the outlines of the government finding on September 8.[23] Finally, on September 26, 1968, the Ministry of Health and Welfare announced both its own findings regarding Minamata and the conclusions of the Science and Technology Agency regarding Niigata. Both were presented as official government conclusions.[24] The finding for Niigata was couched in very tentative terms. The Science and Technology Agency's report said that "the circumstances of the poisoning are extremely complex, and they are difficult to reproduce." It said its research showed that Niigata Minamata disease was caused by consumption of large quantities of fish made poisonous by methyl mercury in the Agano River. However, the only reason the agency concluded that the mercury was probably discharged over an extended period by the Kanose factory of Shōwa denkō was that sufficient evidence was lacking for the other possibilities that it still refused to categorically dismiss—a sudden large discharge from the Kanose factory, waste from other factories on nearby rivers, or even the leakage of pesticides into the river because of the earthquake in June 1964.[25] Shōwa denkō's President Yasunishi Masao adamantly insisted he was still confident that his factory's waste was not the cause of the disease.

The conclusion regarding Minamata, drafted mainly by Ministry of Health and Welfare Pollution Section chief Hashimoto Michio, was far more authoritative in tone but contained a number of inaccuracies. The core of the finding was the explanation of the cause:

Minamata disease is a disease of the central nervous system, a poisoning caused by long-term consumption, in large amounts, of fish and shellfish from Minamata Bay. The causative agent is methyl mercury. Methyl mercury produced in the acetalde-hyde acetic acid facility of Shin Nihon chisso's Minamata factory was discharged in factory wastewater, contaminating fish and shellfish in Minamata Bay. It is recognized that the disease occurred when residents of the area consumed fish and shell-fish containing methyl mercury that had concentrated in their bodies. Minamata disease patients last appeared in 1960, and the outbreak has ended. This is presumed to be due to the fact that consumption of fish and shellfish from Minamata Bay was banned in the fall of 1957, and the fact that the factory had waste-treatment facilities in place from January 1960.

The announcement was accompanied by a chart chronicling the outbreak of Kumamoto Minamata disease: one patient in 1953, 12 in 1954, 14 in 1955, 51 in 1956, 6 in 1957, 5 in 1958, 18 in 1959, and the final 4 in 1960. Of these 111 recognized patients, 42 had died and 12 were hospitalized. The chart also noted that the ministry had provided a total of ¥8,620,000 ($23,900) in assistance for medical costs and ¥217,115,000 ($603,000) to assist in the construction of hospital facilities from 1958 through 1967.[26]

The day before the announcement, MITI instructed the 35 companies using mercury at 49 factories in Japan to avoid pollution. (It had also issued a similar warning in July 1965—years after it should have—and in both 1965 and 1968 the warnings mentioned the Niigata case but not Minamata.)[27] The new president of the Mutual Aid Society, Yamamoto Matayoshi, announced that his group wished to negotiate new compensation. Chisso President Egashira Yutaka promised to accept the government's finding, apologized on behalf of the company for the troubles it had caused (visiting the patients' homes to apologize in person September 28 and 29), and promised to negotiate. At the same time, however, he asked for cooperation from the union and the citizens as Chisso carried out its five-year plan—a not-so-subtle threat that if the company were forced to pay too much in compensation, it would cut operations in Minamata even further, as well as an attempt to persuade the union and citizens to see the patients and their supporters as enemies of the company and the city.

There are conflicting stories of the reasons the Ministry of Health and Welfare issued its finding. Sonoda Sunao later described it as "my recognition [of Minamata disease as a] pollution disease."[28] He recalled that soon after becoming minister, he realized that the 1959 conclusion by the ministry's research committee that organic mercury caused the disease had been kept secret, as had the findings by both Kumamoto University and Chisso's own Dr. Hosokawa that the organic mercury was produced in the factory. "Because of this, as a politician I could not hesitate to make a decision. But there were various pressures. Nevertheless, I asserted my conviction that 'without the support of the people there can be no prosperity for corporations,' and then–prime minister Satō supported me." His suggestion that the government was in danger of losing "the support of the people" implies that the petitions and protests were having an effect. Sonoda may have overestimated his own role in the process, but he was right in describing the finding as "a decision that shook to the roots the 'industry first' philosophy that had been followed since the Meiji era."

One of the key directors of the income-doubling policy was Miyazawa Kiichi, who in 1968 was EPA director and later served as prime minister. The EPA had been in charge of research on Minamata disease since 1960 and had done next to nothing. According to Hashimoto Michio, who earlier had drafted the government finding regarding the cadmium poisoning in Toyama, when Sonoda called Hashimoto to his office in June 1968 and ordered him to draft the finding regarding Minamata disease, Sonoda told him he was doing so at the suggestion of Miyazawa. By having the finding issued by the Ministry of Health and Welfare rather than the EPA, Gotō Takanori believes, Miyazawa was hoping to divert attention from the agency's years of inaction.[29]

The main point of the finding—that organic mercury from Chisso's factory caused Minamata disease—was correct, and official government acceptance of this fact had powerful effects. Yet the rest of the finding perpetuated the false stereotypes about the disease and therefore perpetuated obstacles to fully recognizing and dealing with the problem.[30] First, the disease may not be caused only "by long-term consumption, in large amounts," of polluted fish. Ingestion of high levels of mercury over a short period or low levels over a long period may also result in Minamata disease, but the finding offered no encouragement for research into these possibilities. It implied that only "fish and shellfish in Minamata Bay" were dangerous, but in fact the contamination had spread over a much wider area. Methyl mercury was discharged not only from the acetaldehyde facilities, but also from the vinyl chloride production process, which continued until 1971, and although the amounts from the latter were small, they were not necessarily negligible. The finding stated that "residents of the area," which one might assume meant the Minamata Bay area, were the only ones who developed Minamata disease, but in fact patients appeared throughout much of the Shiranui Sea area. In addition, the outbreak most definitely had not ended in 1960, consumption of fish and shellfish from the bay was never banned, and the factory's treatment facilities did not remove organic mercury from its waste.

The Ministry of Health and Welfare could have made an announcement such as this in the fall of 1959. Had it not shelved the issue then, patients, doctors, researchers, the general public, and the ministry itself would have had a much better understanding of the problem by 1968. Instead, in 1968 it continued its attempts to portray the problem as limited in geographical and chronological extent, making it difficult for those beyond Minamata and immediately adjacent areas, and those who developed the disease after 1959, to be certified. Through the finding, the ministry attempted to minimize the costs to government and Chisso and to promote continued reliance on local, extrajudicial methods of resolution. It encouraged the latter by characterizing the December 1959 solatium agreement, in its summary of "Events to the Present," as a legal "civil settlement" (*minjijō no wakai*). If the 1959 agreement was in fact legally binding, then no suit against Chisso would be possible. In just over six months, the September 1968 announcement, intentionally or not, split the 111 certified patients and their families into two groups over the issue of whether or not to sue.

Nevertheless, official confirmation of the cause of Minamata disease marked perhaps the most important turning point in the incident. It was a great relief to the victims and their supporters. The activists attempting to force Chisso to accept responsibility for the disease were now opposing the government only over whether Chisso had already done so sufficiently, not over whether it was in fact responsible. Most important, patients were given a new sense of dignity. No longer could it be suggested that their sickness was somehow their own fault. Many expressed their gladness at having their suffering recognized by "those above" (*okami*). The frequent use of this term for government officials and others in positions of responsibility throughout the Minamata disease incident by some patients, from the 1950s into the

1990s, cautions against the assumption that all victims saw their polity in terms of democratic rights and egalitarianism. At the same time, the violent objections by other patients (including Kawamoto Teruo and Watanabe Eizō) to this term and the hierarchy it implies show that divisions among the patients sprang not only from disagreements over tactics, or from personality conflicts, but also to a large extent from real differences over interpreting Japan's political and social structure and their own proper place in it.

An End to Solidarity: Leave It up to Others, or Sue?

One symbol of the new official recognition of patients as victims of a pollution disease was the city's sponsoring of a memorial service on September 13 for the 42 people who had died of Minamata disease. Signs of the split among the patients were also visible even before the September 26, 1968, announcement. On September 12, Ueno Eiko of the Mutual Aid Society had announced in a speech to the prefectural branch of the Sōhyō federation of unions that she intended to sue the company. This brought into the open the conflicts within the Mutual Aid Society over whether or not to sue and the society's leaders' suspicion of the Citizens' Council. A special meeting of the society on September 15 declared that the solatium contract with Chisso should be renegotiated and decided on a general strategy. First, direct negotiations with the company would be attempted; if they failed, the society would seek mediation. Only as a last resort, if mediation failed, would they sue. A negotiation committee was chosen along with a new president, Yamamoto Matayoshi. The next day, Yamamoto and Mutual Aid Society Vice President Nakatsu resigned from the Citizens' Council. Not all patients were sure Yamamoto's and Nakatsu's strategy was best, however, and on September 21, Bandō Katsuhiko, a lawyer for the Niigata plaintiffs, discussed compensation issues with some Minamata victims at the invitation of the Citizens' Council.

On October 6, the Mutual Aid Society decided to ask Chisso for ¥13 million ($36,100) for each death and ¥600,000 ($1,670) per year for surviving patients. Two days later, they met company representatives and submitted their demands. On October 24, the company said it had "no basis" for judging fair compensation and preferred to rely on the government to do so. On November 6, society representatives met with Minister of Health and Welfare Sonoda, who agreed to set up a "third-party" body to decide on standards for compensation. Despite this promise from the central government, at their third meeting on November 15, the society accepted Chisso's proposal that Governor Teramoto be asked to mediate, and on December 3 Chisso President Egashira asked the governor to set up a mediation committee.

Governor Teramoto, unlike Chisso, was not willing to repeat the 1959 pattern, partly out of anger at having been deceived by the company about its knowledge of the cause of the disease and about the Cyclator. He repeated his refusal to company executives on December 6 and to the Mutual Aid Society on December 12, and asked the Ministry of Health and Welfare on December 6 and again on December 19 to handle mediation. On December 10, he justified his refusal to the prefectural legislature, saying the company simply intended to add to the 1959 contract. As in 1959, however, the patients were desperate for some sort of compensation before the end of the year and asked Chisso at the fourth meeting, on December 25, to pay each patient ¥10 million ($27,800) as an advance against the new compensation. The company refused.

On January 5, 1969, the Mutual Aid Society decided it would have to petition government ministries to establish standards for compensation. The new minister of health and welfare, Saitō Noboru, responded that ministries could not directly decide on compensation and repeated Sonoda's November promise to set up a third-party board to do so. At the end of January, both the society and Chisso tried one more time to get Teramoto to help, but he continued to insist the matter was in the hands of the central government. The Citizens' Council, hoping to heal its rift with the Mutual Aid Society, demanded on February 15 that Chisso reply directly to the society's demands and also insisted that the company should reimburse the city for the costs of medical treatment for Minamata disease. On February 17, the Citizens' Council held a joint meeting with the Mutual Aid Society to discuss suing, again inviting Bandō Katsuhiko from Niigata. Society President Yamamoto and Vice President Nakatsu refused to attend.

The next day, Chisso notified the Ministry of Health and Welfare it would accept arbitration of compensation. Saitō asked the Mutual Aid Society to submit a "written promise" (*kakuyakusho*) agreeing to accept both the committee to be chosen by the ministry and the decisions of the committee.[31] The society hesitated to accept binding arbitration and decided instead to submit a "request for mediation" (*assen iraisho*). On March 3, the ministry

confirmed its refusal to accept anything less than an unconditional acceptance of binding arbitration, without which it would not appoint a committee. Governor Teramoto refused the legislature's March 14 request that he
persuade the Mutual Aid Society to agree to the Ministry of Health and
Welfare's conditions. On March 18, it was revealed in Diet testimony by
Ministry of Health and Welfare Pollution Section chief Takefuji that the
document the patients were being asked to sign had in fact been written by
Chisso, given to the ministry, and passed on to Kumamoto prefecture and
the Minamata city hall.[32]

On March 17, a group of lawyers in Kumamoto established the Minamata Disease Legal Issues Study Group (Minamatabyō hōritsu mondai
kenkyūkai). Five days later they met with some Mutual Aid Society members and promised to set up a legal team if the patients sued. Yet many patients hesitated to sue because the *haze* tree case (the dispute over whether
the Japan wax trees had been included along with the fields transferred under the postwar land reform program) had taken so long to resolve. When
the Mutual Aid Society met on April 5, Hamamoto Tsuginori remembers,
the discussion was "like a hornet's nest," and President Yamamoto stormed
out of the meeting being held in his own house.[33] The society split into what
became known as the Arbitration Group (Ichininha; literally, the "entrust [it
to others] group") and the Direct Negotiations Group (Jishu kōshōha),
which later became the Trial Group (Soshōha; literally the "litigation
group") (not to be confused with the Direct Negotiations Group formed in
the fall of 1971 by newly certified patients; see Fig. 18). On April 12, the 34
families in the original Direct Negotiations Group requested Chisso to reopen direct negotiations with them.

On April 10, 1969, the 54 families in the Arbitration Group submitted to the
Ministry of Health and Welfare the required written promise to accept
binding arbitration, but saved a bit of face by calling it a "request" (*onegaisho*).
The text, however, was almost exactly as Chisso had written it:

We request the Ministry of Health and Welfare to resolve the Minamata disease
dispute, we entrust it with the selection of committee members who undertake to
do this, and we promise to accept the conclusion the committee reaches by sufficiently investigating conditions in Minamata, by listening carefully to both sides
concerning the situation, and through discussions based on the opinions of both
sides; so we ask your assistance.[34]

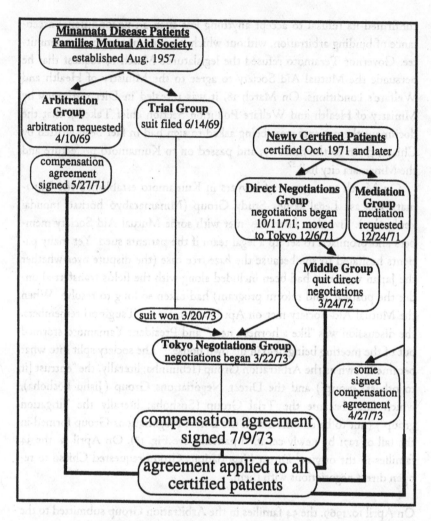

Fig. 18 Minamata disease patients' groups, 1957–1973

The humble tone of the document is impossible to convey in English. The ending *kudasaru* for the verbs *hikiuke kudasaru* (undertake) and *dashite kudasaru* (reach, give out [a conclusion]), for example, indicates an action that is directed downward by a superior benevolently deigning to do something for, or grant something to, an inferior. That Chisso preferred binding arbitration indicates that it believed the Ministry of Health and Welfare was far more likely to take its side than was the Kumamoto District Court. The tone of

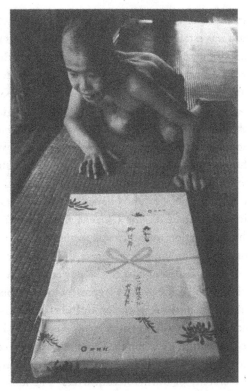

Fig. 19 A congenital Minamata disease patient with
one of the summer gifts given by Chisso to families
choosing arbitration rather than litigation. © Shiota
Takeshi.

the document the company wrote for the patients to sign shows that it was
still incapable of conceiving of them as social equals. Once the patients had
agreed to arbitration, they waited, and the spotlight turned to those patients
who were unwilling to entrust their compensation negotiations to others.

The Direct Negotiations Group had asked Chisso on April 12, 1969, to
resume negotiations with them. When Chisso did not immediately agree,
they met with the lawyers in the Minamata Disease Legal Issues Study
Group the next day and tentatively decided to sue. Chisso finally replied
April 17, insisting the problem should be resolved through a "third party,"
just as with the Arbitration Group. Three days later the Direct Negotiations Group formally decided to sue. At this early date, they were still considering suing both Chisso and the central government.

On the same day, the Association to Indict [Those Responsible for] Minamata Disease was established in Kumamoto City.[35] This group and the network of Association to Indict groups that sprang up throughout the country became the most important sources of support for the activist Minamata disease victims. The founders were Watanabe Kyōji, who had edited the short-lived journal *Kumamoto fudoki*, which had serialized parts of what became Ishimure Michiko's book *Kugai jōdo: waga Minamatabyō*, and Watanabe's friend Honda Keikichi, a high school teacher. Watanabe had spoken with Ishimure and been convinced of the need for support groups for the trial. The Citizens' Council continued its activities in Minamata, but the trial would require publicity and money the Minamata-based group could not possibly generate. Like the Citizens' Council in Minamata, the philosophy of the Association to Indict was to support but not attempt to direct the patients, and to an impressive degree this was adhered to in practice. In both cases this was due in part to the power of Ishimure's example.

Honda was chosen to be the group's "representative" rather than "chairman," since the members of the Association to Indict disliked hierarchy and authority in much the same way as those in the League for Peace in Vietnam. As was the case with the League for Peace in Vietnam, concerned citizens anywhere could form a local branch of the Association to Indict, which had no national hierarchy or official headquarters. The loose network was held together by the monthly journal *Kokuhatsu* published in Kumamoto, by speaking tours and film showings, and by members' journeys to Minamata, Kumamoto, and Tokyo.[36] A third similarity with the League for Peace in Vietnam was the way the group, despite its generally leftist views, distanced itself from the established opposition parties. The Citizens' Council in Minamata, although chaired by a JSP City Council representative, did the same thing, and refused to allow one member to attend meetings when they discovered he had been sent to Minamata from Communist Party headquarters in Tokyo.[37]

This made cooperation with the support groups more directly allied with the parties, especially with the JCP, strained at best. Cooperation with the Prefectural Citizens' Council to Support the Minamata Disease Trial and Eliminate Pollution (Minamatabyō soshō shien, kōgai o nakusuru kenmin kaigi), founded May 24 and affiliated with the Sōhyō labor federation and the JSP, was a bit easier but never entirely smooth. Sharp disagreements over strategy had yet to appear, however, and every new support group was welcomed. In early June, a Student Council to Think About Minamata Disease (Minamatabyō o kangaeru gakusei kaigi) was established at Kumamoto University and began a "caravan" across the nation appealing for support for the suing victims.

Preparations and publicity for the lawsuit speeded up. On May 12, 1969, Watanabe Eizō, the former head of the patients' Mutual Aid Society who was now becoming the spokesman for the trial group, gave a speech to the second conference of the National Alliance for Pollution Countermeasures, where he shared the stage with the head of the Victims' Association in Niigata. On May 18 the Kumamoto Minamata Disease Trial Lawyers' Group was officially established to represent the Minamata patients in the suit they were preparing to file. It initially consisted of 222 members from around the nation (with more added later), but the trial was actually conducted by a core group of ten or so lawyers affiliated to varying degrees with the JCP. Most medium-sized or larger towns and cities in Japan have at least one JCP-affiliated law office, and Manaki Akio, who headed such an office in Minamata, was the most visible of the Minamata disease trial lawyers.

On June 14, 1969, 112 people in 28 families filed suit against Chisso in Kumamoto District Court, demanding ¥642,390,444 ($178,000) in damages.[38] The plaintiffs consisted of 41 patients (17 of them dead and 14 too sick to work) and 71 of their family members. They and their lawyers had decided to sue only the company and not the state, but they still conceived of their struggle as being against both. Watanabe Eizō was the official leader of the plaintiffs and, in a speech outside the courthouse, declared: "Today, and from this day forth, we are fighting against the power of the state."[39] There was no lack of evidence that he was right, including the document signed by the Arbitration Group in April. Yet the Trial Group might never have been able to take its case to court without a recent change in the law that had required all those filing civil suits to pay huge filing fees. Now, unlike in 1959, plaintiffs who could prove they were impoverished could get court assistance. The full filing fee was ¥3,213,300 ($8,930), but the court on July 11 found all but four plaintiffs eligible for assistance and waived the total of ¥3,150,000 ($8,750) in fees for the others.[40]

The Association to Indict published the first issue of its monthly newsletter *Kokuhatsu* on June 25. The lead story was entitled "War Declared On Chisso: Suit Filed in Kumamoto District Court." The journal carried reports of the trial, called for financial assistance, encouraged the formation of support groups elsewhere, and featured columns by Ishimure Michiko, Aka-saki Satoru, and others. In September, to commemorate the first anniversary of the government's announcement that Chisso's mercury caused Minamata disease, the Association to Indict sponsored its first large demonstration in Kumamoto. Without the money and other support raised by the Association to Indict, it would have been difficult to see the trial through to the end.

Yet without another organization established by the Association, the trial could not have been won. No litigation quite like this had ever been attempted in Japan, and so the leaders of the Citizens' Council and Association to Indict were not confident that the eager but inexperienced young JCP lawyers could succeed. The principles of corporate negligence and liability were not at all well established in Japan. The company had not violated any specific legal restrictions on the dumping of mercury; it was no coincidence that standards had been tightened only after the mercury catalyst method for making acetaldehyde was abandoned in Japan in May 1968 (Chisso was one of the last two holdouts). And since before Minamata there had never been a recognized case of organic mercury poisoning through the food chain, the company could argue that the dangers could not have been foreseen. Furthermore, the fact that the litigation was a civil case meant it would be more difficult to force Chisso to disclose confidential documents than in a criminal case. Finally, the Ministry of Health and Welfare had compounded these difficulties by stating in its September 1968 finding that the 1959 solatium contract, which prohibited the patients from demanding further compensation even if the factory was proven to be the cause of the disease, was valid under civil law.

The Association to Indict hesitantly approached several faculty members at Kumamoto University who they felt had the requisite knowledge to develop a successful legal case and strategy. These professors became the core of the Trial Research Group (Saiban kenkyūkai), which was formed September 7, 1969, and changed its name to the Minamata Disease Research Group (Minamatabyō kenkyūkai) in December. Togashi Sadao, perhaps the most important member, was on the law faculty, and an obvious choice. Harada Masazumi of the Medical School was also a logical choice: more than most other doctors he had a good understanding of the patients' lives and homes as well as their disease, and he had never served on a certification committee or other government commission.

The selection of the other members of the Research Group, however, shows the inspiration of the Association to Indict in forming a group that would produce something far beyond a standard legal brief. Maruyama Sadami of Kumamoto University was a regional sociologist and brought to the group an interest in the historical development of relations between the company and the city it created. Ishimure Michiko also joined the group, bringing her unmatched ability to evoke the natural beauty of the Shiranui Sea and use the simple lives of the fishers as symbols of all that was good in pre-industrial rural Japan and, in contrast with this, to make the tragedy of Minamata disease and the responsibility of Chisso all the more stark. Yamashita Yoshihiro (Zenkan), who worked in Chisso's Research Division, was one of several No. 1 union members who provided inside information from the company and participated in the group under assumed names. Ui Jun also attended meetings of the Research Group when he was in Kumamoto.[41]

The families in the Arbitration Group, who had resigned from the Citizens' Council on April 13, 1969, were waiting for the results of the arbitration sponsored by the Ministry of Health and Welfare. The ministry set up a three-member Minamata Disease Compensation Committee (Minamatabyō hoshō shori iinkai) on April 25, and the Minamata City Council agreed to the ministry's request that it pay part of the committee's expenses. It appeared at first that the committee would complete its work quickly. At its first meeting on May 6, it heard from Governor Teramoto and the vice mayor, and on May 13 it questioned patients and Chisso officials. The government issued its first *White Paper on the Environment* on May 1, bolstering the patients' hopes that it would treat the victims of pollution fairly. The committee did little more that year, however, until it called patient representatives to a meeting in Fukuoka on December 25 to ask for more information.

The March 5, 1970, issue of the *Mainichi shinbun* reported that the compensation committee had at last drawn up a plan, requiring Chisso to pay just ¥2 million ($5,600) for deaths and ¥140,000 to ¥200,000 ($390 to $560) per year to living patients. The *Mainichi* article titles and subtitles summarize the patients' responses: "Arbitration Group Strongly Dissatisfied," "Absolutely Will Not Accept," "Hopes Betrayed," "'Absolutely Unacceptable,' Says Yamamoto (Arbitration Group Representative), Voice Trembling," "Patients and Others Shed Tears." Committee Chairman Chigusa Tatsuo, a former Tokyo High Court judge, attempted to limit the damage to the committee's reputation by announcing that the annual payments had not yet been decided and that the final plan would be presented in April.[42]

The Arbitration Group, in the first action it had taken since agreeing to accept arbitration and resigning from the Citizens' Council in April 1969, petitioned the committee and the Ministry of Health and Welfare on March 27, 1970, for a fair and prompt settlement. The Citizens' Council and the trial group also petitioned the committee, protesting against not only the low compensation but also the committee's avoidance of the issue of Chisso's responsibility.[43] Perhaps because of the protests, the committee delayed, and Chigusa announced at the end of April that the revised plan would be presented in late May. On May 4, a *Nishinippon shinbun* scoop confirmed that the committee had been forced to raise the compensation: its latest draft called for ¥3 million ($8,300) for deaths and ¥160,000 to ¥320,000 ($440 to $890) per year for living patients. However, payments made under the 1959 solatium agreement would be deducted from the compensation.

On May 10, the Arbitration Group selected thirteen representatives and gave them full power of attorney to accept compensation. The Trial Group and the Association to Indict, fearing that low compensation for the Arbitration Group would set a dangerous precedent, conducted sit-ins in front of Chisso headquarters in Tokyo, holding photographs of relatives who had died of Minamata disease. When it was announced that the committee would present its plan to Chisso and the patients on May 25, the Association to Indict put out calls for a "May 25 Action" to protest. A flyer was addressed to "friends nationwide who are joined through *Kokuhatsu*":

Although the amounts of money in this decision by the compensation committee are extremely low, the fact that it leaves Chisso's corporate responsibility unclear is absolutely criminal. . . . The compensation committee, in allying with Chisso capital, is attempting to strengthen the criminal 1959 solatium contract. . . . We of the Association to Indict have resolved to dedicate our entire existence to blocking the compensation committee's announcement on May 25.[44]

On the morning of May 25, after listening to speeches by Ui Jun, Honda Keikichi, and others, the demonstrators, including Ishimure Michiko, marched from Hibiya Park to the Ministry of Health and Welfare, where the compensation plan was to be announced to representatives of Chisso and the patients. Some, including Ui Jun and documentary filmmaker Tsuchimoto Noriaki, forced their way into the conference room and read a statement of protest before they were removed by police. Thirteen people were arrested before the committee was able to announce its decision. From ¥1,450,000 to ¥3,500,000 ($4,000 to $9,700) would be paid for deaths. Survivors would receive one-time payments of between ¥500,000 and ¥1,900,000 ($1,400 to $5,300), plus annual payments of ¥170,000 to ¥380,000 ($470 to $1,100). On the same day, according to the *Asahi shinbun*, a settlement in Osaka paid victims of a gas explosion up to ¥19 million ($53,000).[45]

The next day, May 26, a group of Ministry of Health and Welfare employees distributed flyers criticizing the ministry:

The ministry, which should be open to all as the guardian of national health and welfare, closed its doors. Why did we permit the authorities to take this attitude toward the members of the Association to Indict? . . . Let us, having been accused of complicity by the Minamata disease patients, join hands with our accusers and take a hard look at the irregularities occurring around us.

Pollution section chief Hashimoto Michio responded: "We consider the compensation proposal . . . to be the best possible within the framework of the present system. It is highly regrettable . . . that members of the ministry staff should have initiated opposition activities." Their reply was: "The May 25 action was an indictment of thinking in terms of frameworks. Our own actions were entirely in keeping with the spirit of the regulations governing civil servants, who are charged to serve the people. If he considers this regrettable, [Hashimoto] should resign and go to work for Chisso."[46] This internal rebellion by bureaucrats was remarkable. Many of the Ministry of Health and Welfare employees had already been in contact with supporters in Tokyo of Minamata disease patients and became active in support groups as they were founded. The rebellion may have helped persuade government leaders of the need to create an Environment Agency, which was done in July 1971.

Instead of accepting the committee's plan immediately, as they had promised to do, the patients asked that payments for deaths be increased by ¥1 million ($2,800), and that the one-time payments to survivors be doubled. Chisso refused to consider this. The committee was forced to revise its proposal, and while it did, the patients were confined inside the building for two days. The revised proposal was signed by both sides on May 27. Payments for deaths ranged from ¥1.7 million to ¥4 million ($4,700 to $11,100) depending on the patient's age at death, lump-sum payments to survivors from ¥800,000 to ¥4 million ($2,200 to $11,100), and annual payments from ¥170,000 to ¥380,000 ($470 to $1,100). In addition, an extra ¥200,000 ($560) was paid to each patient at the signing. The structure of these compensation payments, if not the amounts, set the pattern for those that were to come.

On May 28 the *Asahi shinbun* carried a revealing discussion between Chigusa Tatsuo, chairman of the compensation committee, Nomura Yoshihiro, a law professor at the University of Tokyo, and Mizukami Tsutomu, a writer:

Nomura: "In this case, in which moral considerations should have been paramount, the settlement was too low." . . .
Chigusa: "But what would have happened if the company had refused to agree to mediation? On what basis do you claim that the settlement is too low?"
Nomura: "Today, ¥10 million [$28,000] is considered the standard compensation for loss of life."
Chigusa: "Why should today's standard be applied to something that happened over a decade ago?"
Nomura: "Couldn't a settlement closer to the norm in terms of both moral and social responsibility have been worked out?"
Chigusa: "The value of money in Minamata is different from what it is in Tokyo. In this case, the minimum annual compensation is ¥170,000 [$470]. People who aren't seriously incapacitated will receive their wages as well. Actually, the compensation seems too high to me."[47]

Chisso's confidence in pushing for binding arbitration had been justified.

On May 27, the day of the signing, the Citizens' Council and the No. 1 union held a protest and memorial service in front of the main gate at the Minamata factory. The union held an eight-hour strike that day, the first strike in Japanese history by a union protesting pollution by its own company.[48] On June 1, the Law Concerning the Settlement of Environmental Pollution Disputes (Kōgai funsō shori hō) was promulgated, and it went into effect on November 1. In the future, arbitration would be carried out by official government bodies, not special committees established for individual issues. On June 5, the *Asahi shinbun* reported that welfare payments to two families had already been cut off because the new compensation was being counted as income.[49]

Kawamoto Teruo and the Uncertified Patients

No one seemed to know or care how many uncertified patients there might be, but one of them, Kawamoto Teruo, forced an end to this ignorance by 1971.[50] Soon after he lost his job in the 1962–63 strike against Chisso, he found work at a new mental hospital not far from his home. He then joined the first class in a new nurses' training program set up by the Minamata doctors' association, working at the hospital in the morning and attending classes in the afternoon and evening, and learned as much as he could about Minamata disease. During his internship at the municipal hospital, he had to inject himself with painkillers in order to be able to work, but sometimes his hands shook so badly he could not draw the liquid from an ampule into a syringe. When his father's condition worsened, Teruo got him admitted to the psychiatric hospital at which he worked and was with Katōta when he died there in April 1965.

On March 24, 1968, the Kumamoto Prefecture Association of Civil Liberties Commissioners (Kumamoto ken jinken yōgo iin rengōkai) announced its belief that the government's failure to clarify the cause of Minamata disease and the low level of the solatium payments were violations of human rights.[51] Thinking this might mean he could get his own and his father's cases reconsidered, Kawamoto approached Ichihara Kiyo, a Civil Liberties commissioner (Jinken yōgo iin) for Minamata, in September. Her reply: "So you want the money that badly?"[52] He then tried to get the prefectural government to release the results of tests of mercury levels in residents' hair, since his father had been one of those tested, but they refused. He persuaded the director of the Minamata Public Health Office to ask the prefecture's certification committee (the prefecture took over responsibility for certification from the Ministry of Health and Welfare in 1964) to change its policy against considering cases of people who had already died, but at their October 8 meeting they confirmed their view that this was medically impossible. Kawamoto wrote letters to all 22 civil liberties commissioners in southern Kumamoto prefecture, but not one replied. He asked the city to exhume and autopsy his father's body, and the clerk told him they did not "dig up bodies so people can get compensation money."[53]

On May 29, 1969, the certification committee recognized five new patients, in its first certifications in five years. Kawamoto, who had applied the previous fall, was among the thirteen whose applications were turned down. The members of this group were notified only that they had been rejected; the board gave no reasons for its decisions and made no suggestions as to what might be the cause of their symptoms, if not Minamata disease. On June 2, Kawamoto sent a list of questions to the chairman of the certification committee, Professor Kita Takeo of Kumamoto University, and to other committee members. He reminded them that in 1956 some patients who had died over two years earlier had been certified and asked why it was not possible to do the same thing now. He also asked whether they felt there was no possibility that the thirteen rejected applicants had Minamata disease and whether the committee had considered the applicants' life histories, especially their consumption of fish and shellfish.

Kawamoto received replies from Kita and from Fuke Masaki, the head of the Minamata doctors' association who would be elected mayor in February 1970. Both said that information concerning individual cases could not be divulged, but that he should come to the municipal hospital if he wished to discuss his own case. The hospital director then called and asked Kawamoto to come in for a private discussion. Kawamoto said he would not do so alone—he wanted all thirteen rejected applicants to come to the hospital together. The director refused, saying each applicant would have to deal directly with the certification committee.

Kawamoto decided to try to persuade the rejected applicants to reapply. He bicycled tirelessly around Minamata in the evenings and on holidays, visiting patients' homes. Before long, he realized that there were a great many uncertified patients, and he broadened his objectives to discovering them and persuading them all to apply for certification. In particular, he tried to get mothers of congenital Minamata disease patients to apply, reasoning that they, and family members of other certified patients with severe symptoms, were most likely to have the disease. He visited most of the mothers of congenital patients, and many of these women told him they had had miscarriages. He often asked people to write, since shaky handwriting was evidence of Minamata disease. Still, many refused to apply. Some said they wanted to avoid, for themselves and their families, the stigma of Minamata disease, which would haunt them at school, at work, in relations with neighbors, and in finding marriage partners. Others feared being criticized as moneygrubbers if they applied for certification for more than one family member.

Their fears were justified, for the ostracism of early patients because they had the "strange disease" was transmuted later into ostracism of patients who rocked the boat by suing or demanding direct negotiations. Sugimoto Eiko, a member of the Trial Group, recalls that neighbors in the hamlet of Modō demanded that she withdraw from the suit. A Chisso executive made the same request, by telephone and in person. When she refused, saying the lawsuit had been her father's last wish, her isolation became complete: neighbors cut her family's nets, boarded and used their boat, refused to speak to her, and threw human feces on her. By this time, there were no more *amiko*. Eiko, her husband Takeshi, and their sons fished from 4:00 A.M. to 7:00 A.M. The eldest son then took his brothers to school and went on to the fish market to sell the morning's catch, arriving back at school two hours late. Eiko did not learn of this until the suit ended, and the boy's teacher spoke to her for the first time about the family's difficulties.[54]

On June 14, 1969, the day the Trial Group filed suit against Chisso, a group of six people met at Kawamoto's house. One of them was Satō Takeharu, with whom Kawamoto had protested the fishing cooperative's refusal to accept Shin Nitchitsu's offer of jobs in 1960. Because he had been hired by Shin Nitchitsu after the 1960 agreement between the company and the co-op (from which he had been expelled), Satō had refrained from applying for certification for his wife. This small meeting at Kawamoto Teruo's home would result in a big change in the Minamata disease incident, adding a third group—uncertified patients—to the equation most people had thought included only the Trial Group and the Arbitration Group. On September 8, Kawamoto delivered certification applications for 28 people to the Minamata Public Health Office. Of these 28, seven were reapplying after having been rejected, seven were mothers of congenital Minamata disease patients, and four were applying on behalf of people who had already died.[55]

On November 14, the certification committee again decided it could not consider applications for those who had died, and on December 6 Kawamoto protested to the District Legal Affairs Bureau and the prefectural civil liberties commissioners that this was a violation of human rights. The commissioners finally responded on January 17, 1970, saying the refusal was not a human rights violation. In the meantime, however, an opportunity for change seemed to have come on December 27, 1969, when a new committee was formed to consider applications from both Kumamoto and Kagoshima prefectures. The Law for Special Measures for Relief of Pollution-Related

Health Damage had been promulgated on December 15, partly because of the lawsuits over the Big Four pollution cases then awaiting resolution in the courts. On December 20, the Ministry of Health and Welfare designated the eastern Shiranui Sea area, from Izumi through Minamata and north to Tanoura, as the area from which patients could be certified as eligible for relief under the law. Under the Relief Law, victims of pollution diseases were to submit applications and results of medical examinations to the governor, who would decide, on the advice of a committee of doctors, whether to certify them. For those certified, the government would pay all medical expenses not covered by insurance.[56] Kawamoto and the other applicants hoped the new system would deal with them more fairly than had the old.

Through 1957, patients had been certified by the Minamata City Strange Disease Countermeasures Committee (Minamata-shi kibyō taisaku iinkai). In 1958 and 1959 their work was continued by a group of eight doctors, chaired by Professor Tokuomi Haruhiko of Kumamoto University. The Ministry of Health and Welfare established an ad hoc certification committee (Minamatabyō shinsa kyōgikai) on December 25, 1959, to decide who would receive sympathy payments from Shin Nitchitsu. On September 14, 1961, this group was superseded by a new ad hoc committee (Minamatabyō kanja shinsakai) under the Kumamoto prefectural Public Health Section. On March 31, 1964, a new Minamata Disease Patients' Investigation Committee (Minamatabyō kanja shinsakai), under the governor of Kumamoto prefecture, took over. This was the first certification committee that was not an ad hoc creation but specifically provided for by law. Now, at the end of 1969, this was replaced by the Kumamoto-Kagoshima Pollution Victims Certification Investigation Committee (Kumamoto-ken-Kagoshima-ken kōgai higaisha nintei shinsakai).[57]

Yet the new system continued to work in much the same way as the old, as Gotō Takanori has explained.[58] The old system, in place since the end of 1959, had existed to decide who would receive sympathy payments from Chisso. The new one was intended to solve some of the problems of the old, and it specifically certified patients to receive government assistance under the Relief Law. It was feared, however, that any newly certified patients would sue Chisso if it refused to extend the solatium agreement to them. The old mentality of protecting Chisso and Minamata by containing the number of certified patients remained. This was especially so because it was the same prefectural bureaucrats who managed the new system, and many of the same people served on the new committee.

The committee, chaired by Tokuomi Haruhiko, met on January 26, 1970, and recertified the 71 surviving patients certified by its predecessors. On February 19, the Citizens' Council and the Prefectural Citizens' Council petitioned the prefecture to make the certification requirements more realistic, to consider applications for those who had already died, and to examine all residents of the affected area. On the next day, however, the discussion at the committee's second meeting suggested that no change was in store: the committee members agreed that because of its relation to compensation, certification was not merely a medical decision, and they would have to proceed cautiously.[59] Its first decisions regarding applicants for certification were announced June 19. Only five of 32 applicants were certified. Decisions were postponed for sixteen, and eleven applicants, including Kawamoto, were rejected.

Instead of applying for a third time, Kawamoto decided to test a new option provided for by the Relief Law, which allowed applicants to file "complaints against administrative acts" (*gyōsei fufuku shinsa seikyū*). Rejected applicants had the right to request, within 60 days, that the minister of health and welfare review the decisions of the certification committee and the governor. Once again, Kawamoto made the rounds of patients' homes, this time with Satō Takeharu, asking them to join him. On August 18, nine of the eleven rejected applicants, including Kawamoto and Satō, submitted a request to the minister of health and welfare.

The complaint by these nine people forced the wheels of bureaucracy to turn, if slowly, and contributed more to changing the actual operation of the certification system than did the passage of the Law for Special Measures for Relief of Pollution-Related Health Damage. In November 1970, the prefecture defended its actions to the ministry, saying its decisions were based on the recommendations of the certification committee, which was the only body capable of making authoritative diagnoses. Around this time, Kawamoto traveled to Tokyo with Trial Group patients Watanabe Eizō and Hamamoto Tsuginori to participate in "Pollution May Day" demonstrations urging the "Pollution Diet" to revise the 1967 Basic Law for Environmental Pollution Control (which it did on December 18, removing the clause that protected the environment only when this did not conflict with economic growth). The many pollution-related laws passed by this Diet session were a successful pre-emption by the LDP and the government of the pollution issue to forestall the opposition from using it to challenge the regime.

In Tokyo at this time, Kawamoto found help in countering the prefecture's response to his complaint. He explained the situation to a meeting of supporters in Tokyo, attended by the lawyer Gotō Takanori and a number of sympathizers from the Ministry of Health and Welfare. Gotō agreed to help, and when Kawamoto took him to Minamata, he was shocked at the number of uncertified patients and the severity of some of their symptoms. He began to prepare a brief to submit to the ministry arguing that the governor's refusal to certify Kawamoto and the others was medically wrong and did not follow legally required procedures. He consulted pollution specialists in Tokyo, as well as Harada Masazumi and Miyazawa Nobuo (an NHK announcer) of the Minamata Disease Research Group in Kumamoto.

In addition to showing why each individual applicant should be certified, Gotō and his team formulated a broad attack on the general view of Minamata disease held by the certification committee. The team showed that the disease began before 1953 and continued after 1960. (The committee implicitly accepted this when in April 1971 it certified one patient who claimed to have developed the disease in 1946 and a congenital Minamata disease patient born in 1961. Applications for certification had started to increase rapidly in early 1971.) They also criticized committee chairman Tokuomi Haruhiko's strict criterion that, to be certifiable, patients had to show all the symptoms of the Hunter-Russell syndrome described by British doctors in 1940 and 1954. Instead, they argued, Minamata disease ought to be defined according to the symptoms of patients in Japan, which was in fact the standard used for certifications in Niigata. The document was completed and submitted on March 1, 1971.[60]

In April, the ministry sent two officials to conduct investigations in Minamata. They visited certified and uncertified patients at their homes and asked about life-styles and diets, heard Harada Masazumi's explanations of symptoms, and visited hospitalized patients. This suggested that the ministry favored considering more than just medical charts describing symptoms, and the officials' meetings with severely disabled patients must have had a powerful impact.

Miyazawa Nobuo had uncovered the results of the prefecture's survey of mercury levels in the hair of 2,700 people from 1960 to 1962. These data enabled Gotō and his team to strengthen their argument against the certification system. Mercury levels in hair are not a reliable measure of total mercury consumption, but they do show recent consumption levels. The data Miyazawa discovered included results for three of the nine people who had filed the complaint against the governor's rejection of their applications. The mercury levels in their hair had ranged from 14.2 ppm to 100 ppm. Kawamoto's father Katōta had registered 35 ppm. One woman in Goshonoura had been found to have had 920 ppm in her hair. It was later discovered that she had died in 1967 after having been confined to bed for ten years. None of the subjects had ever been informed of the results of these tests. All of these results were far higher than the Japanese average of between 5 and 10 ppm. In Niigata, one patient with only 10.7 ppm had been certified.[61]

In May, the Ministry of Health and Welfare called the head of the Niigata certification committee, Tsubaki Tadao, to hearings in Tokyo. Tsubaki believed that certification was much stricter in Kumamoto because no full medical survey of all residents had been done to give the prefecture a clear picture of Minamata disease. As a result, patients were not easily discovered, and those who applied were certified only if their symptoms matched those of Hunter-Russell syndrome, which had been defined on the basis of the symptoms of patients directly exposed to organic mercury rather than on the symptoms of those who ate fish containing mercury that had been concentrated in the food chain. Also, officials in Kumamoto did not recognize that Minamata disease did not always appear in its full-blown form shortly after the consumption of contaminated fish; it could develop later and gradually worsen. In response, Kumamoto committee chairman Tokuomi insisted in meetings with ministry officials in June that Hunter-Russell syndrome did in fact describe the symptoms of Minamata disease patients and that the disease could not develop gradually or long after the consumption of organic mercury.

Tokuomi had been more open to new findings in a private meeting with Miyazawa Nobuo and Ishimure Michiko at his Kumamoto University laboratory four months earlier. Then he had admitted the possibility that Minamata disease cases might have appeared before 1953 and after 1960, that more of the Minamata-area patients with neurological symptoms might have Minamata disease, and that residents of areas beyond Minamata Bay might have the disease. But his reply to the suggestion by Miyazawa and Ishimure that he investigate these possibilities was "I'd like to investigate [these things] someday. But the political problems . . . ."[62] Such "political problems" forced—or enabled—many scientists to acquiesce in perpetuating the narrow and misleading definition of Minamata disease of the government's official finding of September 1968.

The government's decision on Kawamoto's complaint was delayed by the establishment on July 1, 1971, of the Environment Agency under the Prime Minister's Office.[63] The Pollution Section of the Ministry of Health and Welfare was transferred to the new agency and with it responsibility for dealing with Minamata disease. Finally, on August 7, Ōishi Buichi (a doctor), the director general of the Environment Agency, announced that he was overturning the governor's rejections of the nine applications. He also ordered a loosening of certification requirements, the first real change since 1956: if it seemed clear that a patient had been affected by consumption of fish and shellfish containing organic mercury, the cause of his symptoms should be presumed to be Minamata disease, even if other causes were conceivable. Applicants' life-styles and consumption of contaminated fish, as well as the presence of relatives with Minamata disease, would henceforth have to be considered.

Kawamoto and the others demanded that the governor certify them immediately. However, when the committee met on September 3, Tokuomi expressed his dissatisfaction with the Environment Agency's ruling and announced his intention to resign as chair. Ōishi and Governor Sawada Issei met him five days later and persuaded him to stay on. On October 2, the committee announced that henceforth it would merely give its opinion on applicants' symptoms and leave the responsibility for deciding on certification entirely up to the governor. Three days later they discussed the cases of 23 rejected applicants, including Kawamoto's group of nine, and on October 6 Sawada certified sixteen, including Kawamoto and six others from his group. The total number of certified patients was now 150 and certain to rise rapidly. These changes had come about because of the efforts of Kawamoto and his group, which succeeded because of the support they found in Tokyo and elsewhere.

New Forms of Action and a Broadening Base of Support

The assistance Kawamoto and his group received from Kumamoto and Tokyo was indicative of the broadening base of support for Minamata disease patients. By October 1969 there were "Minamata disease discussion groups"

(Minamatabyō o kataru kai) in the cities of Fukuoka and Kitakyūshū.[64] At first most groups, like the Citizens' Council in Minamata and the Association to Indict in Kumamoto, focused on assisting the Trial Group. Anger over the arbitrated settlement signed in May 1970 and the publicity generated by Kawamoto's struggle for certification widened the horizons of the existing groups and sparked the creation of new ones.

Perhaps the most important new support group was the Tokyo Association to Indict [Those Responsible for] Minamata Disease (Tokyo Minamatabyō o kokuhatsu suru kai), established on June 28, 1970, in a meeting at the University of Tokyo, where Ui Jun taught. Ishimure Michiko and Hiyoshi Fumiko attended from Minamata, and the gathering included many people who had taken part in the "May 25 Action" protesting the proposed settlement for the Arbitration Group. One reason behind the founding of the Tokyo Association to Indict was the feeling that they had failed the previous month: "We were able to show the people of the entire nation that this arbitrated settlement was forcibly imposed in the face of opposition. Yet in the end the arbitrated settlement, which we should have prevented, was put in place under the hegemony of Chisso and the Ministry of Health and Welfare."[65] Watanabe Eizō addressed the gathering: "Heaven helps those who help themselves. We victims of Minamata disease are doing our best in our battle against the authorities, but we can't win without your support. Since you might tire if you thought the battle was entirely for the sake of others, make it your own battle too."[66]

Like the chapters of the League for Peace in Vietnam, Association to Indict groups were founded in most of Japan's major cities and universities.[67] There was no official headquarters, although all looked to the original Association to Indict in Kumamoto for inspiration. They were joined in a loose network by the Kumamoto group's publication *Kokuhatsu*, by sponsoring visiting speakers, and by contacts made when members traveled to Minamata, Kumamoto, and Tokyo. The Kumamoto group continued to be the most important because of its publications and its proximity to Minamata and played the leading role in supporting the Trial Group financially and in other ways, especially through its Minamata Disease Research Group. The Tokyo branch took the lead in supporting Kawamoto Teruo and the other "newly certified patients," first in their official complaint to the Ministry of Health and Welfare over the rejection of their applications and later in their sit-in and "direct negotiations" in Tokyo with Chisso. They continued these activities when the Trial Group and Direct Negotiations Group joined forces to negotiate a settlement with Chisso after the court verdict in 1973.

One of the first activities of the Tokyo Association to Indict was to sponsor the "Tokyo-Minamata Pilgrimage Group," led by one of the Association's founders, actor Sunada Akira. Sunada, the leader of the Chikyūza theatrical troupe, had been profoundly moved by Ishimure's *Kugai jōdo*. He and nine others, dressed in white pilgrims' robes, began their journey on July 3, 1970, from Chisso's Tokyo headquarters. Collecting donations for Minamata disease patients in their alms bags, they stopped at several cities on their way west and south, traveling by train between cities. In Osaka they were prevented from entering Expo '70, where they had hoped to collect donations and signatures on petitions.[68] Received in Kumamoto by the Association to Indict and the Citizens' Council on July 9, they turned over to tearful patients the ¥653,144 ($1,800) they had collected.[69] After participating in a demonstration the next day, they took the train to Minamata. There, on July 11, they petitioned the city to carry out medical examinations of all residents and then ended their pilgrimage at Ishimure Michiko's home. In 1971 Sunada wrote a play based on Ishimure's *Kugai jōdo*, and after premiering it in Tokyo in June, he embarked on another "pilgrimage," performing it on the way to Minamata. He and his wife, Emiko, took up residence in Yudō, and he performed his play *Kugai jōdo* in Minamata and throughout Japan thousands of times.[70]

A young photographer named Miyamoto Shigemi accompanied Sunada and his fellow pilgrims to Minamata in July 1970. His photographs, which emphasized the struggles by the victims and their supporters more than the disease itself, reflected and encouraged the new activism. Almost from the start of the Minamata disease incident, photographers have played an important part not only in telling the story but in actually affecting and participating in it. Kuwabara Shisei, who began photographing Minamata disease patients in 1960, had informed and shocked the public concerning the patients' suffering.[71] Shiota Takeshi's work has dealt with both the disease and the movement since he began his Minamata photography in 1968.[72] His photographs of congenital Minamata disease patients are especially powerful.

The best-known and most important photographs of Minamata, of course, are those by W. Eugene Smith and his wife, Aileen Smith, who

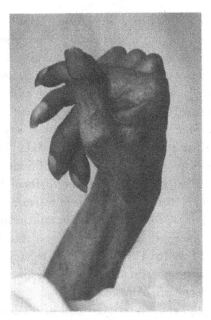

Fig. 20 The contorted hand of Funaba Iwazō, an *amimoto* (fishing net owner) and Minamata disease victim from Tsunagi, immediately north of Minamata. © Kuwabara Shisei.

rented an old house in Tsukinoura near those of Kawamoto Teruo and Hamamoto Tsuginori in 1971.[73] Eugene Smith, who invented the photographic essay while working for *Life* magazine, had already established himself as one of the world's great photographers.[74] Minamata was the culmination of his life's work, and the beating he suffered in the course of photographing the Minamata story shortened both his career and his life. Without the Smiths, Minamata would still have been brought to world attention, but their 1972 *Life* magazine article and 1975 book had a powerful impact.

The qualities that made Eugene Smith's photographic essays great, and that caused so much friction with his editors at *Life* and eventually led to his resignation from the magazine, made him uniquely qualified to tell the story of Minamata to the world. He insisted on spending a great deal of time living in his subjects' worlds, and his essays were always sympathetic, insightful portraits of their lives. More than most photojournalists, he took the time to gain his subjects' consent and understanding before photographing them. He refused to be a neutral recorder of events and never hid his sympathies. He also refused to turn over his negatives to his editors, insisting on keeping them and painstakingly printing his pictures himself so that he could control which pictures were used and exactly how they appeared.

Aileen Sprague, whose mother was Japanese, was 30 years younger than Eugene Smith. She had spent most of her childhood in Japan and dropped out of Stanford to help organize an exhibition of Smith's photographs in New York. It was there that the Smiths heard about Minamata from a Japanese friend. Eugene had wanted to return to Japan since he had done some work for the Hitachi corporation there in 1961, and they decided to go. Without Aileen to interpret (and even she found the Minamata dialect daunting), he could never have lived in and photographed Minamata, but she was much more than an assistant and translator. She took many of their photographs and wrote much of their book.[75]

With Aileen's help, and with a great deal of patience by all involved, Eugene took the one photograph that has come to stand for Minamata disease: Kamimura Yoshiko holding her blind, paralyzed, deformed daughter Tomoko in the bath, the mother's eyes glowing with love and the daughter's staring helplessly. The pose echoes that of Mary holding the dead body of Jesus in Michelangelo's *Pietà*, and in fact Yoshiko described Tomoko as "our treasure child," saying that Tomoko had taken all the poison into herself to save her siblings from suffering. The Smiths were particularly attracted to the congenital patients, and one of the most moving sections of their 1975 book *Minamata* illustrates the life of another girl afflicted with congenital Minamata disease, Sakamoto Shinobu.[76] Sakamoto, born in Yudō in 1956, walks and talks with difficulty. Through great force of will, she was attending junior high school when the Smiths met her, walking up the hill to National Highway 3 to take the bus to school each day. She understood very well who and what had handicapped her, and Aileen Smith wrote in *Minamata* of how Sakamoto hoped for a boyfriend, all the while knowing she would never be able to marry and have children.

In February 1971, six months before the Smiths arrived in Minamata, documentary filmmaker Tsuchimoto Noriaki completed *Minamata: kanjasan to sono sekai* (Minamata: the patients and their world).[77] Over the next six-

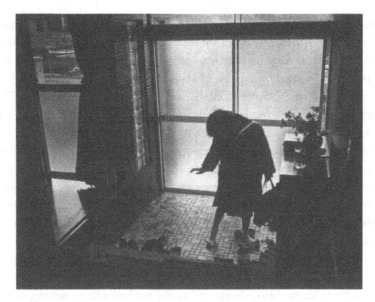

Fig. 21 Congenital Minamata disease patient Sakamoto Shinobu in the entry hall of her home, wearing her school uniform. Photograph by W. Eugene Smith. © Aileen M. Smith.

teen years, he made twelve more documentaries about Minamata and won numerous awards. Tsuchimoto was one of the thirteen people, including Ui Jun and Watanabe Kyōji, arrested at the Ministry of Health and Welfare on May 25, 1970. His film premiered in Tokyo on February 17, 1971, at a showing sponsored by the Tokyo Association to Indict, and it was then shown all over Japan with the cooperation of other Association to Indict groups and helped in raising funds and awareness.

Amateur documentaries were produced by the "Eight Millimeter Group" to which Onitsuka Iwao belonged in the No. 1 union at Chisso.[78] Onitsuka, who had always enjoyed still photography, got his first eight-millimeter movie camera by mail order in the early Shōwa 30s (1955–64). It was a wind-up, spring-operated camera, which he used to take movies of his children playing and of the neighbors. The film had to be sent to Fukuoka for developing, and he showed the movies to the neighborhood children's association and elsewhere. He filmed a little of the wage stabilization struggle, the 1962–63 strike, but soon after the strike the Eight Millimeter Group was formed in the union. At first they filmed union sports days and talent contests, but

when the Citizens' Council was formed in 1968 the group joined it and made
a film of the visit to Minamata by the Niigata Minamata disease victims.
This film, *Minamatabyō I* (1968), was followed by *Minamatabyō II* (1969) and
Ikarenai sekai (A world incapable of anger, 1970). All these were shown by
the union and the Citizens' Council for publicity and fund-raising. The
group also made films recording the exhuming of Kawamoto Katōta's body
in May 1970; the May 27, 1970, strike by the No. 1 union protesting the settlement with the Arbitration Group and Chisso's failure to accept full responsibility for the pollution; Sunada Akira's pilgrimage group arriving in
Minamata in July 1970; and demonstrations in Kumamoto and Tokyo.
Technically, these films are inferior to Tsuchimoto's, and the narration is
melodramatic, but living in Minamata gave the Eight Millimeter Group advantages no outsider could have. They were able to be present at every important event, spoke the language of the victims and other residents of
Minamata (a dialect very different from that of Tokyo), and could take the
time to get to know their subjects, if they did not know them already, before
filming.

The most dramatic moment in Tsuchimoto's documentary *Minamata: kanjasan to sono sekai* is the confrontation between victims and perpetrators of
Minamata disease at the November 28, 1970, Chisso shareholders' meeting.
Gotō Takanori claims to have come up with the idea of the "one-share
movement" while taking a bath at home.[79] His plan was for patients and
their supporters to buy one share each in Chisso in order to be able to confront the company president directly. He bought 10,000 shares at about ¥35
($0.10) each and then proposed the plan to the July 18, 1970, meeting of the
Tokyo Association to Indict. They agreed to try it if the patients were interested, and three days later Gotō met with 30 people from the Trial Group
and the Citizens' Council at the home of Hamamoto Tsuginori and his sister Fumiyo. Kawamoto Teruo, not yet a certified patient, attended but said
nothing. Gotō explained that just one share would entitle its owner to attend the meeting and address Chisso President Egashira, and Watanabe
Eizō said that he thought that would be a good thing. Those present accepted the proposal.

The movement took off rapidly and was publicized in *Kokuhatsu* and reported on by the major newspapers. The trial lawyers, however, opposed it.

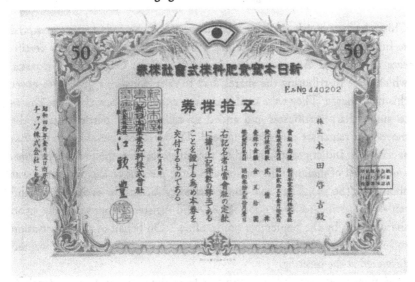

Fig. 22 A certificate for 50 shares of Chisso stock, from the one-share movement. This one was owned by Honda Keikichi, one of the founders of the Association to Indict [Those Responsible for] Minamata Disease (Minamatabyō o kokuhatsu suru kai) in Kumamoto. In the Minamatabyō kenkyūkai collection.

In an explanation of their stand issued on September 26, they argued that the goal for the victims must be monetary restitution, which would come only through victory in court.[80] Furthermore, they believed the victims would probably be unable to confront the president directly at the meeting. Finally, the lawyers said that confusion and violence, if any occurred, at the meeting would invite a backlash by the authorities and turn public opinion against the victims. The Association to Indict responded that any violence or police harassment would harm Chisso in the eyes of the public and in court far more than it would harm the patients. Most important, at the shareholders' meeting it would be possible "to give expression to the feelings that will remain with the patients . . . and to pursue the questions concerning Chisso's responsibility that will remain even after it pays compensation money." Many victims and supporters welcomed the chance to confront Chisso's executives directly, and the lawyers' objections had little effect except to further strain their relations with the Association to Indict.

To attend the meeting, shareholders had to register by the end of September. The stock certificates Gotō had bought were, as is usual in Japan, in large denominations, and had to be exchanged for single-share certificates.

Chisso had previously made such exchanges at no charge but now attempted to hinder the movement by charging a ¥50 ($0.14) fee for each new certificate issued. The Associations to Indict in Tokyo, Osaka, and Fukuoka, which were distributing the shares, had to raise donations quickly to cover this new charge. They were unable to raise enough to convert all the shares to single-share certificates and ended up selling many participants in the movement ten-share certificates instead. The total cost per share to the Association to Indict groups, including the conversion fee, the necessary forms, and the cost of mailing information about the meeting to the purchaser, was about ¥121 ($0.34). They sold single-share certificates for ¥200 ($0.56) and ten-share certificates for ¥1,000 ($2.80) and registered approximately 5,500 shareholders by the September 30 deadline.[81] On behalf of the Association to Indict, Gotō sent Chisso a registered letter, listing questions they wanted answered at the meeting.

Eighteen patients and 35 supporters from the Citizens' Council (including Kawamoto Teruo) and the Association to Indict traveled from Minamata to Osaka for the meeting, dressed in white pilgrims' clothing.[82] Six members of the No. 1 union accompanied them as bodyguards. They stopped in Hiroshima to chant Buddhist pilgrims' hymns at the memorial to victims of the atomic bomb. They were met in Osaka by members of the Osaka Association to Indict, who accompanied them to a protest outside Chisso's Osaka office. After an evening rally of supporters from all over the country, they were put up for the night at the Buraku Liberation League Center. Thus the Minamata victims symbolically identified themselves with the victims of the Hiroshima bombing and with the Burakumin, who are descendants of outcast groups and still subject to discrimination. The logic of linking these three groups of victims—one of discrimination continuing from preindustrial times, one of the first atom bombing, and one of the disease that symbolized the human cost of industrial pollution—was quite obvious to Japanese, who were well aware of how the Burakumin and the bomb victims (hibakusha) had been situated in the democratic movements of the postwar period (and, in the case of the Burakumin, even earlier).

On the morning of November 28, the members of the one-share movement made their way past rightist groups, police, and reporters and entered the conference hall where the meeting was to be held. They found that the seats nearest the stage were already occupied by Chisso employees and by sō-kaiya, gangsters who extort money from companies in return for protecting shareholders' meetings from the disruptions that they themselves threaten to cause if they are not paid.[83] Most companies find the *sōkaiya* a nuisance they can live with and even sometimes make use of, and on this occasion Chisso expected them to earn their pay. The patients and Gotō Takanori found seats on the first floor, and those supporters who managed to get in before the packed hall was closed due to fire regulations sat in the balcony. From the balcony railing, they hung the banners from their demonstrations, with the Chinese character *on*, meaning "rancor" or "bitterness," in white on a black background.

Someone in the audience proposed two minutes of silence in honor of those sacrificed to Minamata disease. Everyone in the auditorium stood, including the *sōkaiya* and the Chisso employees. Tanaka Yoshiaki of Tsubodan led the patients in chanting:

Though we think this world
One long spring,
It is really only a fleeting dream.
Before your departed souls we offer
Sincere and scalding tears
And remember you in sorrow.[84]

The curtain went up to reveal Chisso's top executives seated at a long table on the stage, with Egashira in the center. He stood up and introduced himself, and from that moment on the official proceedings could not be heard because of the commotion from the audience. Hiyoshi Fumiko, ringing her pilgrim's bell, shouted "We want you to let the patients speak!" Through the din, Gotō realized that the executives on stage were "confirming" that there were no objections to their report and were about to declare the meeting closed just minutes after it had begun. He rushed forward and began climbing onto the stage (since no microphones were provided on the floor) to propose an amendment to the financial report, calling for part of the retirement fund to be used to compensate patients and for profits to be used to fund medical examinations to discover uncertified patients. Gotō kicked free of the company employees holding his foot and trying to pull him off the stage, placed copies of his proposed amendment on the table in front of Egashira, and read the amendment into Egashira's microphone. The executives ignored the amendment and declared the meeting closed, as patients and Association to Indict members ascended the stage.

Egashira began reading a prepared response to the questions Gotō had sent him before the meeting. The other executives slipped away, and Egashira was soon surrounded by angry patients, some clutching the memorial tablets of relatives who had died. Kawamoto pulled Egashira down to a sitting position on the stage. One woman pulled out the letter of apology the company had sent patients after the government concluded Chisso's waste had caused the disease and made him read it aloud. One of the last scenes in *Minamata: kanjasan to sono sekai* is of Hamamoto Fumiyo, holding her parents' memorial tablets, confronting Egashira in the middle of the circle of patients:

Aren't you a parent too? Do you understand? Do you really understand? You're a parent, aren't you? My two parents, both parents, no matter what people say they were my parents, do you understand? Do you understand how I feel? What did you say, what did you say when you came to my place [when he visited patients' homes to apologize in September 1968]? You bowed your head three times, have you forgotten? (Egashira: That's why I paid my respects at your Buddhist altar . . . .) You just bowed to the altar; that's not enough! Don't laugh! You laughed! (Egashira: I didn't laugh . . . .) You laughed! I'm not saying anything to laugh at! You laughed, you laughed! My two parents, I'm just a child who wants her parents, just a child who wants her parents! Do you understand, how I feel? A child who wants her parents, parents, those parents, a child . . . . Parents . . . a child. They were old, but old people are important for more than just their bodies. Do you understand, I'm Hamamoto from Detsuki, Hamamoto! Do you understand, how I feel? How I feel, do you understand?

[She grabs him by the lapels.] Do you realize how I've suffered, suffering, how can I explain, it's not something you can explain in words! You can't buy lives with money! My brother's crippled! My parents, my two parents! My brother's crippled and people make fun of him! My parents . . . . [85]

The new tactic of the one-share movement brought the victims' grievances to Chisso more directly and more personally than ever before. It was valuable psychologically, in giving them the chance to fight their own battles rather than leave them to the lawyers. The television coverage of the meeting and Tsuchimoto's film enabled them to appeal directly to the nation, linking their cause to broader political and cultural concerns such as the costs of high growth and the fate of those who were left behind. At Chisso's next shareholders' meeting, on May 26, 1971, guards enabled the company to ignore 554 single-share activists and patients and to close the meeting within

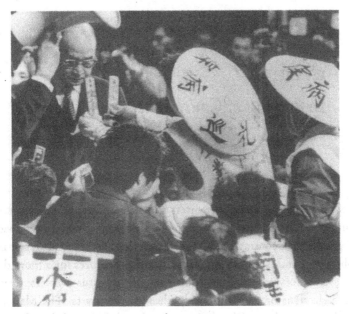

Fig. 23 Patients confronting Chisso President Egashira at the shareholders' meeting, 1970. © The Mainichi Newspapers.

ten minutes, but violence by the guards harmed the company's image further. The one-share movement spread, and the League for Peace in Vietnam used the tactic at the May 28, 1971, shareholders' meeting of Mitsubishi Heavy Industries to protest its arms production. There too, *sōkaiya* were used to attack the protesters.[86] For the Minamata victims, the direct and personal confrontation with the human beings responsible for their suffering set a precedent for the "direct negotiations" Kawamoto Teruo began a year later after his certification and for the "Tokyo negotiations" after the March 1973 court verdict.

EIGHT

In and out of Court: The Second Solution

The efforts of patients and supporters in the second round of responses to Minamata disease led to a "solution," one that represented a moral victory for the patients in contrast with the defeat of 1959. Yet it did *not* result in the establishment and legitimation of regularized procedures for a more democratic system of redress. The Minamata disease issue was not resolved through elections or even, ultimately, through the courts. The March 1973 court victory merely served to legitimate and to shift the balance of power in the informal, direct negotiations that led to the July 1973 agreement replacing the 1959 solatium contract and "solving" the Minamata disease problem again. However, if "postwar democracy" is measured not in terms of regularization of procedures but in terms of the successes of popular action and "struggle" and of shifts in the citizen-corporation-state power balance— measures used by progressive intellectuals and by Minamata's activist patients and their supporters—then this second round of responses certainly extended and enlarged it.

Yet the struggle was costly in many ways and not fully repeatable. Few other groups seeking redress could hope to be blessed with leaders and supporters as creative and effective as Kawamoto Teruo, Ishimure Michiko, and the others, and few could time their problems to coincide with an era of social movements concerned with issues such as theirs, as happened in the Minamata case.

The Leaflet War in Minamata

Kawamoto and other uncertified patients could not take their cases to Chisso until they were certified. After the November 1970 shareholders' meeting, Ishimure Michiko and a group of patients in the Trial Group traveled in pilgrims' garments from Osaka to Kōyasan, the mountain headquarters of the Shingon sect of Buddhism. Rather than joining them to chant hymns, Kawamoto went to Tokyo to seek earthly help in getting certified. When he finally gained certification on October 6, 1971, he believed that, like other certified patients, he had the right to demand compensation. Chisso announced that day, however, that the "newly certified patients," as they came to be known, had been certified according to standards that were different and unclear; compensation for the new patients could not be handled in the same way as that for the old. Chisso's assumption, which was in fact shared by many of the patients certified earlier, was that the newly certified patients were not as sick and therefore not entitled to the same level of compensation. This complicated their struggle, as did the divisions that appeared along lines similar to those in the Mutual Aid Society, which was composed of patients certified earlier. Although some of the newly certified patients stuck with Kawamoto in his attempts to negotiate directly with Chisso, within months of their certification, others would choose government mediation, and a few would abandon all attempts to obtain compensation.

Kawamoto and the fifteen others certified by the governor of Kumamoto on October 6, plus the two certified by the governor of Kagoshima on October 8, met at Ishida Masaru's home in Yudō and decided to negotiate directly with Chisso rather than accept government mediation. They had their first meeting with Chisso on October 11, 1971. These "direct negotiations" would continue for seventeen months and then for four more months when the Direct Negotiations Group joined with the Trial Group to negotiate with Chisso after the March 1973 verdict.

Chisso insisted at this first meeting in October 1971 that it had no "yardstick" for determining compensation because the new certification standards were different from the old. Compensation, it said, should be determined by the Council for Control of Environmental Pollution (Chūō kōgai taisaku shingikai), which had replaced the Minamata Disease Compensation Committee when the new Law Concerning the Settlement of Environmental Pollution Disputes took effect on November 1, 1970. Some of the new patients chose to accept the board's arbitration; others stuck with Kawamoto.

As in past confrontations, all groups in Minamata took sides, and some new groups were formed. Despite the suspicion with which some previously certified patients regarded the new patients, the Citizens' Council, the Association to Indict, and the No. 1 union supported Kawamoto's group. His assistance with the one-share movement may have helped secure this support. The Association to Indict held a demonstration and sit-in at the factory on October 25 demanding that Chisso agree to negotiations with the new patients.

On Chisso's side, in addition to the No. 2 union, were two newly formed groups of "concerned citizens." On October 20, the Minamata Citizens' Pollution Countermeasures Association (Minamata shimin kōgai taisaku kyōgikai) was established, led by Ikematsu Nobuo (an executive of Shin Nihon kagaku, a Chisso subsidiary) and Watanabe Katsuichi (a prefectural assemblyman). The next day, others led by Tokutomi Masafumi (who chaired the local branch of the LDP) formed their own group. These two conservative citizens' groups launched a petition campaign to avoid the "social unrest" they feared as certifications increased. They urged that the patients receive proper care (preferably at national government expense), that the government rank patients according to their symptoms (presumably as a way to achieve the preceding goal at minimum cost), that the bay be dredged and partly filled in, and that the name of Minamata disease be changed because it "darkens the image of Minamata and gives the impression of misery."[1] (This was neither the first nor the last campaign to remove the name of the city from the name of the disease, but a Ministry of Health and Welfare committee had decided in December 1969 that "Minamata disease" should be the official name of the disease, and it has remained so ever since.)

On October 28, Kawamoto and seventeen other newly certified patients issued an "open letter" to Tokutomi's group, accusing them of trying to mobilize public opinion to isolate the patients. This marked the beginning of the "leaflet war" fought through newspaper inserts and handbills. He accused the group of being a "mouthpiece for the company" and asked "Why do you not mention a thing about the company's responsibility for Minamata disease? . . . Has even one of you met with patients [to learn] how severe their symptoms are, how they are suffering, . . . what they think, and what they want most?" He quoted Governor Sawada's statement that there was no difference between the old and new certifications, and cited the Environment Agency's rulings to show that the new standards were clear. What caused the "social unrest" the conservatives feared, he said, was not the current increase in certifications but the previous policy of "Don't wake a sleeping child"; in other words, intentionally ignoring the existence of uncertified patients.[2]

"Part 2" of the open letter, addressed to "citizens of good sense," followed on October 30.

We have not become Minamata disease patients because we wanted to.

It is because of the mercury waste Chisso spewed from 1932 on. . . .

We will never forget that there are people who say, "You ate the fish you like and didn't care about getting the strange disease. You get money, so you can't complain about anything." . . . In our long months and years of suffering, we've learned well how to see into people's hearts.

Whether they like fish or not, what else could fishers and people who live by the sea have eaten to survive so long up to now, except for the fish they caught? . . . Why does becoming patients mean we have to be treated like people who have done something wrong? . . .

In December 1959 [we were forced to accept] ¥300,000 [$830] as the price of a life, and ¥100,000 [$280] for adults and ¥30,000 [$83] for children as the price of health.

And since then we have suffered difficulties concerning work, marriage, and friends.

And then when [Minamata disease was recognized as a] pollution disease in 1968 and when the compensation committee was established and the suit was filed in 1969, . . . we were said to be darkening the image of Minamata.

At the time of the arbitrated settlement [in May 1970], patients felt just as they had in 1959 about the annual payments they were forced to accept. . . .

One person is now in the hospital, getting the maximum of ¥380,000 [$1,100] per year. He says he wants to leave the hospital and live at home. Unfortunately he cannot live without nursing care. He could get about ¥10,000 [$29] per month for nursing expenses, but is there anyone who would be willing to do this for ¥10,000 a month for someone living on only ¥380,000 per year? . . .

We ask [the Tokutomi group] to reply publicly by November 3. . . .

Unfair though it may be, if there is no reply, although we know it will trouble you, we will visit each and every one of you at home.[3]

The Tokutomi group sent a written reply to each of the eighteen people in Kawamoto's group, but it did not directly answer any of the questions raised in the open letters. Members of the group insisted that they were acting on their own initiative and not on behalf of the company or a party.[4]

On November 1, 1971, the patients met with Chisso again, and demanded compensation of ¥30 million ($86,000) per person. This figure was taken from a pamphlet Chisso had produced and distributed to high schools in Kyūshū (causing a great deal of protest from the teachers' union). According to the pamphlet, the company estimated that the maximum paid to any one patient covered by the May 1970 arbitration agreement over his or her life-time would be "over ¥30 million."[5] Executive Director Kuga Shōichi responded to the patients' demand for ¥30 million each by saying: "If that's what you want, we won't pay even ¥10,000," and walked out.[6] The angry patients borrowed a tent from the No. 1 union and began a sit-in at the factory gate that evening. Kawamoto went on a hunger strike but ended it on doctor's orders the next day. The protesting patients were verbally and physically harassed.[7]

The propaganda war escalated, with flyers coming out daily from all the groups involved. A JSP-affiliated group joined the fray, and the JCP put out at least one flyer, but most of the groups competing for public support kept their distance from party organizations. The most intense part of the battle began with a flyer inserted in the morning newspapers on November 6 by a group of "Citizen Volunteers," asking "What's wrong with joining a petition drive (citizens' movement)?"[8] This appallingly mean-spirited, right-wing group reminded its opponents that it had just as much right as the patients and their liberal supporters to use "democratic" methods. The flyer made the crudest attacks yet on the patients, suggesting that they did not want to get well or to find appropriate work, that their tactics were unpleasant reminders of the 1962–63 strike, and that they were being used by the No. 1 union in its struggle against management. Their November 9 flyer, entitled "Patients, What Do You Think Will Be Left in Minamata If You Ruin the Company?," went even further in blaming the victims when it pretended to quote a concerned citizen: "No one has anything good to say about their demand for ¥30 million, either. It's exorbitant, people are saying, much too much to get for simple neuralgia or alcoholism." The same flyer went on to say:

In your eagerness to bring down Chisso, in your greed for money, you have traveled around the country dressed like pilgrims and made a fuss at a Chisso shareholders' meeting, creating the impression that Minamata disease still exists. *You must realize that your tactics have merely served to turn not only Chisso but also the citizens of Minamata against you. Your excessive demands are hurting other people....*

Be warned: No matter who supports you, no matter what your reasons, the citizens of Minamata will rise up as one to thwart your attempts to destroy Chisso.[9]

The Minamata Citizens' Pollution Countermeasures Association claimed on November 7 to have collected 14,111 signatures.[10] Supporters

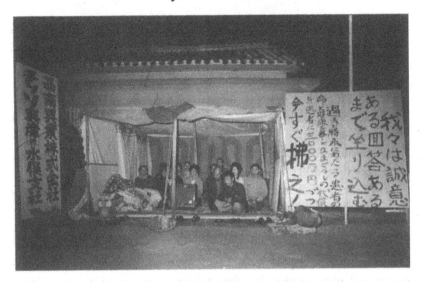

Fig. 24 Kawamoto Teruo (third from right) and other newly certified patients during their November 1971 sit-in at the factory gate, before moving to Chisso's headquarters in Tokyo. © Shiota Takeshi.

from Fukuoka and Kitakyūshū had a flyer distributed with the November 10 newspapers calling on citizens not to harass the protesting patients. A November 11 flyer from the Citizen Volunteers told the writers of the flyer from Fukuoka and Kitakyūshū to mind their own business: "The over 20,000 citizens who have signed [petitions] cannot understand those who dream of an anti-establishment movement and socialist reforms."[11]

On November 12, the two main conservative groups announced they would merge at a rally on November 14, forming the Citizens' Assembly to Brighten Minamata (Minamata o akaruku suru shimin renraku kyōgikai). The announcement said they had collected a total of 27,000 signatures (the Tokutomi group collecting 12,000, and the Ikematsu group 15,000). The mayor, who had urged them to merge, would submit their petitions to the prefectural and national governments. The new group would "absolutely exclude all political parties and factions" and serve as "an umbrella organization to promote pure citizens' groups."[12] On November 14, 500 supporters of the Direct Negotiations Group rallied outside the factory, and 1,500 people attended the founding ceremonies of the Assembly to Brighten Minamata. The vice chairman of the Arbitration Group, Nakatsu Miyoshi, attended and thanked the assembly for its concern. Chisso President Shimada Ken'ichi (who had taken over from Egashira Yutaka when Egashira moved up to become chairman July 27) also spoke, thanking the group for its support. The previous day he had announced Chisso's intention to donate ¥91 million ($261,000) to the city for the construction of new facilities for Minamata disease patients and, after the trial and compensation issues were resolved, another ¥300 million ($860,000) for a culture center.[13] Mayor Fuke Masaki declared at the rally: "Even if the opinion of the whole country is against us, we shall protect Chisso."[14]

The next day Shimada, continuing his attempts to improve Chisso's image during his visit to Minamata, visited Trial Group patients for the first time and then visited the protesters' tent. (Shimada was accompanied on this Minamata trip by two advisers from the Dentsū advertising agency.)[15] He asked them to let the Council for Control of Environmental Pollution decide their compensation and offered them an advance of ¥100,000 ($290) each against future compensation if they would agree, but they refused.[16] On November 24, Chisso asked the Council for Control of Environmental Pollution to have the eighteen families seeking direct negotiations sign agreements to accept arbitration, but the board, probably remembering the criticism of the forms signed by the Arbitration Group, hesitated.

Direct Negotiations in Tokyo

The Direct Negotiations Group finally decided it was making no progress in Minamata and would have to take the struggle to Tokyo. There, at Chisso's headquarters and the headquarters of the national government and media, away from Minamata where the balance of power still seemed to be against them, the group hoped to get results quickly. Six members, including Kawamoto and Satō Takeharu, would go to Tokyo, and the others would remain in Minamata to occupy the sit-in tent at the factory.

Two of the original eighteen families had already dropped out of the Direct Negotiations Group. The remaining members of the group had considered trying to join the plaintiffs in the trial in Kumamoto but decided that their presence would complicate the trial dangerously since Chisso insisted on treating them differently. When another patient suggested going to Chisso's head office in Tokyo, Kawamoto and Satō resisted at first, since they both had jobs in Minamata and were continuing to work during the protest. Satō, in fact, still had the Chisso factory job he had gotten after the 1960 agreement between the fishing cooperative and the company. Kawamoto changed his mind after making a short trip to Tokyo and meeting supporters there, including a group holding a sit-in in front of Chisso's headquarters, and he and five others left for Tokyo on December 5, 1971. Togashi Sadao of Kumamoto University saw Kawamoto on his way to Tokyo and remembers that Kawamoto was so confident of finishing the negotiations quickly that he had not even brought a change of clothes.[17]

On arriving at Tokyo Station the next day, Kawamoto's group and the supporters who met them at the station marched directly to Chisso's headquarters in the Tokyo Building, almost immediately outside the station exit.[18] They met briefly with Shimada on December 7, and what they expected would be substantive negotiations began in a fourth-floor conference room on the morning of December 8. Some 150 supporters, most from the Associations to Indict in Kumamoto and Tokyo, were sitting in the hall outside the meeting room. The patients restated their rejection of arbitration and their insistence on direct negotiations. Shimada, obviously concerned about the cost of compensating the growing number of certified patients and confident the Council for Control of Environmental Pollution would keep compensation levels down, repeated his insistence that the new patients were certified according to different standards and that only the review board could set appropriate compensation levels.

Kawamoto then made a dramatic gesture symbolic of the primary goal of the Direct Negotiations Group, who wanted to be recognized as human beings entitled to sit down and discuss compensation with Chisso executives as equals. He took out a razor and proposed that they cut their fingers and sign a pledge in blood to come to a sincere agreement as fellow human beings. A photograph by Miyamoto Shigemi shows Kawamoto squatting next to Shimada's chair, holding the razor, while Shimada looks away as if hoping to see a way out. Hamamoto Tsuginori of the Trial Group, there to support the new patients, holds his chin in his hand, exhausted. In the background, standing against the wall and looking over the whole scene, is Ishimure Michiko.[19]

Shimada refused, and Kawamoto, Satō Takeharu, and Ishida Masaru cut their fingers and wrote in blood: "Letter of Request: We request a sincere

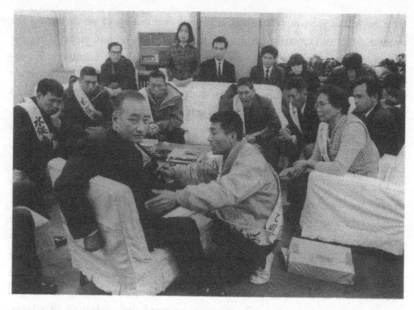

Fig. 25 Kawamoto Teruo (kneeling) holding a razor and asking Chisso President Shimada to cut his finger and sign a pledge in blood to come to agreement as equals. Seated at the extreme left, with his chin on his hand, is Hamamoto Tsuginori, one of the trial group patients. Standing at the rear is Ishimure Michiko. © Miyamoto Shigemi.

answer." The fruitless discussions continued past midnight, and some of the patients became exhausted and were examined by the four doctors among their supporters. Shimada collapsed from hypertension and was removed on a stretcher and taken to the hospital in an ambulance. As Shimada was carried out, Kawamoto clung to the stretcher, crying and telling the president how his father had died in a mental hospital. Later Kawamoto and Satō took flowers to Shimada in the hospital.[20]

The patients expected other executives to take charge of negotiations while Shimada was hospitalized, but Managing Director Irie Kanji and Executive Director Kuga Shōichi announced that only Shimada could negotiate. He would do so in Minamata when he recovered, and the patients should go home. Instead, the patients and their supporters occupied the hallway outside the president's office. On the afternoon of December 10, 1971, two squads of riot police arrived and carried the supporters out to the sidewalk, arresting three of them. Kawamoto remained in the corridor and began a hunger strike, but ended it on doctor's orders two days later. With supporters continuing to demonstrate outside, the patients decided to continue their sit-in inside the building. Letters and telegrams of support arrived from all over the country, thanks to the extensive media attention. Nearly 50 articles appeared from December 9 through December 15 in the *Asahi shinbun, Mainichi shinbun,* and *Yomiuri shinbun* about the events at Chisso headquarters, out of a total of more than 80 articles relating to the Minamata disease incident during the same period.[21] No progress had been made with Chisso, but coming to Tokyo had brought the Direct Negotiations Group far more media attention than they had ever received in Minamata.

On the same day that the Mediation Group applied to the review board, December 24, 1971, at Kuga's orders 200 employees from Chisso's Goi plant forcibly removed the 30 people who had joined the patients in their sit-in at company headquarters. Only Kawamoto and Satō, along with Ishimure, were left inside, the other patients having tired and returned to Minamata, and the two patients found themselves surrounded. Kuga appeared holding an envelope and asked them to take the money it contained to buy tickets back to Minamata. Kawamoto said he would do so only if Kuga would sign a promise to set compensation through direct negotiations. At 10:00 that night, Personnel Section chief Kawashima Tsuneya, in charge of security, ordered employees to toss Kawamoto, Satō, and Ishimure out on the street. It looked as though they would have to return home emptyhanded, just as the fishing co-op members had in 1960 when their Tokyo sit-in failed.

But things had changed since 1960. Kawamoto and Satō spent the night in the tent set up by supporters outside the Tokyo Building. The next day, they and two other patients in the tent, Komichi Tokuichi and Egoshita Kazumi, delivered a "statement of protest" to Chisso, expressing their "intense anger" and vowing never to forget.[22] They and the sit-in group in Minamata continued to demand negotiations. A group of 33 writers, critics, editors, professors, and other intellectuals, including the sociologist Hidaka Rokurō and the commentator Tanigawa Ken'ichi (from Minamata, brother of the writer Tanigawa Gan who had headed the JCP cell in Minamata), issued a statement of support for the patients on December 29. Some of them, along with the patients, Ishimure Michiko, and Honda Keikichi of the Kumamoto Association to Indict, forced their way into a meeting with Kuga that day and read a statement of protest. Two of the intellectuals, the writer Ueno Hidenobu and Harada Naō, editor of the journal *Tenbō,* staged a

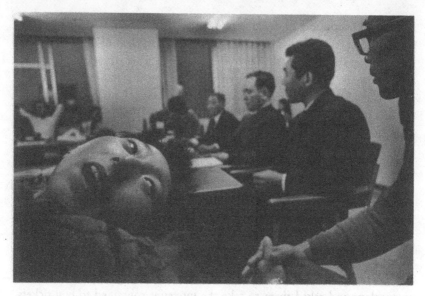

Fig. 26 Congenital victim Kamimura Tomoko was brought by her parents to court sessions, demonstrations, and meetings. Photograph by W. Eugene Smith. © Aileen M. Smith.

hunger strike in front of the Tokyo Building from December 31 to January 3.[23] Kawamoto's wife, Miyako, came to Tokyo with their two children to spend the holidays with Teruo, and they pounded *mochi* (traditional New Year's sticky rice cakes) at the protest tent. Satō's wife, Yae, confined to a wheelchair, also came up to Tokyo soon after the new year began.

And more and more often, patients in the Trial Group joined in demonstrations in Tokyo. Dr. Harada Masazumi told the parents of Kamimura Tomoko, shown being bathed by her mother in Eugene Smith's famous photograph, not to bring Tomoko to demonstrations in Tokyo and to court sessions in Kumamoto. Yet they decided they knew better and told Harada that this was the only way Tomoko could contribute to the cause. And she did have a great effect on company and government officials, as well as on the public who saw her in news reports.[24] This new stage in public visualization of the patients illustrates the growing role of the media in Japan's citizen politics.

Neither side in the direct negotiations, however, was able to find an advantage and break the stalemate. President Shimada recovered and went to Minamata on January 3, 1972. The patients protesting there insisted he must negotiate with Kawamoto and the others in Tokyo. Governor Sawada refused Shimada's request that he persuade the patients to accept mediation by the Council for Control of Environmental Pollution. He told Shimada that the newly certified patients had Minamata disease just as surely as did the old and that he ought to negotiate with them. Shimada told the press he would never again meet with the Direct Negotiations Group, either in Tokyo or in Minamata.

Kawamoto decided to meet with Natsume Hideo, the leader of the union at the Goi factory, whose workers had expelled the protesters from the Tokyo Building on December 30. Natsume agreed to meet him at Goi at 11:00 A.M. on January 7, 1972. Kawamoto, fourteen supporters, and ten reporters including Eugene and Aileen Smith went to Goi for the meeting. They waited outside the gate for two hours. Natsume never appeared, and the guards refused to let them in or to accept the petition Kawamoto asked them to deliver to Natsume.[25] Eugene Smith tells what happened next:

A newsman demanding to use a telephone to meet a deadline suddenly vaulted the iron gate. The patients' supporters, triggered by this, rushed forward. The guards, I believe, suddenly opened the gate, and the heat cooled. More waiting. More bad faith. Now it was claimed [Natsume] . . . was on his way to Tokyo. Kawamoto . . . got a promise that Natsume would telephone upon his arrival in Tokyo, at 3 o'clock. . . .

Suddenly, a mob of workers rounded a factory building to converge on the gatehouse. . . .

They hit. They hit me hardest, among the first. After my cameras, perhaps. . . . Then four men raked me across an upturned chair and thrust me into the hands of six who lifted me and slammed my head against the concrete outside, the way you would kill a rattlesnake if you had him by the tail. Then a toss outside the gate. . . .

They had made a serious mistake. The beating of a respected American journalist loosed an avalanche of unfavorable publicity upon Chisso, and it gave increased respectability to Kawamoto and the Minamata cause: if Chisso were really like this, people said, maybe the patients were right.[26]

Kawamoto was injured as well. According to Gotō Takanori, the attack was ordered by Kawashima Tsuneya, the same person who had had Kawamoto, Satō, and their supporters tossed out of the Tokyo Building two weeks earlier. Shortly after the incident, Goi union leader Natsume visited Gotō's office to explain that the workers had merely been trying to protect themselves.[27]

On January 8, the day after the Goi incident, a thousand people attended a "Minamata Disease Citizens' Assembly" (Minamatabyō shimin shūkai) called by outraged intellectuals to hear and cheer Kawamoto and the other patients and then demonstrated through downtown Tokyo, led by Satō Yae in her wheelchair.[28] Three days later, when patients and supporters went to Chisso's fourth-floor offices in the Tokyo Building, they found that the elevator no longer stopped at the fourth floor and Kawashima had had the corridor blocked off by a door made of iron bars two inches in diameter. He undoubtedly was trying to fulfill his responsibility to defend the company from angry protesters, but the bars could not protect it from ridicule. The protesters immediately printed a flyer proclaiming: "New Famous Site Appears In Tokyo!—Chisso Zoo."[29] They made good use of the bars for public relations, setting up an altar outside them for those who had died of Minamata disease and intoning prayers. Mitsubishi Real Estate, which owned the building, asked Chisso to remove the bars, since they had been installed in a public area and without permission. Chisso refused, saying they were necessary to protect its employees.

In 1959 the organized left had been distracted by its single-minded focus on opposing renewal of the United States–Japan Mutual Security Treaty and, like most of the nation, had not considered the Minamata issue significant. But now the publicity finally pushed the left-wing establishment—the Communist and Socialist parties and the Sōhyō labor federation—to move more decisively to support the Minamata activists. On January 11, Sōhyō officials called on Chisso to negotiate and asked the Environment Agency to help. The suggestion that the established opposition might try to make the Minamata issue its own prompted the government to take pre-emptive action. On January 12, Director General Ōishi Buichi of the Environment Agency announced his desire to mediate a resumption of negotiations. Chisso responded with a new tactic: if it was forced to pay more in compensation than it could afford, it wanted the government to provide financial assistance.

Kumamoto Governor Sawada Issei, having been asked by the legislature to help end the stalemate, came to Tokyo and met first with Kawamoto and Satō and then with Shimada. Ōishi met with Shimada and then with Kawamoto and Satō, who agreed with some reluctance to accept mediation by Ōishi and Sawada. Chisso then withdrew its official request that the Council for Control of Environmental Pollution arbitrate compensation for Kawamoto and the other members of the Direct Negotiations Group.

The first meeting was held at the Environment Agency on February 23, 1972, with Sawada acting as chairman and Ōishi saying little. Chisso expressed its desire for a settlement along the lines of the one accepted by the Arbitration Group in May 1970. The patients objected to that settlement's low compensation, its ranking of patients, and the fact that it did not formally acknowledge Chisso's responsibility for Minamata disease. Kuga said that Chisso's willingness to discuss compensation for the newly certified patients, even though their certification did not automatically entitle them to it, ought to convince them of the company's goodwill.

At the second meeting of the Direct Negotiations Group and Chisso, at the Environment Agency on March 8, the patients asked for an advance on compensation of ¥1 million ($3,300). Shimada responded the next day with an offer of ¥200,000 ($660), and the patients refused. On March 21, however, they reversed themselves and accepted the ¥200,000 offer. The reason for the aboutface was that events in Minamata were weakening the patients' bargaining position.

Defections and Confrontations

The Direct Negotiations Group's leverage against Chisso had been reduced by what one might expect would have strengthened them, the certification on December 16, 1971, of 29 more patients. One of the 29 was Ishida Masaru, who was in Tokyo with Kawamoto and until now had been negotiating only on behalf of his certified son. Another was Maeda Noriyoshi, who was an active LDP member and a relative of one of the people in the Arbitration Group. He persuaded 24 of the 29 to request the Council for Control of Environmental Pollution to set their compensation, and they were joined by six of the 18 certified at the same time as Kawamoto, including Kaneko Naoyoshi, who had joined the sit-in in Minamata and had been the first to suggest the move to Tokyo.

The review board established a three-member Minamata Disease Compensation Mediation Committee (Minamatabyō hoshō chōtei iinkai) on December 28. Chisso gratefully paid these more cooperative patients an advance of ¥200,000 ($570) each, and they formed a group called the Meisuikai. They became known as the "Mediation Group" (Chōteiha). Now the "new" patients, like the old, were divided into two groups. On March 2 and

3, 1972, the review board's Minamata Disease Compensation Mediation Committee visited Minamata and confirmed it was planning a settlement similar to that of May 1970.

Another split occurred in March 1972. The Minamata Fishing Cooperative had decided on February 23 to petition the government to change the name of Minamata disease. At the same time, it began to move toward expelling Ishida Masaru of the Direct Negotiations Group because it disapproved of the activists. (Neither Kawamoto nor Satō was a member of the fishing co-op.) Kawamoto received word from Minamata that Ishida would do something serious (presumably meaning he would drop out of the direct negotiations) if he (Kawamoto) did not accept Chisso's offer.

On March 24, most members of the Direct Negotiations Group met at Ishida's home in Yudō to decide whether or not to continue. The reasons for the break between those in Minamata and those in Tokyo are complex.[30] The most important was probably that the patients minding the store in Minamata felt more pressure and received less support. Ishida, in particular, very much wanted to remain in the fishing co-op, which was threatening to expel him if he did not quit the direct negotiations. He and the others in Minamata were jealous of the financial support Kawamoto and Satō were getting from backers in Tokyo, who were sending money to their families in Minamata to help make up for their lost salaries. (Kawamoto's family was receiving ¥40,000 [$130] per month from Tokyo, and Satō's ¥60,000 [$200], since he had four children and had received a higher salary.) In addition, Chisso had been treating Ishida and others of the Direct Negotiations Group in Minamata, as well as some people from the Trial Group, to visits to hot spring resorts. Kawamoto and Satō returned to Minamata for the meeting but failed to persuade Ishida and the others to stay the course.

Only Kawamoto and Satō, it seemed, were left. They returned to Kawamoto's home after midnight and opened a bottle of shōchū (a distilled liquor that is especially popular in southern Kyūshū, where it is too warm to brew sake). After talking and drinking much of the night, Satō insisted that they should continue the negotiations, even if it was just the two of them, but that they should try to get the others to reconsider.[31] He went from house to house the next day arranging another meeting for March 28. Twelve people attended and decided to continue the negotiations. Only four people, including Ishida and his son, stuck with their decision to give up. These dropouts had been defeated by the pressures brought to bear on them in Minamata and became known as the "Middle Group" (Chūkanha), pursuing neither direct negotiations nor mediation. So the "newly certified patients" were now divided into *three* groups.

The patients continuing negotiations decided to reduce their demand for ¥30 million to bring it more in line with the amounts demanded by the Trial Group patients. They asked Chisso for ¥18 million ($59,400) for patients, ¥6 million ($19,800) for spouses, and ¥3 million ($9,900) for children of patients. The company refused to discuss specific amounts, insisting on the need for a ranking system. The talks at the Environment Agency were effectively ended when Ōishi canceled the next scheduled meeting due to Chisso's inflexible attitude. Governor Sawada agreed on July 19 with Koyama Osanori, who replaced Ōishi as head of the Environment Agency when the Tanaka Kakuei cabinet took office July 7, to officially suspend the talks.

The company believed, with good reason, that the Council for Control of Environmental Pollution's Minamata Disease Compensation Mediation Committee would give it the best possible settlement. With certifications continuing—21 new certifications on June 3 brought the total to 202, with 41 more July 27, 49 on October 6, and 52 on December 5—and no response to its suggestion that the government might need to help it pay compensation, Chisso was especially concerned to keep compensation levels low.[32] The Direct Negotiations Group maintained its presence and daily pressure on Chisso, but from the spring of 1972 the focus shifted to the mediation committee and the trial. If the committee finished its work first, the company hoped, and the activist patients feared, that the lower compensation levels it was certain to set would hold down the amounts those in the Trial Group and Direct Negotiations Group would receive. Equally important, if the mediation committee's solution set the pattern, Chisso's responsibility for causing the disease might not be clarified in the settlements.

The Trial Group and the Direct Negotiations Group began cooperating more closely, holding a joint demonstration for "victory in the Minamata disease struggle" with the Citizens' Council and the Association to Indict on July 2 in Minamata. Part of the reason for this increased cooperation was that many of the patients now being certified were relatives of members of the Trial Group. With the end of the trial in sight—testimony finished on October 14, 1972—a number of these newly certified patients joined the Direct Negotiations Group rather than joining the plaintiffs in the trial.

In Tokyo, minor incidents of violence between Chisso employees and the patients and their supporters increased, perhaps out of the frustration both sides felt. On July 19, a toe on Kawamoto's left foot was broken. In another struggle on July 21, Kawamoto removed the splint from his toe and hit Personnel Section chief Kawashima on the head with it, giving him a contusion. The company filed charges against Kawamoto and published a pamphlet entitled "The Truth about the Direct Negotiations Group and Their 'Supporters'" with photographs and text to show that Kawamoto and his group had used violence against Chisso employees.[33] The patients, of course, pointed to the Goi incident and the mercury poisoning itself to argue that the serious violence had been committed by the company.

Both carrots and sticks were used by Chisso. At the urging of Environment Agency director Koyama, it met once more with the Direct Negotiations Group on October 19, when Kawamoto asked for an advance compensation payment of ¥200,000 ($660) per patient. Surprisingly, on November 20 the company paid the money to all 158 "newly certified patients" without requiring the patients to promise anything in return. On October 31, however, Kawamoto was forcibly taken to the Marunouchi police station for questioning concerning Chisso's charge that he had attacked Kawashima (who had a fifth-level black belt in *judō*). The police then searched the Tokyo supporter's home in which Kawamoto was staying, as well as Kawamoto's home in Minamata, and seized the splint as evidence. On November 14, Kawamoto was called to the Tokyo District Public Prosecutor's office and told to take down the tent and go home.

Kawamoto remained in Tokyo, and on December 27, 1972, he asked Miki Takeo, the new Environment Agency director (and future prime minister, December 1974 to December 1976) to mediate a reopening of negotiations with Chisso. Miki promised to intercede. The public prosecutor indicted Kawamoto that same day, charging him with four counts of inflicting bodily injury on Kawashima and other Chisso employees between July 19 and July 21 and one count of inflicting bodily injury on Kawashima on October 25.

The Mediation Group and the Forgery Incident

As of the end of 1972, 328 Minamata disease patients had been certified in Kumamoto prefecture and 16 in Kagoshima.[34] It was looking more and more likely that the mediation committee (whose parent organization, the Council for Control of Environmental Pollution, had been replaced by the Environmental Dispute Coordination Commission [Kōgai nado chōsei iinkai] on July 1) would complete its compensation plan before the trial ended, and the Trial Group and Direct Negotiations group saw no way to prevent this. In August, the Mediation Group patients and Chisso had agreed to the committee's suggestion that the patients be ranked for compensation purposes according to their symptoms. On December 12, the committee announced that its proposed settlement would be ready early in 1973. This meant the agreement with the Mediation Group might well be signed before the Kumamoto District Court issued its verdict.

A discovery by Kawamoto prevented this and thereby guaranteed that the court verdict, and not the mediation plan, would set the pattern for compensation.[35] On December 11, 1972, when the mediation committee was at the Minamata city hall holding hearings with patients in the Mediation Group, Kawamoto, other members of the Direct Negotiations Group, and some from the Trial Group went to city hall to request a meeting with the committee. They intended to petition them not to issue their compensation plan before the verdict. Their concern was that if there were two different sets of standards for compensation, Chisso would use this as an excuse to appeal the court verdict, and so resolution would be delayed and the final settlement would be lower than that ordered by the court. When the committee left the room for lunch, Kawamoto noticed that the documents they had left on the table were the official requests from patients for the committee to mediate their compensation. He noticed that all the names were written in the same handwriting. Kawamoto asked several people who had applied for mediation to look at the applications, and all said they had never seen such documents.

On December 28, 1972, the day after his indictment, Kawamoto visited Gotō and asked him to go to the Environmental Dispute Coordination Commission to investigate the apparently forged documents. They went on January 10, accompanying two patients who had applied for mediation and who now asked to see the applications and the forms giving representatives power of attorney to accept a settlement. After seven hours of negotiations, the two applicants and Gotō, acting as their lawyer, were allowed to see the documents while Kawamoto waited in a separate room. Not only were the names of all the applicants written in the same handwriting (which could simply have meant that someone had filled out the forms for them), but there were mistakes in many names and addresses, some names had been blacked out, and in some cases no seal had been affixed next to the names. Gotō had brought samples of some of the applicants' handwriting and seals and could see immediately that many of the documents had been forged. The forms designating representatives for 147 patients gave power of attorney to twelve people, including Maeda Noriyoshi. They were given power to conduct "all procedures, including withdrawal of applications and acceptance of the proposed settlement."[36] In fact, each of the twelve representatives was empowered to do all of these things his own. One of the patients with Gotō, Ogata Shizue, said she had no memory of filling out either form and announced on the spot that she wished to have her application withdrawn. The other patient said he had never affixed his seal to the documents.

On January 22, Kawamoto, Gotō, and four patients in the Mediation Group pushed their way into a meeting of the executive committee of the Environmental Dispute Coordination Commission. They found the committee had documents by which 80 other patients had supposedly given power of attorney to five representatives. On these documents, too, some of the names lacked seals, and there was even one person listed as having applied after his death. Kawamoto was so angry that Gotō had to restrain him. The chairman of the committee, Igarashi Yoshiaki, finally agreed to go to Minamata to investigate.

The investigation showed that of 144 applicants, 115 confirmed that they had designated representatives to negotiate on their behalf, but nineteen of these said they had not intended to give their representatives the power to decide on compensation levels by themselves. Sixteen applicants said they had never given anyone power of attorney, and eleven said they did not know if they had. It was later discovered that the applications and power-of-attorney forms had been forged at the committee's direction by the Pollution Section in the Minamata city hall. The committee maintained that even if the patients had not filled out the forms themselves, the papers still represented the wishes of the patients, and that sympathetic officials had only filled them out on behalf of the patients to save them trouble. As Gotō points out, however, since each patient had received ¥200,000 ($660) from Chisso in return for filing an application, even those whose applications were legitimate had been under financial pressure to submit them. Furthermore, most did not intend to grant their representatives such broad rights and did not realize they had done so.

On January 23, the same day the committee began its investigation in Minamata, the Kumamoto District Court announced that it would hand down a verdict March 20. When Ozawa Fumio replaced Igarashi as chairman of the committee on February 3, the committee sent a letter to all applicants for mediation saying it would not be able to prepare a mediation proposal before the March 20 verdict. So because of the bizarre incident of the forged documents, the committee had failed to do what it had been established to do: quiet the fuss over Minamata disease by compensating most of the victims at a relatively low level, without trumpeting the company's responsibility for the disease, before the court verdict.

The Trial: Proving Negligence

The trial took place, as trials normally do, in a controlled atmosphere according to prescribed procedures, conducted by lawyers as proxies for the company and patients. It stretched from June 14, 1969, to March 20, 1973, and was rarely as dramatic as the direct negotiations, the one-share movement, and the other events in Minamata and Tokyo. Yet it was at least as important in determining the shape of the settlement ultimately put together in the summer of 1973. And despite the trial lawyers' views, actions outside the court undoubtedly helped the Trial Group win its case.

There were three points at issue in the trial. First, was Chisso guilty of negligence in discharging the organic mercury that caused Minamata disease? It was not difficult to prove in court what the government had finally acknowledged in September 1968: that Chisso had discharged the mercury, and that the mercury had caused the disease. But could and should the company have anticipated what would happen, and was it legally at fault for not taking steps to prevent the tragedy? Second, even if Chisso had been negligent in causing Minamata disease, was the December 30, 1959, solatium agreement a legally binding contract that prevented the victims from demanding further compensation? Finally, only if these first two points were decided in the plaintiffs' favor could a third point be argued: what sort of compensation, and how much, should Chisso be required to pay the victims?

The weakness and narrow scope of the plaintiffs' lawyers' first brief, filed on July 31, 1969, worried many of the patients and their supporters in the Citizens' Council and the Association to Indict. The young lawyers had chosen not to make a broad attack on Chisso and its responsibility for the tragedy it had caused, knowing that corporate negligence was difficult to prove and that only after Minamata disease was discovered had strict legal limits been imposed on factory waste. Instead, they charged Chisso with violating the Law for the Control of Poisonous and Powerful Substances.

Such a strategy might bring a victory, but if it brought financial compensation without a clear and sweeping indictment of Chisso for the disaster it had perpetrated and perpetuated, the patients would not feel vindicated. It would not be the *moral* victory they wanted as much as money, after suffering for so long physically, economically, and socially. The team within the Citizens' Council in charge of assisting the Trial Group patients and lawyers considered the brief weak and consulted legal experts who agreed. These concerns prompted the Citizens' Council and the Association to Indict to decide a study group was needed to provide the expertise necessary for a strong legal case against Chisso. Watanabe Kyōji of the Association to Indict visited Togashi Sadao of Kumamoto University's law faculty in August and asked him to help.[37]

A Trial Research Group was formed on September 7, 1969, and changed its name to the Minamata Disease Research Group in December. Except for Harada Masazumi, most members of the group had little direct knowledge of Minamata disease, and they began their work by studying Ui Jun's collection of materials covering the Minamata disease incident up to 1968 (published in 1969 by the Association to Indict), and medical reports from Kumamoto University.[38] They began working on a report that became the basis for the successful court case, dividing themselves into teams with responsibilities for different areas, as had the Citizens' Council in Minamata. The whole group met in the evenings three times per month or so and had to work quickly. *Corporate Responsibility for Minamata Disease: Chisso's Illegal Acts* (Minamatabyō ni tai suru kigyō no sekinin: Chisso no fuhō kōi; 385 pp.) was published by the Association to Indict in August 1970. It was far more than a dry legal brief, and in fact it was the contributions by others that made law professor Togashi Sadao's argument for Chisso's negligence so forceful.

Corporate Responsibility begins with a section entitled "The Frightful Facts of Minamata Disease." The first chapter is a medical description of the disease by Harada Masazumi. This is followed by an eloquent description of the patients' lives by Ishimure Michiko, whose writings had helped Harada to see his patients as more than names on medical charts. In March 1970,

Ishimure refused the first Ōya Prize for her book *Kugai jōdo*, explaining that she was too busy working on *Corporate Responsibility* and did not want to appear to be profiting from the patients' suffering.

The second part of *Corporate Responsibility* is a scientific explanation of the cause of Minamata disease, based on the research by Kumamoto University. In the third part, Togashi Sadao carefully makes his case for Chisso's negligence.[39] The most fundamental cause of Minamata disease, he says, is the fact that "Chisso is a model of a corporation than ignores safety. The sort of results that can be expected when a company such as this operates an inherently dangerous chemical factory is shown by the industrial accidents at the Minamata factory and its past history of environmental pollution. Because of this, the occurrence of Minamata disease was inevitable." Chisso did not conduct the research necessary to ensure safety, even after the disease was identified and the factory was suspected to be the cause, even though the need for waste treatment was already well understood at the time and it was already known that poisons could be concentrated in the food chain. "Yet even after Minamata disease was officially discovered and became a serious social issue, Chisso continued to insist that it could not have been foreseen." It continued to discharge its waste untreated, installing treatment facilities only when forced to. These did not remove the poison, which continued to be discharged until acetaldehyde production ended in 1968. The company argues that it used better waste-control technology than was standard at the time, but whether this is true or not, it does not excuse Chisso of the responsibility it had for foreseeing and preventing the harm it caused.[40] The fourth and final section of *Corporate Responsibility* shows how Chisso not only neglected to investigate the cause of Minamata disease but intentionally hindered, confused, and delayed the efforts of outside researchers, particularly those from Kumamoto University.

Proving Chisso's negligence required what Togashi calls a "paradigm shift" in established Japanese legal interpretations, but Togashi could find no models for his new concept.[41] He finally hit on one when he read about the debates in the 1950s over banning atmospheric testing of nuclear weapons. Some scientists and the United States government had argued that low-level atmospheric radioactive pollution posed no significant danger to human health. Japanese scientists and citizens were naturally quite concerned with the issue, because of the bombings of Hiroshima and Nagasaki and because of the 1954 "Lucky Dragon incident." A Japanese fishing boat, the *Lucky*

Dragon no. 5 (Dai go Fukuryū maru), had been showered with radioactive fall-out from a U.S. hydrogen bomb test at Bikini Atoll. The issue was resolved in a way remarkably similar to what had happened in Minamata in 1959: the United States gave a sympathy payment of ¥1 million ($2,800) to the widow of the one crewman who had died and ¥2 million ($5,600) to the Japanese government to compensate for all damages caused in this and other incidents, without officially admitting responsibility.

A well-known Japanese theoretical physicist named Taketani Mitsuo had argued that the effects of long-term, low-level exposure to atmospheric radiation were unknown and that the possibility of danger could not be denied.[42] Taketani reversed the argument that the tests were allowable as long as there was no proof at the time that they were dangerous. He asserted that if there were no proof that they were safe, then they were unacceptable. Reading these arguments, Togashi realized that a similar logic could be applied to the Minamata case, and in *Corporate Responsibility* he attempted to give it a legal foundation. Only this kind of indictment of Chisso's negligence, he believed, would not just convict Chisso and make it pay but also create a precedent for the future protection of Japanese citizens and their environment.

Drafts of the Minamata Disease Research Group's report were shown to a number of people, including the trial group's lawyers. The lawyers, who had earlier criticized the research group as "a bunch of Trotskyites," asked the Association to Indict not to publish it. Here the division of opinion was the same as that over the one-share movement: the trial lawyers wanted the struggle controlled and confined to the court, whereas the Association to Indict insisted that the fight must be waged on the larger battleground of the public sphere. They published 5,000 copies of *Corporate Negligence* in August 1970. The lawyers then submitted a fourth brief that plagiarized, errors and all, the draft of *Corporate Negligence* and then quickly withdrew it. Nevertheless, the research group report set the terms of the courtroom debate and the lawyers' strategy.[43] The trial lawyers simply lacked the expertise and creativity of the research group. *Corporate Negligence*, they reluctantly recognized, provided a winning strategy and the detail to support it.

The first testimony in the case was not heard until October 15, 1969. The patients entered the court carrying pictures of family members who had died of Minamata disease, and later there was a demonstration. This was the usual pattern of activity for them throughout the trial. They testified, but much of their time in court was spent simply listening. Since the main issues were whether Chisso had been negligent and whether the solatium contract prohibited the patients from demanding further compensation, the most important testimony came from Chisso executives and workers. How or whether Judge Saitō Jirō would accept the arguments concerning Chisso's negligence was uncertain at first. The Supreme Court sponsored a conference in Tokyo of judges in pollution cases on March 12 and 13, 1970, and on March 20 a Supreme Court official announced that the courts would admit testimony concerning involuntary corporate negligence, opening the way for the lawyers to use Togashi's arguments.[44]

Perhaps the most dramatic and damaging testimony for Chisso was by Hosokawa Hajime, who testified from his hospital bed on July 4, 1970, as he was dying of cancer. He told of his cat experiments, including the one in which cat no. 400 developed Minamata disease after being fed acetaldehyde waste in 1959. He stated that this confirmed that factory waste caused Minamata disease and that he had informed factory executives of this. He also said he had opposed the 1958 switch in the acetaldehyde waste outfall from Minamata Bay to the mouth of the Minamata River.[45] Hosokawa died three months after his testimony.

Other testimony from Chisso attempted to refute Hosokawa, but in June 1972 a doctor who had worked with him, Kojima Akikazu, supported Hosokawa's testimony by saying they had both been relatively certain that cat no. 400 had Minamata disease, and that company officials had ordered Hosokawa to halt his experiments in the fall of 1959. In August 1970, Chisso was forced to submit documents on approximately 1,000 cat experiments conducted from 1957 to 1962. However, in a pamphlet printed in July 1970, mainly for internal circulation, it resurrected the theory that pesticides had caused Minamata disease.[46]

Testifying in February 1971, however, former factory manager Nishida Eiichi admitted that the methyl mercury in the acetaldehyde factory's waste had caused Minamata disease. A month later, he testified that he had known by around 1954 that there was a causal connection between the factory waste and the damage to fishing but had not investigated. In May, he admitted that working conditions at the factory were dangerous because it put profits ahead of safety and that it should have been more careful with mercury. In August, former Chisso president Yoshioka Kiichi testified that the company had promoted the theory that explosives caused the disease even though it knew that the idea was unfounded. A former assistant section chief in the Research Division even testified in April 1972 that company researchers had found in March 1962, before the newspaper reports of Kumamoto University's similar discovery, that methyl mercury was produced in the production process.

Part of the explanation for these rather remarkable admissions is tactical: Chisso expected to lose the case and may have hoped that by showing some openness and contrition it could prevent the settlement from being too punitive. Japanese courts tend to give much lighter punishments to those who confess their guilt and show contrition. But there may also be a psychological explanation: as with the "conversion" (tenkō) phenomenon of arrested Communists repudiating their beliefs before and during World War II, one confession may have triggered another.

Former governor Teramoto Hirosaku was called to testify on June 26, 1972, about the December 1959 solatium agreement he had helped bring about and spoke of how the company had withheld information: "We put together the mediated settlement without knowing the facts. Looking back on it now, it was not enough."[47] Despite its efforts in court to appear to be no longer hiding anything, Chisso still seemed unwilling to divulge how much mercury it had dumped. Kumamoto prefecture asked for statistics from the company, and on August 3, 1972, Chisso reported that between 1945 and 1968 it had used 856.8 metric tons of mercury, losing 57.4 tons of this, in acetaldehyde production (which had begun in 1932). It also said that in vinyl chloride production from 1941 to 1970, it had used 132.2 tons of mercury and reclaimed all but 215.2 kilograms. After the legislature expressed its dissatisfaction with these figures and moved to investigate, on September 22 Chisso revised its figures. It now said that in producing 456,352 tons of acetaldehyde from 1932 to 1968, it had used 1,185 tons of mercury and discharged 81.3 tons of it into the ocean. In producing 509,725 tons of vinyl chloride from 1941 to 1971, it had used 132 tons of mercury and lost 212.2 kilograms.[48] MITI, which is not known for exaggerating the magnitude of pollution by Japanese factories, estimated in July 1973 that Chisso had lost a total of 224.4 tons of mercury.[49] Other estimates have ranged up to 600 tons.

The revelations inside and outside the court, the shifting of public opinion to favor the patients, and especially the September 29, 1971, victory of the Niigata patients all made it seem likely that the Kumamoto patients would win. The awards to Niigata patients were ¥10 million ($28,600) to deceased and congenital patients, between ¥1 million and ¥10 million ($2,860 to $28,600) to surviving patients (divided into five ranks according to symptoms), ¥400,000 ($1,145) to people found to be contaminated with a significant amount of mercury, and ¥300,000 ($858) to women who had been "advised" to have abortions due to the danger mercury posed to their fetuses. The Niigata verdict is often cited as crucial to the Kumamoto trial because it set a precedent for court acceptance of the concept of negligence. As explained earlier, however, it was much easier to prove negligence in the Niigata case since the disease had been discovered in Minamata first. Nevertheless, it would have been difficult for any judge to refuse compensation to the patients in Minamata after those in Niigata had been awarded it.

Toward the end of the trial, concern focused on the amount and type of compensation that would be awarded to the patients if they won. Harada Masazumi testified in September 1972 that it was medically difficult to rank patients according to the severity of their symptoms. A specialist from Niigata testified that the symptoms of the certified patients in Kumamoto were worse than those of Niigata patients and that previously unknown patients were not being discovered, examined, and certified in Kumamoto nearly as well as in Niigata. The two sides finished their closing arguments by mid-October 1972. Chisso bowed to pressure and promised on March 18, 1973, two days before the verdict, that it would not appeal and would obey the ruling.

As the verdict approached, the split between the lawyers on the one hand and the Trial Group patients, the Direct Negotiations Group, and their supporters in the Citizens' Council and the Association to Indict on the other hand widened and became more public. On January 20, 1973, the lawyers filed a second suit in the Kumamoto District Court on behalf of 141 patients and family members. Among the plaintiffs were 34 uncertified patients, the first time uncertified patients had gone to court. There were also ten "newly certified patients," meaning that there was now a third group among the new patients—in addition to the Mediation Group and the Middle Group—that had decided not to follow Kawamoto in his direct negotiations. On March 12, the Association to Indict resigned from the Prefectural Citizens' Council, which remained closer to the lawyers.

The split, which until very late had not been visible even to close observers such as the Smiths, became clear in the two weeks before the verdict.[50]

On March 8, the Trial Group and Direct Negotiations Group met with the lawyers to discuss post-verdict strategy. The itai-itai disease patients in Toyama had negotiated a compensation agreement directly with the Mitsui Metal Mining Company after their court victory, and patients in Niigata were negotiating one with Shōwa denkō. After the Kumamoto verdict, negotiations would have to be conducted with Chisso to finalize a compensation agreement and to try to get the agreement applied to both the Trial Group and the Direct Negotiations Group. The lawyers preferred to conduct the negotiations themselves, perhaps with the support of Diet members. To the Trial Group, this sounded too much like the mediation procedures that led to the 1959 solatium agreement. They had sued precisely to keep matters in their own hands and avoid repeating that experience. Likewise, the Direct Negotiations Group existed because its members were unwilling to delegate authority to outsiders to negotiate their compensation. On March 15, the Trial Group patients met and voted to conduct the negotiations with Chisso in Tokyo directly and not through the lawyers.

There was great relief but little celebration among the patients at the Kumamoto District Court when they won their suit on March 20, 1973. That Togashi's argument in *Corporate Negligence* had carried the day was evident from the verdict read by Judge Saitō:

The defendant's factory was a leading chemical plant with the most advanced technology and facilities. As such, the defendant should have diligently researched the relevant literature and should have assured the safety of its wastewater. . . . Also the defendant should have cast a watchful eye on the environmental conditions of the area. . . . Defendants should have made sure that no harm whatsoever came to the residents in the area. . . . It would have been possible to foresee the risk from the discharged water. . . . The defendant could have prevented the occurrence of Minamata disease or at least have kept it at a minimum. We cannot find that the defendant took any of the precautionary measures called for in this situation whatsoever. . . . We cannot find even one measure taken by the defendant that was either adequate or satisfactory. . . .

The presumption that the defendant had been negligent from beginning to end in discharging wastewater from its acetaldehyde plant is amply supported. Even if the quality of wastewater was within legal and administrative standards and the facilities and methods of treatment . . . were superior to those of other factories in the same industry, it is not enough to overcome this presumption. . . . The defendant cannot escape liability for negligence. . . .[51]

The solatium agreement was found to be invalid, and a violation of public order. Chisso was ordered to make one-time payments of ¥18 million ($66,000) for each deceased patient and from ¥16 million to ¥18 million ($59,000 to $66,000) to each surviving patient, for a total of ¥937,300,000 ($3.44 million)—the largest compensation that had ever been awarded by a Japanese court.

After the Verdict: Negotiating from a Position of Strength

The importance of the court victory for the patients in the Trial Group went beyond financial compensation. To them, the court victory meant recognition that their complaints were just and that they were owed restitution by a system that had no right to exclude them. To some of the patients, the victory meant that they had used its own laws to force an oppressive capitalist system, which had attempted to exclude them and to sacrifice them on the altar of growth, to recognize their existence and compensate them. This was certainly the way Watanabe Eizō had spoken of the trial from the day the suit was filed; it was also the view presented by Ui Jun in *Kōgai no seijigaku*. Other patients, or perhaps even some of the same ones at different times, saw the victory as recognition by "those above" (*okami*), in a hierarchical society, that the victims had suffered unjustly. All felt that their honor and dignity had been restored, but none could ever forget that their disease could not be cured.

The day of the verdict, the Association to Indict distributed a flyer announcing its break with the lawyers. Among other accusations, the Association to Indict charged the lawyers with publishing patients' testimony without their permission. Their first brief had foolishly charged Chisso with violating the Law for the Control of Poisonous and Powerful Substances, even though that law had not covered mercury until later. The fourth brief, withdrawn soon after it was submitted, had plagiarized from a draft of *Corporate Responsibility* that the Minamata Disease Research Group had asked the lawyers to comment on. This was done despite the fact that the lawyers had opposed the research group's activities and asked it to keep *Corporate Responsibility* secret. Their second brief, too, had plagiarized parts of an interim report by the research group. The lawyers had done a poor job of choosing and questioning witnesses, attempting, for example, to ask factory workers about upper management decisions. Former factory manager Nishida had been called to testify only because of a suggestion by someone outside the lawyers' group. The Association to Indict continued:

We could give numerous examples of how we have had to bite our tongues and keep silent over the past four years. . . . We have endured the unendurable so as not to disrupt the trial while it was in progress. And now after the trial, without consulting the patients and their families, the lawyers are planning to force their way into the patients' group negotiations and divert the Minamata disease struggle. We cannot help feeling the Minamata disease struggle is in grave danger of being destroyed, as the lawyers' stand continues to be one of guiding the "ignorant patients," even after the verdict. And the Prefectural Citizens' Council thinks the same way as the lawyers.

This is the reason we had to leave the Prefectural Citizens' Council. We reject interference by those who would attempt to guide the Minamata disease struggle. . . . We . . . oppose attempts to bring the Minamata disease struggle under the control of a particular party or faction.[52]

As their decision on March 15 indicated, the patients did not see the trial victory as the final resolution of their complaints. In a way, it was the beginning, since they did not intend to accept only the compensation ordered by the court. Instead, they felt the verdict had proved them right and Chisso wrong and therefore gave them the legal, political, and social power and right to negotiate a fuller settlement directly with Chisso by themselves, without lawyers or compensation committees taking control of the process.

Chisso, too, had to accept this premise, and to negotiate jointly with the Trial Group and the Direct Negotiations Group, because the company was in a relatively weak position.[53] It had agreed not to appeal the verdict partly because the Minamata Disease Compensation Mediation Committee had not completed its plan in time. Had it done so, Chisso could have argued that the court-ordered settlement was unreasonably large by comparison. Instead, Mediation Group patients had told the press that they, too, would ask Chisso to negotiate compensation directly, and on March 27 they officially voted to do so. Even the Arbitration Group, which had accepted a settlement in May 1970, announced that it would demand to be paid the difference between its settlement and the amounts given to the Trial Group, and on March 24 Chisso agreed to pay them the compensation the court had ordered.

The Trial and Direct Negotiations groups formed a Minamata Disease Tokyo Negotiations Group (Minamatabyō Tokyo kōshōdan) immediately after the verdict and chose Tanoue Yoshiharu to lead it. Tanoue, one of the first designated patients in 1956, was a childhood friend of Kawamoto. The negotiators and their supporters left that night for Tokyo. The patients' position was that the court-ordered payments were compensation only for past suffering. Chisso should also pay all their living expenses and medical costs from now on and should compensate all certified patients, not just those in the Trial Group.

The negotiations began on the morning of March 22, 1973, at company headquarters in Tokyo.[54] Because the patients had been victorious in court, the atmosphere was different from past meetings, but as before, patients, supporters, and reporters crowded the room. Tsuchimoto Noriaki was there also, holding a microphone near the company president while a cameraman filmed the discussions. The first few days saw some of the most dramatic scenes of the entire Minamata disease incident. Tanoue Yoshiharu began by reading aloud a "pledge" (seiyakusho) that Kawamoto had written the previous night for President Shimada to sign: "The Chisso Corporation has declared that it will not exercise its right to appeal the March 20, 1973, verdict of the Kumamoto District Court. Therefore, based on the verdict we admit our full responsibility, and hereafter we will in good faith make compensation for all matters relating to Minamata disease."[55]

Tanoue asked Shimada to stamp the pledge with his seal and sign his name. For a moment it looked as if he would, but Executive Director Kuga Shōichi, who was at Shimada's side, stopped him. They consulted and then suggested adding the words "to the best of our ability" after "make compensation." Congenital Minamata disease patient Sakamoto Shinobu picked up a pen in her bent fingers and tried to hand it to Shimada, bowing her head and begging "Please!" Kuga wiped the sweat off Shimada's brow.

In a reversal of the behavior Minamata and its citizens had been accustomed to for 65 years, the executives used exceptionally polite language, and the increasingly angry patients spoke plain, direct, and even rude Japanese. For this short period after the trial, the tone of the discourse reflected a reversal rather than an elimination of the hierarchy between the two sides. The patients were addressed as superiors and the executives as inferiors. Kawamoto Teruo was one of the few who rarely changed his speaking style: he spoke to Shimada in a plain, direct manner, as an equal, even though Shimada continued to address Kawamoto in an honorific manner.

The stalemate continued through the afternoon, with Shimada and Kuga insisting that unless they could qualify their pledge, the company might go bankrupt and then be unable to compensate the patients who would be certified later. They finally gave in when Hiyoshi Fumiko, the head of the Citizens' Council, begged Shimada to sign, bowing low and saying: "No one in Minamata wants to bankrupt the company. . . . You've never trusted us, have you? Just this once, show that you trust us. Then no one will ask you to do anything impossible. . . . Everyone in Minamata really likes Chisso." At this, some members of the Association to Indict walked out, incensed that anyone should have groveled before Shimada. But Hiyoshi's tactic worked, and the tension was temporarily relieved. Shimada signed the pledge as originally worded, bowed his head to the patients, and said: "I'm sorry to have caused you so much trouble."[56]

The next day, March 23, the negotiations were held on the fourth floor. Symbolizing the new mood, the iron bars protecting the offices had been removed, and the elevator once again stopped at the fourth floor. Patients hoped an agreement could be reached quickly, but when they presented their specific demands, the negotiations quickly came to another impasse. The patients wanted Chisso to compensate all patients, to pay all their medical costs, and to pay each patient an annuity of ¥720,000 ($2,600) per year to cover living costs. Kawamoto forced some progress the next day when he got Shimada to agree to pay compensation for a deceased patient who had had to withdraw from the suit because he had not been certified. He had died before being certified, but the head of the certification committee, Takeuchi Tadao, had just announced that an autopsy showed that the patient had in fact had Minamata disease. Shimada's agreement to pay compensation for this patient set a precedent for compensating the "newly certified patients" such as Kawamoto.

Kawamoto pushed Shimada further on March 25 when he asked him to pay compensation, according to the court verdict, for two of the newly certified patients who had died. Kawamoto sat in front of Shimada for hours, at times sitting on the table directly in front of him, and spoke quietly about his work since 1969 trying to find uncertified patients and persuade them to apply. More than any other patient, Kawamoto seemed intent on forcing Shimada to understand his suffering and treat him as an equal. He asked Shimada about his religion (Zen Buddhism), his wife's religion (Catholi-

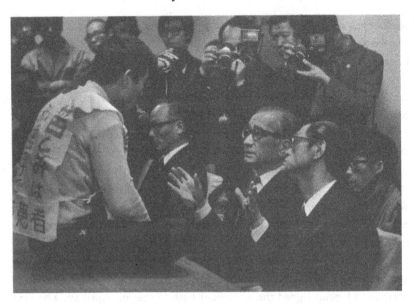

Fig. 27 Kawamoto Teruo (on table) speaking with Chisso President Shimada in the "Tokyo Negotiations," 1973. Photograph by Aileen M. Smith. © Aileen M. Smith.

cism; Shimada, too, was later baptized a Catholic), and his children and their hobbies. He asked him what sort of religious books he read, and whether the ideas in the books had anything to do with the deaths of these two patients.

Shimada asked Kawamoto to wait until March 28 for an answer, but Kawamoto insisted he should explain why a delay was necessary. At 4:00 the next morning, Shimada finally asked for a break. He and Kuga went out to discuss things, and when they returned over two hours later, Shimada announced that the families of each of the two deceased patients would be paid ¥18 million ($66,000), the amount prescribed by the court for the trial patients. Now it seemed that Chisso would have to agree to compensate all patients, from all groups, in the same way.

The next hurdle was the question of living expenses. Chisso held fast to its insistence that it would make only the one-time payments required by the court. On April 5, the company announced what it said was its final offer: it would pay all certified patients the ¥16–18 million mandated by the court decision, but not annuities or medical costs. It continued to maintain this stance even after the Industrial Bank of Japan and other banks it dealt with promised the company long-term, low-interest loans. The negotiations were suspended after April 15.

On April 25, the Minamata Disease Compensation Mediation Committee finally announced its much-delayed, and now much more expensive, plan. It suggested that ¥18 million ($66,000) be paid for each death, between ¥16 million and ¥18 million ($59,000 to $66,000) to each surviving patient, and between ¥1 million and ¥4.5 million ($3,700 to $16,600) to each family with a severely afflicted patient. It also proposed that patients be paid between ¥180,000 and ¥720,000 ($660 to $2,600) per year for living expenses. Rather than proposing a plan that undercut the court verdict, the committee now had been forced to produce one that expanded on it. It could hardly suggest lower figures than the court, and the committee members may well have felt that they could take the lead in resolving the dispute by proposing annual payments, which now seemed unavoidable. Thirty patients from the Mediation Group signed the agreement with Chisso on April 27. The next day, all of the certified patients suing Chisso in the second trial withdrew from the suit, turning the trial into one of only uncertified patients versus Chisso. Those who withdrew signed an agreement with the company that it would compensate them according to the verdict in the first suit.

The company was still unable to make an agreement with the Trial and Direct Negotiations groups, and on May 5 Chisso literally tried to run away from the bargaining table. Without notice, the company vacated its headquarters offices and began operating from temporary office space in several locations in Tokyo. The Negotiation Group then occupied the empty company offices, while Chisso tried to save itself by finding a sympathetic mediator, a tactic that had worked well for it in the past. Miki Takeo, still head of the Environment Agency, began trying to work out a settlement.

In the meantime, public concern was heightened by a scare over a "third Minamata disease," which the May 22 issue of the *Asahi shinbun* reported had broken out in the Ariake Sea to the north of the Shiranui Sea. The cause was believed to be an acetaldehyde plant in Uto. Although many experts still believe Minamata disease did in fact occur in the area, the government eventually concluded it had not. However, on June 18, the scare and the news of the compensation Minamata victims were getting prompted 30 fishing cooperatives in the Shiranui Sea area to demand new compensation from Chisso for Minamata disease. On June 25, they accepted an advance payment of ¥750 million ($2.76 million). The Minamata Fishing Cooperative demanded ¥1,360,000,000 ($5 million) on July 5 and blockaded the factory. Before long, the blockade forced the factory to shut down. The blockade ended when the co-op accepted ¥400 million ($1.47 million) on July 20. The 30 Shiranui Sea cooperatives then blockaded the factory on August 7 and forced it to shut down again. They ended their blockade on August 29 when Governor Sawada agreed to mediate, and they signed an agreement with Chisso for ¥2,280,000,000 ($8.38 million) on November 20. On December 6, three coops from Kagoshima prefecture, including the Izumi co-op, reached an agreement with Chisso for ¥700 million ($2.57 million) in compensation.

In Tokyo, Chisso softened, ever so slightly, its resolution not to pay medical costs when it announced on May 31 that it would help pay for treatment at hot springs. The Tokyo Negotiations Group refused the offer, but met with Environment Agency Director Miki on June 15 and agreed to accept the general outlines of the Minamata Disease Compensation Mediation Committee plan as the basis for compensation, in return for Miki's agreement to set up a system for ranking the patients according to their symptoms. The Niigata patients finally signed an agreement with Shōwa denkō on June 21: Shōwa agreed to pay ¥15 million ($55,000) for each deceased and severe patient, ¥10 million ($37,000) for other patients, and a living allowance of ¥500,000 ($1,800) per year. The agreement gave the Niigata patients everything they had demanded when they began negotiations in April 1972.

Miki put together a plan that gave the Minamata patients most of what they had asked for, although they had to accept ranking by symptoms. The agreement was signed at the Environment Agency on July 9, 1973.[57] One-time payments were ¥16 million, ¥17 million, or ¥18 million ($59,000, $63,000, or $66,000; equivalent to 15.4, 16.4, or 17.4 times per capita annual GNP). Monthly payments for living expenses were ¥20,000, ¥30,000, or ¥60,000 ($74, $110, or $221; equivalent to yearly payments of 23 percent, 35 percent, or 69 percent, respectively of per capita annual GNP).[58] (These, but not the one-time payments, have since been regularly adjusted for inflation.) Chisso also agreed to cover medical expenses. A ¥300 million ($1.1 million)

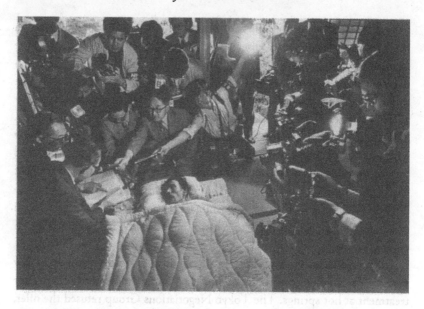

Fig. 28 Miki Takeo, director general of the Environment Agency, visiting a Minamata disease patient. Photograph by W. Eugene Smith. © Aileen M. Smith.

fund was set up, with the interest used to cover the costs of such things as diapers, hot spring treatments, and acupuncture and moxibustion. All patients certified in the future would automatically be covered by the agreement if they wished. Later, all the other certified patients' groups—the Arbitration Group, the Mediation Group, and the Middle Group—signed identical agreements with Chisso.

Because of the rapid economic growth in the years since 1959, the 1973 compensation amounts were not as much of an increase over the 1959 solatium payments as they seemed. Certainly the one-time payments under the 1973 agreement, which ranged from 15.4 to 17.4 times per capita GNP for 1973, were a great improvement. The solatium agreement included no one-time payments except for deaths, and those had been only 2.24 times the 1959 per capita GNP. But the monthly payments under the 1973 agreement were actually *lower* in relative terms than those paid to adults under the solatium agreement. The amounts accepted in 1973 for living expenses ranged from 23 percent to 69 percent of per capita GNP that year, whereas the annual solatium payments to adults had been 70 percent of the per capita

GNP for 1959 (the solatium payments for children had been only 21 percent of per capita GNP).

But the important difference in 1973—far more important than the new one-time payments—was the moral victory for the patients. Chisso had been found legally responsible for Minamata disease and had been forced to accept this responsibility and to apologize.[59]

On July 12, 1973, the tent on the sidewalk outside Chisso's offices was taken down. Altogether some fifty supporters had lived and worked in it since December 1971. They had collected signatures and donations from over 50,000 people and over ¥30 million ($110,000) to support the Direct Negotiations Group.[60] On July 13, twelve patients including Kawamoto Teruo, Satō Takeharu, and Tanoue Yoshiharu boarded a train for home. In the process of forcing a second settlement to the Minamata disease issue that contrasted in every way with that of 1959, they and their supporters from throughout Japan had, in various ways, tested and extended the possibilities of postwar democracy. Yet as the course of the Minamata disease struggle since 1973 shows, this second settlement was still incomplete, and postwar democracy remained, in practice, a system that was ad hoc rather than regularized.

PART V

Since 1973

NINE

Minamata and the Tragedy of Japan's "Modernity"

Remembering: Tales and Lessons of Minamata

On March 2, 1994, sixteen patients including Tanoue Yoshiharu, Hamamoto Tsuginori, Hamamoto Fumiyo, Satō Takeharu, Kawamoto Teruo, and Ogata Masato presented a petition to the newly elected mayor of Minamata, Yoshii Masazumi, asking that land reclaimed from Minamata Bay be made a place of prayer. They wrote of how the bay had been "the treasure house of the sea." "Industrial civilization," however, had "poisoned to death all living things, from sea life to human beings. This original sin is a historical fact that cannot be erased" and will remain "forever in the history of the sins of humanity." Therefore, they wished "to place on this land reclaimed from the bitter sea a large number of stone statues (small Buddhas)" as reminders of the "depth of humanity's sins" and to make it a place "of continual prayer that the souls [of all the living things killed by the poison] may be saved."[1]

The 58 hectares of reclaimed land had been created between 1983 and 1990 by dredging every area of the bay whose sludge had a mercury concentration of over 25 ppm, dumping the sludge in the inner, worst polluted area of the bay, and covering it with a thick sheet of plastic and then "clean" dirt. Chisso was required to pay most of the ¥48.5 billion ($335 million) cost. This small area had become, in the 1990s, symbolic of the question of how to remember Minamata disease and its victims. The group that petitioned Mayor Yoshii wanted the reclaimed land to be a monument and not tennis courts, parks, or golf driving ranges.

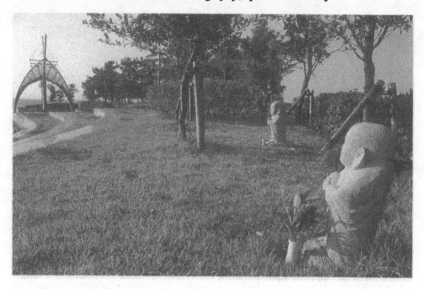

Fig. 29 Stone statues placed by patients on land reclaimed from the most polluted parts of Minamata Bay, 1996. © Timothy S. George.

Precedents were found elsewhere in Japan for city sponsorship of such memorials without violating the principle of separation of church and state. In June 1996, the city and prefecture agreed to the placing of statues (which all sides were usually careful to call just "stone statues" to play down their religious significance), although not nearly as many as the patients hoped. The first two were in place by the fall of 1996, the year the city's third general plan (1996–2005) called for making Minamata into "a city of industry and culture that values environment, health, and welfare" within ten years.[2]

As is obvious to anyone who has read Ishimure Michiko's works, the patients' petition was written in consultation with her. Both she and her husband, Hiroshi, were active backers of the plan. Her writings have made her memories and interpretations of the Minamata disease incident the dominant narrative. She has also helped make Buddhism central to Minamata protests and petitions. For Ishimure, Minamata condenses the tragedy of Japan's "modernity," in which Minamata disease was only the crowning blow in the destruction of the traditional community and of a life-style in harmony with the sea and all of nature. She paints this destruction as already well under way in the difficult days she remembers from her childhood in the 1930s. (She was born in 1927.) Poor farming and fishing families had to send most of their children away (a practice known as *kuchiberashi*, or "reducing the number of mouths" to be fed) to work in brothels or mines. The mines of the Chikuhō area in Kyūshū, she says, were the "blood vessels of capitalism," where human beings were "burned as fuel." The poverty she knew in southern Kyūshū was also the rule for "people on the periphery" elsewhere in Japan, she believes, and their suffering continued in the postwar period when they were "ground in the gears of high growth."[3]

The dominant narrative of the Minamata story has been created not only by Ishimure but also by others in, allied with, or strongly sympathetic to the Citizens' Council and the Association to Indict. Ui Jun, Harada Masazumi, Togashi Sadao, Gotō Takanori, Tsuchimoto Noriaki, Hamamoto Tsuginori, and Onitsuka Iwao all more or less share Ishimure's views. So do Irokawa Daikichi and most of the scholars in his research group, who studied Minamata from 1976 to 1980.[4] Those more closely allied with the traditional left, such as the lawyers in the first court case, would offer different interpretations of and prescriptions for activism and use slightly different terminology, but they, too, would put the Minamata disease incident in a somewhat similar framework. It represents, for them, the destruction of traditional society and the oppression of the poor under capitalist development.[5]

The traditional left would not, however, agree with Irokawa's belief in the importance of "small leaders," such as Kawamoto Teruo. For Irokawa, the struggle is not against capitalism or modernity in general but more specifically against the state and its tentacles that reach into the community. He puts more emphasis on key individuals, his small leaders, who come from within rather than above the common people but at the same time serve as their vanguard. His interpretation of the Minamata disease incident, then, may romanticize the pre-industrial past almost as much as Ishimure's, but because of the possibilities represented by the small leaders, it is more optimistic about the present and the future.[6]

There is no doubt that individuals such as Kawamoto Teruo and Ishimure Michiko played key roles in the course of the Minamata disease "incident." After 1973, although Minamata was rarely in the spotlight, they and others continued to do so.

Events Since 1973: Toward a More Complete Solution

The 1973 settlement resolved the two most urgent issues in the Minamata disease incident by finding Chisso legally responsible and providing relatively reasonable compensation for all certified patients. Yet it was by no means a complete solution, as the title of a 1985 book by Harada Masa-zumi—*Minamata Disease Is Not Over (Minamatabyō wa owatte inai)*—reminded his readers. Thousands of patients remained uncertified, and the question of the legal responsibility of the central, prefectural, and city governments was left unresolved. In addition, the higher payments to larger numbers of patients worsened Chisso's already declining financial situation, and it became necessary to find ways to keep the company from going bankrupt so that it could continue paying compensation. These three problems—certification, government responsibility, and financial support for Chisso—were the three major issues after 1973.[7]

Two other legal issues remained to be resolved when the 1973 settlement was put in place. Kawamoto Teruo's trial for assaulting Chisso employees went all the way to the Supreme Court and was not finally resolved until the end of 1980. Partly as a response to the indictment of Kawamoto, patients managed to have Chisso executives tried for homicide for their part in the mercury poisoning, particularly the switching of the acetaldehyde waste from Minamata Bay to the mouth of the Minamata River in 1958.

In addition to all these issues, other less easily solved problems remained. The disease itself remained the most intractable. Minamata disease is incurable. Although the body can slowly rid itself of mercury, the damage it causes to the brain and central nervous system is largely irreversible. By 1980 Hamamoto Tsuginori had tried physical therapy, acupuncture (regular and electric), moxibustion, massage, boiled herbs, Chinese medicine, chiropracty, ultrasound, vitamins, ointments, hot springs, injections, and hot compresses. Yet he was rapidly losing muscle strength and control in the lower half of his body. He could walk only a few steps with a cane, and because he had to use the toilet fifteen or more times per day, he could never sleep well.[8] By the early 1990s he could not walk at all and had to use a catheter to drain his bladder.

And beyond the physical destruction, there is the psychological damage caused by the suffering of the disease itself, by ostracism, and by the inability of many patients to work or to care for themselves. Families, communities, and human relationships were often severely damaged, at times seemingly beyond repair. As patients aged, they required more care, and the congenital Minamata disease patients faced the prospect of having to get by without their parents' assistance.

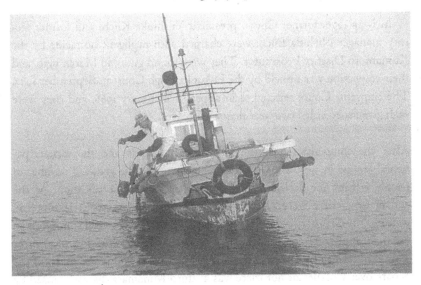

Fig. 30 Raising an octopus pot, 1994. Members of the Minamata fishing cooperative continued fishing outside the bay until the fish in the bay were declared safe in 1997. © Timothy S. George.

Even though the majority of families in the city were not touched by Minamata disease, all residents were affected by the financial decline of Chisso and the city, the falling population, the poor image of Minamata, the exodus of young people unable to find jobs in Minamata, and the blow to civic pride. Such problems are common to many small cities in rural areas of Japan, and indeed to virtually all of Kumamoto prefecture outside the capital city, but were intensified by Minamata disease and its repercussions. In January 1975, the Tokyo District Court found Kawamoto Teruo guilty of assault and battery.[9] He and his lawyer Gotō Takanori appealed to the Tokyo High Court, hoping it would accept their argument that the indictment itself was illegal because the government had been biased in favor of Chisso from the very beginning of the Minamata disease incident. In June 1977 the High Court agreed, marking the first time in Japanese legal history that a court had dismissed an indictment as illegal. Kawamoto and Gotō had succeeded in turning the trial into a detailed indictment of Chisso and of the role of the government itself in protecting Chisso and neglecting the victims. Chisso appealed, but the Supreme Court upheld the High Court's decision on December 17, 1980.

In May 1976, former Chisso president Yoshioka Kiichi and former factory manager Nishida Eiichi were charged with negligent homicide by the Kumamoto District Prosecutor. They were found guilty in March 1979, and their conviction was upheld by the Fukuoka High Court in September 1982. The Supreme Court rejected their appeal in February 1988, and they were each given suspended two-year prison sentences.

After the compensation agreements between Chisso and the various patients' groups in 1973, the next major problem was the growing number of people waiting for decisions on their applications for certification. At the end of 1973, there were 2,007 applicants from Kumamoto prefecture still waiting.[10] In February 1974, the prefecture established a special committee to examine applicants to speed up the process. The certification committee members' terms came to an end that April, however, and in the midst of the debate over whether or not there was a "third Minamata disease" caused by factory waste in the Ariake Sea (north of the Shiranui Sea), the prefecture found it impossible to appoint a new committee. By the end of 1974, 2,725 applicants were awaiting decisions, but it was not until May 1975 that a new committee was appointed and began considering applications.[11] In December 1974, 406 applicants sued the governor over the delay. When they won in December 1976, the governor officially apologized, and it appeared that he would have to do something to speed up the certification process.

What he did was not what the victorious patients expected. Governor Sawada Issei was under pressure not only from the patients demanding certification but also from Chisso, which was asking for financial help to avoid bankruptcy. Petition drives in Minamata by various groups, including both unions at the factory, urged government help for the company. Sawada asked the central government to help with certification and to back the prefecture in issuing bonds to raise money to lend to Chisso. By the end of 1977, 4,460 patients were awaiting certification, and Chisso seemed ready to go under, but the government was unable to decide whether it would, or even could, help the prefecture help the company.[12] Aiding Chisso would violate the "polluter pays principle" (PPP) and might not be legal under the laws governing prefectural finances.

Sawada found a way to increase the pressure on the national government. In April 1978 he reversed what had been an established pattern and began certifying far fewer applicants than he rejected. He and Tokyo then worked out a compromise plan that was approved by the Cabinet in June and passed by the Diet in October. The Environment Agency set up its own certification system, so that both it and the prefecture could certify patients, and the national government assisted the prefecture in issuing 30–year bonds to aid Chisso. The national government bought 80 percent (60 percent at first) of these bonds, and the rest were sold to financial institutions. The prefecture then lent the money to Chisso, which used it to pay compensation to patients.

For the government, Minamata has always been first and foremost a question of damage control, but the new certification and bond systems marked important turning points. Guidelines issued by the Environment Agency in 1977 and 1978 made certification standards stricter; indeed they nearly revived the pre-1971 standards, which required the classic Hunter-Russell symptoms. The facts that these standards were set by the Environment Agency rather than the Ministry of Health and Welfare and that they were so regressive confirmed that certification remained a political and financial issue more than a medical one.

By providing financial assistance to Chisso, the government abandoned the polluter pays principle and might even be said to have tacitly accepted some responsibility for Minamata disease. The system was extended in September 1994 when Chisso was unable to pay the interest it owed. The government further subsidized the loans to Chisso so that the interest rates could be lowered. At the same time, a five-year Minamata-Ashikita Regional Development Foundation was established. The prefectural government sold bonds to fund the foundation (with the central government again buying 80 percent of them), and the foundation lent the money to Chisso. If Chisso could not repay the loans, the government promised it would do its best to rescue the prefecture.

The government attempted to protect Chisso through the Ministry of Education's textbook-screening process as well. Tokyo University sociologist Mita Munesuke quoted from Ishimure Michiko's *Kugai jōdo* in a 1981 high school textbook he wrote. The ministry asked the book's publisher to remove the name "Chisso" from the quote. Both Mita and Ishimure refused to allow this, and the ministry finally backed down.[13]

There have been nearly 30 court cases surrounding Minamata disease, including the trial of fishermen for the October 1959 riots at the factory, the first suit by patients, and the trial of Kawamoto Teruo for assault and battery.[14] The largest of these cases were civil trials in which uncertified patients sued Chisso, or Chisso along with the prefectural and national governments, for certification and compensation. Rulings on government responsibility for Minamata disease were mixed, and in the one such case that reached the Supreme Court, the lower court's ruling in favor of the plaintiffs was nullified, and the case was returned to the lower court. There were also suits over rejection of applications and over delays in processing them. One suit was an unsuccessful attempt to stop the dredging and landfill operations in Minamata Bay that began in 1977 and were completed in 1990.

The number of patients being certified dropped to a handful in the 1990s, but the many court cases surrounding certification and government responsibility threatened to worsen the plight of Chisso and thereby of the prefectural and national governments. The government and the prefecture could hold down costs by holding down the number of certifications, but only if they could withstand the political pressure from the groups of patients demanding certification. As patients aged—those suing for certification and compensation averaged well over 70 years old by the mid-1990s—their cases became more urgent, and the public relations harm to the government of denying them certification increased. Combined with its fear that the judicial system, which it could not directly control as it could the certification system, might order the certification of thousands of patients in one fell swoop, the rising pressure to give the patients something before they died pushed the government toward an accommodation.

In January 1993, the Fukuoka High Court, instead of issuing a verdict on the "third Minamata disease suit," proposed a *wakai*, a court-mediated out-of-court settlement that is common in Japan. The suit had been filed in 1980 and was the first to ask that not only Chisso but also the prefectural and national governments be found responsible for Minamata disease. The plaintiffs won the case in Kumamoto District Court in March 1987, but all three defendants had appealed to the High Court. In January 1993 the High Court proposed a *wakai* dividing the patients into thirteen ranks and giving them one-time payments of between ¥2 million and ¥8 million ($18,000 to $72,000).[15] Chisso and Kumamoto prefecture, along with nearly all patients' groups, were willing to accept, but the LDP and the Environment Agency insisted on waiting for the court to decide the case and then appealing to the Supreme Court if necessary.[16]

This was quite different from the situation that had prevailed up to this point. The government strategy had always been one of stalemating. Earlier, the best way to do this had been to attempt to keep the issue out of the courts. Now this was no longer possible, and the government had to make the best of the situation by *using* the judicial system. The best way now was to utilize the slowness of the process to delay a final settlement. The patients in the 1990s felt a great deal more time pressure than they had in 1969 when the first suit was filed. They had also found in the *wakai* what they considered a much fairer mediation system than one relying on local bosses and government-appointed arbitration committees. Yet the government refused a *wakai*, and the Fukuoka High Court refused to issue a verdict.

The stalemate was broken when a Socialist, Murayama Tomiichi, took office in June 1994 as prime minister at the head of a coalition government including the LDP. Murayama was in many ways an ineffective prime minister, handicapped by his coalition partners and his own party's identity crisis. Yet he announced that as a Socialist, there were several issues he especially wanted to resolve. Three of them related to World War II: an official government apology on the fiftieth anniversary of the end of the war, compensation of the sex slaves ("comfort women") forced to serve soldiers in East and Southeast Asia, and better compensation and care for victims of the atomic bombings of Hiroshima and Nagasaki. The fourth was a political settlement of the Minamata disease issue. In return for cooperation in other areas and in the face of growing recognition of the need for at least token progress in all these areas, Murayama's conservative coalition partners agreed that the government should work toward solutions to these four issues. In each case something was achieved, but in no case was it all that Murayama, or the victims, had hoped.

When the LDP and the Environment Agency ended their opposition to a *wakai*, negotiations began among the relevant government agencies, Kumamoto prefecture, and the victims' groups. By late 1995 a deal had been worked out that was acceptable to nearly all sides. The aging victims felt they needed to accept what they could get while the coalition was still in office. The Cabinet passed the plan December 15.[17] Eligible uncertified victims would receive ¥2.6 million ($27,700; 67 percent of per capita GNP in 1995) each. To be "certified" as eligible for compensation under this scheme, they would have to show loss of sensation in all four limbs and agree to withdraw their court suits and requests for certification. Approximately 8,000 people were expected to receive compensation, and all but a handful of those pursuing restitution through the courts were expected to withdraw their suits. In addition, five victims' groups would be given a total of ¥4.94 billion ($52.6 million), and Chisso would be provided with ¥26 billion ($277 million) more in financial aid. Finally, although the agreement would not constitute legal recognition of government responsibility, the prime minister would apologize for the government's role. Murayama did so the day the Cabinet accepted the plan, issuing a statement of "regret" for the suffering of the victims and emphasizing the need for the government to "reflect honestly" on its slow response.[18]

Like the war apology resolution passed by the Diet in the summer of 1995, Murayama's statement was seen by the victims as less than a clear and full apology. In other ways, too, this third "full and final solution" to the Minamata disease issue, like those of 1959 and 1973, was less than complete. Because it left out an unknown number of victims, Kawamoto Teruo said:

The "settlement" is fake, and has no relationship to the reality of Minamata disease.

Patients are becoming older, and the power of the victims as well as the energy of their supporters is decreasing. The social environment is worsening as well. I think these factors led the Minamata movement to accept the "settlement."

Our organization called it an "honorable retreat," but in my opinion it was rather a "shameful retreat." We were defeated by the politicians and bureaucrats.[19]

Social pressures against applying for compensation remain very strong. Nishi Yasunori, a 40-year employee at Chisso, explained his own reasons:

As the "final settlement" was nearing, many people advised me to apply.... I do experience occasional convulsions, but I never bothered to apply, thinking that perhaps the convulsions are a result of my age. I have not let my family apply either, though my wife has an occasional convulsion too....

People still face social sanctions for receiving compensation from the company, and I can manage my life despite the effects of Minamata Disease....

I was seeing a doctor until last year, but he told me there was nothing he could do for me. I no longer enjoy my meals because I have no sense of taste or smell. I do not need to eat very much any more.[20]

Even though 10,353 people—well above the initial estimate of 8,000—were compensated under the new agreement by 1999, many victims were still left uncompensated, and a few others refused to accept it. Moreover, it left the question of government responsibility legally unresolved. In fact, in an echo of the 1959 solatium contract, this third "solution" required those who accepted it to agree not to pursue the question in the courts. Yet, although this solution was not complete, it will probably be the last, given the ages of the victims.

Painfully Slow Healing

All the various participants have tried to tell their versions of the story of Minamata and to tell the nation what lessons should be learned from the tragedy. In many ways these efforts are part of their attempts to solve, or to live with, the legacies that could not be solved through certification and compensation. Until very recently, however, each group was preaching mainly to itself, since those in opposing camps largely refused to speak to each other. Not only would patients and their supporters refuse to speak with city government officials; even members of different victims' groups and support groups kept their distance from each other. Only in the early 1990s did the walls begin to come down.

A central symbol of the change in the character of the Minamata disease incident after 1973 is the completion in 1974 of the Minamata Disease Center Sōshisha. As the end of the trial neared, Ishimure Michiko and other supporters realized the need for a new type of organization that would support patients in their daily lives, provide a place for them to meet, and collect and preserve documents.[21] Ishimure decided to accept the Magsaysay Prize for her writings in August 1973 and used the prize money to help build the Sōshisha in the hills of Fukuro, overlooking Detsuki, Tsukinoura, Yudō, and the Shiranui Sea.

Many fishing families who were able to work had turned to growing mandarin oranges and Watson's pomelo (*natsu mikan,* or "summer oranges"). A number of them, like Hamamoto Tsuginori, began to do so with few or no chemicals, not wishing to poison others the way they themselves had been poisoned by Chisso. Tanoue Yoshiharu, who had led the Tokyo Negotiations Group, set up a mostly organic, mostly self-sufficient farm, Otomezuka nōen (Virgin Hill Farm), on the southern edge of Minamata. He named his farm in memory of Kamimura Tomoko, the congenital patient who was immortalized in W. Eugene Smith's famous photograph "Tomoko in the Bath" and who had died in 1978.

The actor Sunada Akira and his wife, Emiko, moved into a home near Tanoue and built a meeting hall that could be used by patients, Minna no ie (Everyone's house). This is where patients and their families have met and held memorial services annually since the early 1980s, on the anniversary of the 1973 trial victory. Sakamoto Fujie, the mother of congenital patient Sakamoto Shinobu, says: "We use the occasion to discuss the government's various attempts to 'resolve' the Minamata disease affair. By 'resolve' we assume they mean 'forget.'"[22] In the hall is a stage for performances, decorated by a mural depicting victims of Minamata disease, painted by the husband and wife team Maruki Iri and Toshi. The Marukis, who became known for their Hiroshima murals, have done murals of Auschwitz, the Rape of Nanjing, the Battle of Okinawa, and Minamata.[23] On the hill above Minna no ie is a monument to all living things that have died of Minamata disease. Next to it is a sculpture by Kinjō Minoru of Okinawa. On the base is an English inscription explaining that it shows "a mother holding her dying child in her arms," with the admonition: "Remember Nangking [sic] slaughter, Okinawa and Gulf War. No more Hiroshima, Nagasaki, and Chernobyl. Never forget Minamata, Vietnam, and Bhopal. Otomezuka, the memorial monument. Memorial services are held for all human and non-human victims of Minamata disease."[24]

A number of the most active victims had their perspectives and concerns similarly broadened by their experiences. Hamamoto Tsuginori helped form a group called the Conference Linking Minamata and Asia (Ajia to Minamata o musubu kai). Although he now uses a wheelchair, this former fisherman with only a junior high school education travels throughout Japan and much of east and southeast Asia, warning that Minamata should not be repeated. He tells listeners that World War II, Hiroshima, Nagasaki, Okinawa, and Minamata must be remembered as "minuses" resulting from Japan's modernization. He wants to make them "pluses" by making people aware of them and using them to argue that further tragedies, such as nuclear power plant accidents, must be prevented by citizen action. We live in a high-consumption, high-production, high-waste society, he says, but "Let's finally give it up. Let's finally graduate from this."[25] Unlike many other patients and supporters, Hamamoto cooperated with the city in 1993 when it opened a museum and document center devoted to Minamata disease at Myōjin, where Harada Masazumi encountered congenital Minamata disease patients in 1961. In 1994 he began working there, telling visitors his story.

Minamata disease patients continue to confront discrimination and prejudice. Araki Yōko recalls that when her family used some of the com-

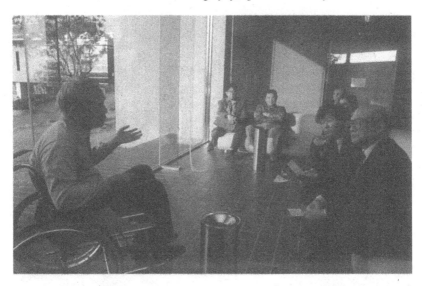

Fig. 31 Hamamoto Tsuginori telling his story at the city's Minamata Disease Museum, 1994. © Timothy S. George.

pensation money they received in 1973 to repair their roof, a neighbor re-marked: "Look at that nice roof. I think I'll get Minamata disease too."[26] This attitude was exemplified in remarks by two prefectural assembly members in August 1975 that there were many "false patients" (*nise kanja*) among those applying for certification. Two patients and two supporters were charged with assault after a struggle during a protest against the remarks. All four were found guilty and given suspended sentences, and appeals to the Fukuoka High Court and Supreme Court failed to overturn the verdict. In the meantime, patients sued the two representatives for slander. The two politicians were found guilty in March 1980, and the governor was required to take out advertisements to apologize.

One of the two patients found guilty of assault in the protest against the "false patient" remarks was Ogata Masato of Meshima, north of Mina-mata.[27] Ogata was born in 1953, the year certified patient no. 1 (Mizoguchi Toyoko) became sick. His brothers participated in the November 2, 1959, riot at the factory, and the death later that month of their father, Fuku-matsu, helped confirm the spread of the disease beyond Minamata. In 1985 Masato withdrew his application for certification, which had been submitted

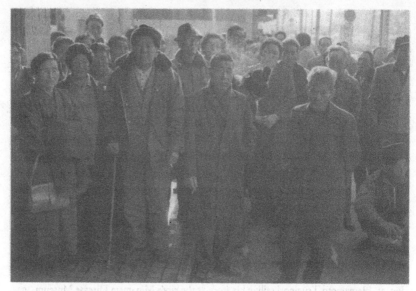

Fig. 32 Patients protesting remarks about "fake patients," 1979. © Akutagawa Jin.

in 1974 and was still pending. For the next two years, he conducted a series of solo sit-ins at the factory gate and asked some disturbing questions. In a January 6, 1986, open letter to the president of Chisso, he explained his action: "I no longer see the significance in the term 'recognition' nor in my application for 'recognition.' I have come to think that my Minamata disease has to be affirmed by myself and recognized as such."[28] Ogata describes the "system" of applications, certification, and compensation as one devised to trap patients, to obfuscate the issue of true responsibility, and to avoid treating people as human beings. He even admits to wondering: "If I think about it, if I had been in Chisso or the government, wouldn't I have done what they did?"[29]

For many years after 1973, the city government and most residents of Minamata preferred not to think about—or were pathologically incapable of facing—Minamata disease and the problems it brought, hoping that the issue would simply go away if it were ignored. Ostracism and less severe forms of discrimination against patients faded slowly but have by no means disappeared. Discussions of Minamata disease are almost taboo. Children from Minamata on school trips to other areas have reported being avoided by people who still think Minamata disease is contagious. Many people, young and old, are reluctant to admit they are from Minamata, and tell people they are from Kumamoto prefecture or from Yatsushiro.

One reminder of the bitter divisions in the city came in 1975 in the form of a speech by a female student attending evening classes for part-time students at Minamata High School.[30] The girl's main point was that the word "Minamata" ought to be removed from the name "Minamata disease," because of the discrimination it brought on the citizens of Minamata. She suggested that not all of those applying and being certified as patients really had Minamata disease and said she was envious of people who simply had to hold their hands out to get money, rather than sweating in the hot summer or working in the cold winter. She also referred to a fight that had broken out when she was an elementary school student on a school trip to Kumamoto. The Minamata students were approached at an inn by a group of students from Hiroshima, one of whom yelled "Minamata disease!" A boy from Minamata shouted back, "What do you mean, atomic bomb disease!"

The speech won first prize in the school-wide contest, and the girl went on to the prefectural competition as one of the representatives from Minamata. Because of its objectionable content, however, the speech was omitted from the published proceedings of the prefectural contest. In response, the Minamata High School evening school printed the speech in the graduation edition of the newsletter distributed to the parents of all evening students in the spring of 1976.

The prejudice evident in the speech is partly explained by its social context: citizens near the bottom of the economic and social order turning their frustrations on others—Minamata disease patients—who were below them.[31] Unlike graduates of Japan's elite urban schools, few students from Minamata High School—and virtually none from its night school—go on to universities. Many of the night school students worked during the day at Chisso, where they had no chance of being promoted to upper management positions, and saw little prospect of finding good jobs in Minamata. And Minamata disease patients were still stereotyped as being from hamlets populated by poor fishing families, outsiders (*jigoro* in the local dialect) who were poor immigrants (*nagure*), mostly from Amakusa.

The furor was immediate. In June a group of young patients met with Principal Tsukuda Tameyoshi and handed over a list of questions and a demand for an apology.[32] Tsukuda refused to apologize and insisted that he and all the teachers believed there was no prejudice in the school against Minamata disease patients. Within a few days, however, Tsukuda, along with the head teacher of the night school and the head of the teachers' union, was persuaded to visit the homes of several patients and to meet with congenital patients. The teachers' union head was shocked into apologizing: "Even though I drive back and forth on this National Highway no. 3 almost every day, not once have I set foot in the hamlet just one step below this highway. I wonder just how many of the teachers at our school know about the Minamata disease in the hamlets just off this highway. Have they tried to learn about it?"[33] The principal issued a detailed reply to the young patients' questions, admitting that discrimination against patients existed in the school and promising to strengthen "environmental education."

The city has yet to find a solution to its declining economy and population. A semiconductor company, Hara denshi, built a small factory that by the early 1990s employed more workers than the Chisso factory, which had only 680 employees at the beginning of 1994. One mayoral candidate in the 1994 election proposed building a koala zoo to attract tourists. Like other rural cities, the city campaigned to have a planned bullet train line and expressway run nearby. Strong opposition to the bullet train plan was led by Matsumoto Tsutomu, who had been one of the leading members of the Citizens' Council.

A bit of healing for the community, and a great morale boost for the youngest patients, came in 1978 when a group of eight congenital Minamata disease patients decided they wanted, for once in their lives, to do something big and meaningful and to do it themselves. Most of them had recently turned 20, the age of majority in Japan. They decided to put on a concert by Ishikawa Sayuri, a popular singer about their age who happened to be from Kumamoto.[34] Takishita Masafumi and other young patients traveled to Tokyo and persuaded the head of Ishikawa's production company to stage the concert at cost. Sakamoto Shinobu and others made posters and sold tickets. The congenital patients visited remote fishing villages in the Amakusa islands, meeting victims they did not know and bringing them invitations and gifts. On the day of the concert, three of the patients met Ishikawa at the Kumamoto airport. From there she visited Meisuien, the facility at which the most serious patients are hospitalized.

Before the concert began, the eight organizers stood on stage to greet the full house of 1,200 people, many of whom had never had any contact with Minamata disease patients. Takishita struggled to force out words that would impress on the audience that he and his fellow patients had realized their goal by working together. He said that he hoped the people of Minamata realized this and that they would remember the patients in Meisuien. Onitsuka Yūji had a severe headache, as many patients often do, and when he groaned in pain and began to suffer convulsions, Harada Masazumi stepped up to help. As they left the stage to let Ishikawa begin her show, most were crying, as were many people in the audience.

In Minamata's fishing hamlets, another reason attitudes toward patients began to soften ever so slightly by the late 1970s was the fact that the number of certifications increased so rapidly. By 1978, 34 percent of families in the hamlets of Tsukinoura, Detsuki, Yudō, and Modō included at least one certified patient. Sugimoto Eiko felt less ostracized when in Modō 77 of 132 families included a certified patient. Nearly 35 percent of the hamlet's population had been certified.[35]

In the early 1990s the city government and a growing number of citizens came to acknowledge that Minamata disease had much to do with the city's problems and that these problems could be addressed only if the disease and its legacies were openly discussed.[36] In 1993 the city began sponsoring "citizens' forums to discuss Minamata disease" (Minamatabyō o kataru shimin kōza). In the first four, Hamamoto Tsuginori, Ishida Masaru, Kawamoto Teruo, and Hashiguchi Saburō (the leader of the plaintiffs in the third Minamata disease suit) each spoke to and then fielded questions from audiences of 50 to 100. Minamata was certainly no longer Chisso's "castle town." But it was not at all certain what it had become.

At the end of 1993 a city official, Yoshimoto Tetsurō, and Yoshinaga Toshio, the director of the Minamata Disease Center Sōshisha (the support group and museum introduced above) established an informal discussion group, the Minamata Research Group (Minamata kenkyūkai).[37] The group brought together city and prefectural officials, members of victims' support groups, the Junior Chamber of Commerce (which in Japan involves business people well into their forties), and farmers. Although their monthly discussions were unofficial, they had a significant impact on city and prefectural plans and policies. For example, they helped bring about cooperation between the city and victims' support groups in organizing both a joint exhibition at the city's Minamata Disease Municipal Museum, and the annual "Get in Touch with the Environment in Minamata" (*Kankyō fureai in Minamata*) festival that the prefecture and city have sponsored each fall in Minamata since 1993. The city museum and the Sōshisha even managed to agree on the contents of a pamphlet giving basic information about Minamata disease that was distributed at their joint exhibition.[38] Such cooperation did not come easily and was not without its critics on both sides, however. Yoshinaga wondered: "Was being called 'antiestablishment!' easier?"[39]

The election of Yoshii Masazumi as mayor in 1994 took the city another step forward in acknowledging the legacies of Minamata disease.[40] Yoshii, an LDP member, was in the lumber business and lived in a rural inland area of the city. He had no strong connections either to Chisso or to patients and their support groups. At an annual memorial service for victims of Minamata disease on May 1, 1994, held on land reclaimed from the most polluted parts of Minamata Bay, he became the first mayor to formally apologize on behalf of the city. He acknowledged the "defamation, prejudice, and discrimination" the victims had suffered and said "it is extremely regrettable that we were unable to take proper measures for those who were victims of Minamata disease." Finally, he said all the citizens of Minamata should join together, from that day, to begin *moyainaoshi*, a local term meaning to start over or make things right (literally, "to re-moor a boat," or "to reconnect two boats lashed together for fishing").[41]

But *moyainaoshi* soon became the buzzword not for citizens' reconciliation but for an expensive government construction program. The 1995–96 "political resolution" of the Minamata disease problem, besides compensating uncertified patients and providing further financial support for Chisso, included a plan to promote economic recovery and development in the region. In postwar Japan this has usually meant pouring funds into local construction projects. By 1998 the Minamata Moyainaoshi Center, the Southern Minamata Moyainaoshi Center (Orange Hall), and the Ashikita Moyainaoshi Center had been completed, giving the area an embarrassing surplus of meeting halls.

In his 1994 speech of apology, Mayor Yoshii referred to the "movement to place prayers and vows on [the land reclaimed from Minamata Bay] in the form of stone statues." His willingness to accommodate the petitioning

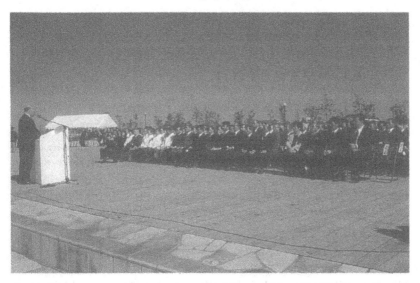

Fig. 33 The 1994 memorial ceremony at which Minamata Mayor Yoshii Masazumi apologized to the victims on behalf of the city. © Timothy S. George.

patients by allowing them to place Buddhist stone statues on part of the land was a remarkable change from the stance of earlier administrations. But he was neither able nor willing to allow the patients to determine the fate of the entire 58 hectares. The Ministry of Construction, the prefecture, and the city had been trying to work out details concerning jurisdiction and plans for the reclaimed land while waiting for it to settle enough to be built on (it will never be able to support large buildings). It is now occupied by a park and bamboo garden, athletic fields, a port, a restaurant, and a shop selling local products to tourists.

In 1993 the city built its Minamata Disease Museum on a bluff overlooking the reclaimed land, and the prefecture built an environmental education center next to the museum. After an international contest to choose the design, the Minamata Memorial was dedicated between these two buildings in the fall of 1996. On multilevel terraces, looking out over the Shiranui Sea, are numerous stainless steel spheres representing the souls of victims of Minamata disease or the lights of fishing boats on the sea. On the highest terrace is the Prayer Fountain, and suspended from a frame over the fountain is a bronze Memorial Chest. Inside the chest, out of reach and unseen, are plates engraved with the names of those who have died of Minamata disease, still hidden in death as they often were in life.

CONCLUSION

Minamata and Postwar Democracy

This thing called democracy contains a paradox. This is that democracy is given true life only by the political activity of people who do not make politics their primary career or their purpose.

—Maruyama Masao

Minamata tells us a great deal about the potential, changes, and limitations of democracy in postwar Japan. It shows the processes as well as the legal and institutional infrastructure of democracy and is a case study of citizen organization at the local, regional, and national levels and how these levels interact. It shows the ways and extent to which citizens' political participation has affected policymaking and been made regular and legitimate. Despite important changes over the postwar decades, there have been two overriding constants: citizen democracy in postwar Japan has been ad hoc, and it has been constrained.

The second and third postwar decades were critical, as the differences between the first (1956–59) and second (1968–73) rounds of responses to Minamata disease show. The first decade after the war was one of recovery and rebuilding. By the end of 1955, the year before Minamata disease was discovered, the basic building blocks of the postwar structure were in place: the constitution, the military and economic alliance with the United States, the Self-Defense Forces, the education system, the police, labor unions, the government administrative structure, and the "1955 system" dominated by the LDP, government bureaucrats, and big business. The questions then became how these building blocks would be arranged and rearranged, who would do this, and what tools they would create, or appropriate from the past, to do the job.

The complex Minamata story shows that Japan was not simply ruled from 1955 on by an unresponsive "iron triangle" of business, bureaucracy, and the LDP. The changes that occurred in the crucial decade from the late 1950s to the late 1960s made it possible for the second round of responses to Minamata disease to play a major role in the development of new forms of social citizenship. The LDP did remain in power for another twenty years after 1973, and Chisso continues to exist thanks to government assistance. But the ruling elites were undeniably put "on a shorter leash," in James White's phrase.[1] They were forced to employ to the utmost their talent, evident throughout modern Japanese history, for pre-emptive response and co-optation.

Although the Minamata disease incident did not shatter the tense equilibrium of the postwar Japanese polity, it helped change not only the point of equilibrium among the various forces but also the way in which that equilibrium was reached. In other words, political scientists are correct in noting a significant change in the early 1970s in the personnel, process, and outcomes of policymaking. But the role of pressure from outside both the ruling conservative coalition and the established opposition parties is much more important than is usually recognized. The citizen-corporation-state relationship was changed at least temporarily, as citizens forced the government to make significant policy changes and the courts to take on policymaking roles when the government would not. The 1973 court decision on Minamata showed that the judge felt a sense of crisis facing Japan (a sense that faded from later decisions); he was affected by the mood, opinions, and activities of citizens. Citizens devised patterns of political action such as the one-share movement that were truly new, quite unlike peasant rebellions, rice riots, or tenant unions.

This was done through patterns of organization and action separate from the established opposition parties. Only because the dominant stream of the Minamata movement was independent of the parties was it able to build a sufficiently broad base of support. Because it did, its contributions to postwar democracy were more important than those, for example, of the struggle by farmers and radical student sects against the construction of the New Tokyo International Airport in Narita, a struggle which alienated many Japanese with its violence and radical ideology. The outside supporters in Narita were far less willing than those in Minamata to let the victims speak for themselves.[2]

There was one important similarity between the Minamata and Narita movements, however. Both, at their peak, avoided domination by what

Patricia Steinhoff calls "a national protest cartel, formed by a few political *zaibatsu* [mainly the JSP and JCP], that monopolizes a large share of protest markets and eagerly swallows up new movements whenever possible."[3] But whereas the radical students in Narita proceeded to "swallow up" the farmers' protest for their own purposes, the Minamata movement, like the consumers' movement, was able to attract more mainstream support. But because the Minamata coalition was ad hoc and not incorporated by the established parties, it was temporary. And after 1973, most of this coalition, unlike established opposition groups such as the JCP, disappeared.

The Minamata movement's stress on autonomy from the established parties was by no means something new. Since the inception of political parties in the early 1880s, few Japanese have enthusiastically identified with them. The dominant conservative parties have often been perceived as corrupt, self-interested pyramids of local, regional, and national bosses, rather than channels through which public opinion can be made public policy. The leftist opposition parties have often been seen as rigid hierarchies driven by ideology, unwilling to deal with local issues except when they can be controlled from above and used to further their impractical ideological ends. This persistent distrust of political parties helps explain not only the ease with which the parties were removed from power in the 1930s and dissolved in 1940 but also the attraction of the New Left and the dominant groups in the Minamata movement.

Likewise, the co-optive responses of the conservative rulers were an extension of techniques skillfully practiced throughout Japan's modern history by leaders reacting to problems they did not expect, problems that have often been unintended results of their own policies. Marginalized groups, when they move to center stage with their complaints, have frequently been recognized, compensated, or co-opted just enough to partially remarginalize them without a full acceptance of their demands. This was the response to the Freedom and Popular Rights movement in the early 1880s, to the challenge posed to the oligarchs by the parties in the first decades of the Meiji constitution, and to tenant unions in the 1920s and 1930s.

Such a solution was applied to Minamata in 1973: the elite leadership, at the price of becoming more responsive and less complacent, was successful in remarginalizing challengers by partially compensating them for damages and to some extent recognizing their grievances. Pluralism was expanded, but still highly constrained. This incompleteness—in which neither side completely won or lost, and the issue was never completely resolved—meant the Minamata incident did not lead to revolutionary changes in the postwar political system. Yet it brought citizens more tools with which to act, and the political system itself was made somewhat more sensitive and open to popular concerns. It showed ways that average citizens *could* be active, and even confrontational, participants in politics, and that there was a wide range of channels and patterns for conflict.

Although there were great advances in terms of both participation and compensation from the first to the second round, processes for redress of citizens' grievances and for political participation in general were *not* significantly regularized or legitimated. Many of the new patterns of action and organization were costly and difficult to sustain or repeat. Certainly they were also less necessary after the 1973 settlement, but the aging Minamata disease victims and their shrinking support groups found it difficult to use the new tools developed from 1968 to 1973 effectively enough to resolve the remaining issues. What remained of the movement seemed mostly reactive and no longer aimed at having a significant influence on policy.

Other groups, of course, used some of the same techniques used by Minamata activists, but none was able to match the impact of the Minamata movement at its peak. The victims of poisoning by PCBs in Kanemi brand rice oil are one example.[4] The Kanemi Company of Kitakyūshū, like Chisso, was at the leading edge of its industry and denied responsibility and refused direct negotiations with patients as long as possible after its contaminated oil killed animals and sickened people beginning in 1968. Kanemi, like Chisso, signed an agreement paying some victims but denying responsibility. Victims were split between those who sued and those who did not, as well as between those willing to accept support from opposition parties and those who wanted to keep their distance from the JSP and JCP. Suits continued into the 1980s over certification, compensation, and responsibility, but they ended in 1989 when the last plaintiffs accepted a *wakai* that foreclosed all further chances to confirm government responsibility.

Reflections of the Minamata movement can also be seen in consumer activism and the anti–nuclear power movement.[5] No other "incident" or movement, however, has caught the public's attention or come to symbolize the dark side of high growth or been seen as a crucial test of postwar democracy to the extent that Minamata has. None, of course, has matched Minamata in scale or been as photogenically tragic or painfully drawn out. None has had the fortuitous timing of the second round of responses to Minamata, coming as it did between 1968 and the oil shock of 1973. None has been blessed with a writer such as Ishimure, a filmmaker such as Tsuchimoto, or photographers such as Kuwabara, Shiota, Akutagawa, Miyamoto, and the Smiths. The dominant stream of the Minamata movement stayed far more independent of the established opposition than most other movements did, thanks to the support groups in Minamata and Kumamoto. And the Minamata patients have been blessed with creative and persistent small leaders (as Irokawa calls them) within the community, such as Kawamoto Teruo and Ogata Masato.

It might even seem that Japan's citizens' movement has almost disappeared. It does seem to have lost much of its ability to grab headlines, as well as many of the links among local groups nationwide. The speculative boom of the late 1980s and the economic stagnation of the 1990s were not fertile soil for citizen action. But another reason the citizens' movement has partially disappeared from view is that much of it has dropped down to a local level, concerned with very local issues. Matsumoto Tsutomu of Minamata, for example, decided that the one hope for true democracy in Japan lay in the sort of "direct democracy" possible only at the community level.[6] If this means that he, and others like him, have given up hope that the system as a whole can change enough to be truly democratic, it is not an encouraging sign.

So Minamata does not offer a simple answer to questions about the nature of postwar democracy and whether it has "progressed." Institutions and procedures for pluralism were not made permanent by Minamata. But if democracy is measured instead by the effects of popular concerns and pressures on public policy, then Minamata did in fact strengthen democracy, at least in the early 1970s. If it is measured by the extent and vigor of popular political action and struggle (as progressive intellectuals and activist victims measure it), then the answer is also that Minamata did in fact advance the cause of democracy, but again more so during the second round of responses than later. And Matsumoto Tsutomu is not the only discouraged activist who has gone from believing that democracy at the national level can and must be built from the grass roots to the conclusion that the system at higher levels can never change enough to meet his standards for democracy.

The second round in the Minamata incident showed the value of the courts as venues for dispute resolution and compensation for those who lacked other channels of access, but the decisions in the courts were greatly influenced by the protests outside. And the courts did not dictate the terms of the solutions: patients used the court decisions to strengthen their hand in the negotiations resulting in the final compensation agreements. So Minamata undermines—but only partly—the stereotype of Japan as a society based on harmony, consensus, and informal dispute resolution. The Tokyo negotiations in the spring and summer of 1973 and the *wakai* agreement that resolved the Minamata issue for the third time might be called "formalized informal" dispute resolution—more public and better refereed than was the case in 1959, but still the result of direct, out-of-court negotiations.

By no means, therefore, did Japan inaugurate a permanent golden age of citizen activism in the late 1960s. Even if Japan's rulers today remain more responsive than in the 1950s, citizens' movements are weaker and more fragmented than in their heyday in the early 1970s. The 1973 Minamata settlement, in its very incompleteness, symbolizes both the possibilities and the *limits* of postwar democracy. This incomplete, ad hoc, constrained nature is not unique to Minamata; it can be seen in the anti–security treaty protests of 1960, the New Left, the antiwar movement of the 1960s and 1970s, and perhaps even the labor movement.

Minamata also offers a glimpse across the "criteria gap" in evaluations of Japan's postwar democracy. To draw the distinction broadly, Japan's governing elite, as well as most political scientists and most Americans, tend to focus on the infrastructure, whereas Japan's progressive intellectuals emphasize thought and behavior. We often say Japan is a democracy because it has a constitution, political parties, free elections, a free press, and popular rights. Such criteria are natural for Americans, who live with the legacies of the fight for the right to build this infrastructure for themselves. Indeed, when we do discuss thought and behavior in relation to our own democracy, we quote a foreign observer, de Tocqueville.

For Japan, it was Maruyama Masao who in the early postwar era exemplified the stress on the internalized patterns of thought and action essential for Japan to be truly democratic. Although some proclaimed him irrelevant after 1960, or 1968, in a general sense Maruyama's view of democracy remained widespread, as did his suspicion of parties and politicians, voiced in the quote that begins this chapter. Such a view is quite natural for people who have had a democratic system, and an imperial system before that, imposed on them from above.[7]

Minamata victims and supporters made this same point to the general public: there is more to democracy than the institutional/procedural definition used by political scientists whose criteria are representative government, free and fair elections, and constitutional guarantees of rights.[8] The Minamata movement exemplifies a much broader procedural definition: if democracy means government by the people, then no definition of democracy can ignore popular thought and action.[9] This latter definition is closer to the one used by scholars who emphasize questions of access to power and decision-making and of control of dispute resolution.[10] So Minamata might be seen as a struggle between these two definitions of democracy: a narrow institutional/procedural definition and a much broader procedural definition.

Both sides justify their views by recourse to a third definition of democracy, a substantive or distributive definition that stresses results. Japan's leaders pointed to the nation's dramatic growth and the relatively even distribution of its fruits compared to that found in the other industrial powers. Minamata disease victims argued, often very explicitly, that a democracy must be judged by whether minority voices are heard and respected when they demand compensation for their suffering. Neither view triumphed over the other, of course, but by challenging Japanese to judge their democracy by their own thought and actions as well as by the structure and functioning of their government, Minamata has had a significant effect.

In sum, then, despite the formal legal and institutional infrastructure, "postwar democracy" as defined and practiced by Japanese citizens and exemplified by responses to the Minamata disease incident has remained quite ad hoc: it is creative, exciting, and full of tools for citizens to use but always dependent on continual definition and redefinition in practice. Minamata has left a legacy not of regularized procedures and institutions for expanded pluralism but of possibilities.

EPILOGUE

Restless Spirits

"From this place, from Minamata as a miniature portrait of modern civilized Japan, I cry out from the bottom of my heart for the souls' return."

—Ogata Masato

On an early fall evening in 1996, Sugimoto Eiko stood on a patch of bare ground outside Shinagawa station in Tokyo, dressed in a white robe. Around her were other patients from Minamata. Invisible, but just as present and far more numerous, were the spirits of the people and all living things killed by Minamata disease. In the brisk wind Sugimoto tearfully welcomed the souls of the dead. Behind her was the *Nichigetsu maru*, an old wooden fishing sailboat known as an *utasebune* that had brought the spirits from the Shiranui Sea to Tokyo on a voyage captained by Ogata Masato. The large boat, which would never sail again, was dwarfed by the huge cranes behind it, building new skyscrapers as the city expanded farther out into Tokyo Bay.

The occasion was the opening of the Minamata Tokyo Exhibition, a striking example of the continuing hold of Minamata on public memory 40 years after the discovery of the disease. Earlier that evening there had been a different ceremony, by and for the organizers and staff of the exhibition. Irokawa Daikichi had talked of the significance of Minamata disease and the exhibition. Kan Naoto, who had begun his political career in citizens' groups and recently as minister of health and welfare had forced bureaucrats in his ministry to "discover" supposedly lost documents regarding the scandal in which hemophiliacs contracted HIV through contaminated blood products, had been expected to appear. But Kan was too busy preparing for the upcoming election, in which the new Democratic Party he cofounded did

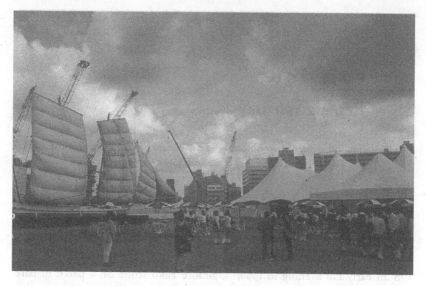

Fig. 34 The Minamata Tokyo Exhibition, visited by 30,000 people in the fall of 1996. At left is the *Nichigetsu maru*, sailed to Tokyo for the exhibition. © Timothy S. George.

poorly. The outgoing director general of the Environment Agency had arrived with his security men and driver and spoken of the *wakai* being put in place.

But the second ceremony was by and for the victims, living and dead. I had been asked to participate but declined, uncomfortable with being more than an observer of something that seemed so painful and private. Standing at the back of the group, I looked to my right and saw next to me the eminent sociologist Ishida Takeshi. To Ishida's right were Irokawa Daikichi and Ueno Chizuko, a feminist sociologist. These three were among the many public figures who had called for the holding of the exhibition, yet they too seemed to feel they belonged outside the circle of patients.

Soon, however, we and the others who had been standing moved forward and sat on the ground behind the patients. We joined in the chanting of a sutra for the restless souls from Minamata, reading the text by candlelight.[1]

The Minamata Tokyo Exhibition officially opened the next morning, and continued for sixteen days.[2] With its huge white tents and the white sails of the *Nichigetsu maru*, the site was clearly visible from Shinagawa station and the passing trains. Nearly 30,000 people attended. In addition to the *Nichigetsu maru*, the exhibition featured interpretive displays, showings of seventeen documentary films, five photo and art exhibits, four music and drama performances, a bookstore, and booths selling Minamata products—including seaweed and dried fish. There were 26 panel discussions and lectures by patients, scholars, writers, critics, activists, government officials, members of the media, and others.

A reproduction of the 1980 mural *Minamata* by the husband and wife artists Maruki Iri and Maruki Toshi was on display, and Toshi was present to show and comment on Tsuchimoto Noriaki's documentary film of the making of the mural. Photographs by the Smiths, Kuwabara Shisei, Shiota Takeshi, Miyamoto Shigemi, and Akutagawa Jin were shown. Aileen Smith joined a panel discussion on the significance of the photographs she and Eugene Smith took. A drama group from Minamata High School performed a play, and a choir sang a work with words by Ishimure Michiko.

For the first time, slices of the brains of Minamata disease victims were displayed in public. The brains were spongy, full of holes where cells should have been. One was from Tanaka Shizuko, who had become sick in April 1956 and helped prompt Hosokawa Hajime to recognize the disease. She had died in January 1959 at the age of eight.

The most powerful exhibit was a display of some 500 photographs of deceased victims of Minamata disease. Tsuchimoto Noriaki and his wife had spent over a year in Minamata collecting the photographs from relatives of the victims, and the difficulties they encountered are enlightening. To begin with, he wanted a list of names and addresses of certified patients who had died of Minamata disease. Amazingly, only Chisso had such a list, necessary because it pays compensation to certified victims. When a patient dies, Chisso sends a condolence letter to relatives and stops payments. Chisso refused to make the list public, ostensibly out of concern for the privacy of relatives, but the result is that even in death victims cannot escape the company that poisoned them. The Ministry of Health and Welfare, the Environment Agency, and Kumamoto and Kagoshima prefectures claim to keep only statistics, not complete lists of names and addresses.[3]

As a result, Tsuchimoto was not able to contact the relatives of all of the approximately 1,200 certified patients who had died. Even more surprising than Chisso's monopoly on the names of deceased victims were the reactions Tsuchimoto often encountered to his requests for photographs. He had been making films of Minamata for 30 years, always strongly on the side of

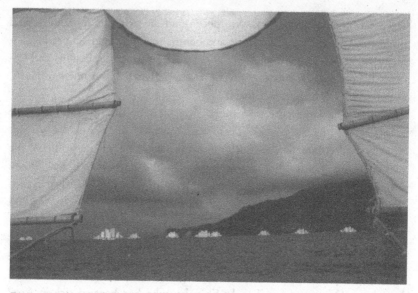

Fig. 35 *Utasebune* (sail-powered fishing boats) on the Shiranui Sea. These are similar to the *Nichigetsu maru* sailed to Tokyo in 1996 for the Minamata Tokyo Exhibition. © Akutagawa Jin.

the patients. Yet only two-thirds of the families he asked were willing to let him copy and display their relatives' photographs. In more than one case, people who had married into the family were dumbfounded at his request; until then they had not known that an in-law had been a victim of the disease.

And at the end of the exhibition, the fate of the photographs, powerful reminders that real people had suffered and died from the disease, was uncertain. Tsuchimoto offered the negatives to Mayor Yoshii, but some of the families had agreed to their display on the condition that they never be shown in Minamata or Kumamoto. As long as this need to hide the disease continues, says Tsuchimoto—and it is something he has seen ever since he first filmed in Minamata in 1965—the community will not have fully recovered.[4]

The *Nichigetsu maru*, too, was without a home at the end of the exhibition. Most of the few remaining Shiranui Sea *utasebune* are now used for tourist cruises. There was no need, and no money, to bring this one back home. It had already cost a great deal to repair and refit it for the voyage to Tokyo through open seas for which it was not designed and to have it hauled out of Tokyo Bay and brought to the exhibition site. But it had carried the spirits of the victims of Minamata disease to Tokyo. It could not simply be scrapped. Finally, the operator of an incinerator not far from Shinagawa agreed to handle the boat separately from the garbage he usually burned. Another ceremony—this time a funeral—was held for the boat and the memories and souls it had carried, and the *Nichigetsu maru* was reduced to ashes.

Reference Matter

Notes

For complete author names, titles, and publication data for works listed here in short form, see the Bibliography, pp. 339–64.

Introduction

1. Hamamoto tells his story in Saishu Satoru, ed., *Detsuki shiki.* The book consists of Hamamoto's reminiscences, recorded at his home on cassette tapes and transcribed and edited by Saishu. I have supplemented this with information from talks by Hamamoto and interviews with him, particularly an interview on Feb. 11, 1994. Hamamoto also briefly summarizes his own story in "Our Environment and Healthy Bodies Will Never Be Restored."

2. Saishu, *Detsuki shiki,* p. 100.

3. Ibid., p. 101.

4. Ibid., p. 107.

5. Ibid., p. 109. Yen amounts throughout this book are converted to dollars at then-current exchange rates. For 1945, however, no dollar conversion is attempted. Sources for exchange rates: for years through 1941, Bank of Japan, Statistics Department, *Hundred-Year Statistics of the Japanese Economy,* pp. 318–23; for 1971–72, *Japan: An Illustrated Encyclopedia,* p. 1746 (based on data from Bank of Japan, *Gaikoku keizai tōkei nenpō*); for 1973–95, *Asahi Shimbun Japan Almanac, 1995,* p. 104 (based on data from Bank of Japan, *Keizai tōkei nenpō*). From December 1949 to December 1971, the exchange rate was officially fixed at ¥360/$1.00; from December 1971 to February 1973 it was fixed at ¥308/$1.00 ±2.25 percent.

6. Shin Minamata-shi shi hensan iinkai, ed., *Shin Minamata-shi shi,* 1: 665–66.

7. Interview, Feb. 15, 1994; Kawamoto Teruo, "Tsubodan," in Akutagawa Jin, photographs, and Yanagida Kōichi, text, *Minamata: genson suru fūkei,* p. 175. According to Kawamoto, the group was very small (with seven or eight, perhaps as many as twelve, members), but the group disappeared around 1955 as more young people left Minamata for jobs elsewhere. *Seinendan* is usually translated as "young men's group," but Kawamoto's group included women.

8. Saishu, *Detsuki shiki*, pp. 63, 64.

9. Tsurumi Kazuko, "Man, Nature, and Technology: A Case of Minamata," p. 14.

10. Miyake Reiji, "Fukumeisho," in *MBJSS*, 1: 79–81.

11. Saishu, *Detsuki shiki*, p. 64.

12. "Neko tenkan de zenmetsu," *Kumamoto nichinichi shinbun*, Aug. 1, 1954; Minamata Disease Center Sōshisha, *Illustrated Minamata Disease*, p. 138.

13. Kitamura Masaji et al., "Minamata chihō ni hassei shita gen'in fumei no chūshū shinkei kei shikkan ni kan suru ekigaku chōsa seiseki," *Kumamoto igakukai zasshi* 31, no. 1 (Jan. 1957); reprinted in *MB* (an excellent annotated collection of primary sources, especially articles from newspapers and medical and scientific journals), p. 11.

14. When Eugene and Aileen Smith moved to Minamata in 1971, they rented a small house from Mizoguchi Toyoko's parents (W. Eugene Smith and Aileen Smith, *Minamata*, pp. 58–59).

15. On perceptions of disease and concepts of purity and impurity, see Emiko Ohnuki-Tierney, *Illness and Culture in Contemporary Japan*.

16. Harada Masazumi, "Minamatabyō igaku kenkyū no ayumi to konnichi no kadai," in Arima Sumio, ed., *Minamatabyō*, p. 6. See also W. Eugene Smith and Aileen Smith, *Minamata*, pp. 74–75.

17. Kumamoto-ken Minamata hokenjochō [Itō Hasuo] to [Kumamoto-ken] Eisei buchō, "Minamata-shi aza Tsukinoura fukin ni hassei seru shōni kibyō ni tsuite," May 4, 1956, in *MBJSS* 1: 473–74; "Kumamoto-ken Eisei buchō denpō (Kōseishō, Kōshū eiseikyoku bōeki kachō ate)," Aug. 3, 1956, in *MBJSS* 1: 474.

18. "Kono hito kono michi," *Kumamoto nichinichi shinbun*, April 25, 1976, quoted in Maruyama Sadami, "Kaisetsu," in *MBJSS* 1: 103.

19. Hosokawa's medical report on Egoshita Kazuko is given in part in Harada Masazumi, *Minamatabyō*, p. 4.

20. W. Eugene Smith and Aileen Smith, *Minamata*, pp. 10–11. Egoshita Kazuko was the first Minamata disease victim to be autopsied.

21. Saishu, *Detsuki shiki*, p. 112.

22. Hamamoto Tsuginori, interview, Feb. 11, 1994; lecture, "Uchi naru Minamata ni mimi o katamukeru," May 8, 1995.

23. Saishu, *Detsuki shiki*, pp. 112–26; Hamamoto Tsuginori, interview, Feb. 11, 1994; W. Eugene Smith and Aileen Smith, *Minamata*, pp. 76–81.

24. A wonderful exception is Norma Field's evocative *In the Realm of a Dying Emperor*. Through case studies of three nonconformists—an Okinawan supermarket owner who burned the rising sun flag, a Christian widow opposed to the Shintō enshrinement of her husband, who had been a member of the Japan Self-Defense Forces, and a mayor of Nagasaki who suggested that the Shōwa emperor bore some responsibility for the war—Field depicts a "system of coercive consensus" (p. 29).

This system, still symbolized for her by the emperor and reinforced by taboos and economic incentives, encourages an "unreflective prosperity" (p. 46) that rewards sacrifice, hard work, and docility and penalizes independent thought and action with ostracism and even bullets.

Field's emphasis on the importance of the free-thinking individual echoes the ideas of Maruyama Masao's classic early postwar essays stressing the need for "subjectivity" in casting off the psychological fetters of the emperor system and fascism. For Maruyama, Japanese after the war had to escape an "all-pervasive psychological coercion" through "an inner or spiritual revolution" (Maruyama Masao, "Theory and Psychology of Ultranationalism"). Maruyama, and others who shared his non-Marxist, "modernist" views such as Ōtsuka Hisao and to a lesser extent Ishida Takeshi, focused much more on the social structure and internalized patterns of thought and action necessary for democracy than on its legal and institutional infrastructure. In the early postwar period, they tended to see the traditional village community as a closed, hierarchical, feudal bastion of support for the emperor system and fascism and as highly resistant to change (Ishida Takeshi, "Sengo shakai kagaku to sonraku shi kenkyū," p. 35). In other words, the modernists' concern was less with constitutional or policymaking issues than with making Japanese into the kind of autonomous individuals on whom democracy depended in the West. (Many writings by Maruyama, Ōtsuka, and Ishida are available in English. In addition to the collection cited above for Maruyama, see especially Ōtsuka Hisao, "The Formation of Modern Man"; and Ishida Takeshi, Japanese Political Culture. On Maruyama, see also J. Victor Koschmann, Revolution and Subjectivity in Postwar Japan; and Rikki Kersten, Democracy in Postwar Japan.)

A compelling critique of the modernists (and Marxists) comes from Irokawa Daikichi and the "people's history" (minshūshi) school. (On the people's history school, see Carol Gluck, "The People in History.") Irokawa, greatly influenced by the ethnologist Yanagita Kunio, finds in the traditional village community (kyōdōtai) not oppressive hierarchy and a foundation for feudalism and militarism, but cooperation and egalitarianism and a strong source of resistance to state power and of an indigenous form of democracy. (Ishida Takeshi criticizes Irokawa's "romantic" view of the village community in "Sengo shakai kagaku to sonraku shi kenkyū," p. 37.) Since the early Meiji period, the village community has fought a "survival struggle" against centralized control, unbridled capitalism, and imperial ideology (Irokawa, "The Survival Struggle of the Japanese Community"). Irokawa (who is an activist as well as a scholar and has taken a particular interest in Minamata) has a more optimistic view than the Marxists or modernists because of the village-based movements he sees arising from among the people, from the early Meiji Movement for Freedom and Popular Rights to the present. Although I do not always agree with the "people's history" school's characterization of the traditional village, its emphasis on the local community, on real individuals, and on documents and oral history that other historians ignore has helped and inspired me.

25. Curiously, more work has been done on this topic by historians of imperial Japan; see especially Carol Gluck, *Japan's Modern Myths*; Sheldon Garon, *The State and Labor in Modern Japan*; Sheldon Garon, *Molding Japanese Minds*; Andrew Gordon, *Labor and Imperial Democracy in Prewar Japan*; Gregory James Kasza, *The State and the Mass Media in Japan, 1918–1945*; and Louise Young, *Japan's Total Empire*.

One exception for the postwar period is an essay by Sheldon Garon and Mike Mochizuki that takes issue with prevailing policymaking interpretations in two ways. First, they argue that rather than skillfully undercutting the opposition through pre-emptive adoption of its demands, the conservative coalition was in fact forced by strong pressures from below and outside and by a broad social consensus to negotiate "social contracts" with small business and labor. Second, they see no "unraveling of the 1955 system" in the early 1970s, arguing instead that Japan's rulers have had to negotiate such "social contracts" throughout the postwar period (see Sheldon Garon and Mike Mochizuki, "Negotiating Social Contracts," pp. 147–48, 164–65).

Two others with wider views of postwar politics are Susan Pharr, who has studied social protest groups, and Margaret McKean, who has analyzed anti-pollution residents' movements (see Pharr, *Losing Face: Status Politics in Japan*; and McKean, *Environmental Protest and Citizen Politics in Japan*). Pharr (*Losing Face*, p. xii) shows how protest groups may have little incentive to become highly organized or institutionalized because they have little hope of gaining a seat at the tables of power. Instead, they seek one-time "concessions" from "paternalistic" authorities. McKean's residents' groups, too, have as their immediate objectives specific, local policy decisions rather than permanent membership in the policymaking circles they find distant and distasteful.

26. T. J. Pempel ("The Unbundling of 'Japan, Inc.'") has argued that after the first fifteen years of the "1955 system," the system of rule by conservative elites symbolized by the unbroken reign of the Liberal Democratic Party (LDP) from its creation in 1955 until 1993, power leaked from top bureaucrats in key ministries to a somewhat broader range of elites, including party leaders, Diet members, and even foreign actors pressuring Japan. The result was by no means grass-roots democracy, but an increased, if still narrowly circumscribed, pluralism that made the system governing Japan far too complex by the 1980s to be called "Japan, Inc."

Kent Calder describes postwar Japanese political history as alternating between periods of calm and periods of crisis, both within the ruling conservative coalition and between it and the opposition. He concludes that "the Japan of noncrisis periods . . . appears much less democratic than when crisis pertains" (Calder, *Crisis and Compensation*, p. 473). During the crisis periods, despite the "deeply rooted anti pluralist bias to much of Japanese political structure and culture" which has "discouraged the assertion of citizen rights against the state," conservative rulers find it necessary to at least partially translate some opposition demands into policy (ibid., pp. 470–71). The third of the crisis periods Calder identifies was from 1971 to 1976, and it therefore overlaps with both the period of significant change identified by Pempel and the second round of responses to Minamata disease.

Gary Allinson, too, sees this period as critical. For him the early 1970s were the time when "specialist elites"—including career politicians within the LDP, "policy tribes" (*seisaku zoku*) of LDP Diet members interested in particular policy areas, and new types of leaders in business—replaced "bureaucratic elites" in the dominant position within the ruling elite (Allinson, "The Structure and Transformation of Conservative Rule," pp. 127, 137–39).

Chapter 1

1. Aston, *Nihongi*, p. 198; Shin Minamata-shi shi hensan iinkai, *Shin Minamata-shi shi*, 1: 140.

2. Shin Minamata-shi shi hensan iinkai, *Shin Minamata-shi shi*, 1: 141–43; Irokawa Daikichi, "Shiranuikai minshūshi," pp. 244–45.

3. Irokawa, "Shiranuikai minshūshi," p. 246. For a detailed look at the Sagara and the areas they controlled, see Nobukuni Masafumi, *Shin Sagara shiwa*.

4. Irokawa, "Shiranuikai minshūshi," pp. 252–53. In one rebellion, the home of journalist Tokutomi Sohō's *shōya* (village headman) grandfather was surrounded but not damaged. Tokutomi Sohō was Minamata's most famous native son (see Pierson, *Tokutomi Sohō*). On Tokugawa peasant rebellions, see Bix, *Peasant Protest in Japan*; Vlastos, *Peasant Protests and Uprisings in Tokugawa Japan*; and Walthall, *Social Protest and Popular Culture in Eighteenth-Century Japan*.

5. Irokawa, "Shiranuikai minshūshi," p. 249.

6. Shin Minamata-shi shi hensan iinkai, *Shin Minamata-shi shi*, 2: 29.

7. Irokawa, *Minamata*, p. 46. As Neil Waters (*Japan's Local Pragmatists*) has shown for the Kawasaki area, local notables in the early Meiji period were often able to modify or weaken the effects of the new government's policies on their areas and on their own power.

8. Okamoto Tatsuaki and Matsuzaki Tsugio, *Kikigaki Minamata minshūshi*, is an oral history of Minamata from Meiji to just after World War II, compiled over twenty years of interviews and editing. For Saiki's comment, from an interview, see 2: 217.

9. Shin Minamata-shi shi hensan iinkai, *Shin Minamata-shi shi* 2: 154–56; Irokawa, "Shiranuikai minshūshi," p. 276. On the lives and work of those producing salt, see the section on the salt industry in Okamoto and Matsuzaki, *Kikigaki Minamata*

minshūshi, 1: 117–30. On salt production in the Fukuoka area during the Tokugawa period, see Kalland, *Fishing Villages in Tokugawa Japan*, pp. 91–95.

10. Shin Minamata-shi shi hensan iinkai, *Shin Minamata-shi shi*, 2: 154, 157. Tobacco had been made a government monopoly in 1904, also to help pay the costs of the war.

11. Irokawa, "Shiranuikai minshūshi," p. 276; Shin Minamata-shi shi hensan iinkai, *Shin Minamata-shi shi* 2: 154. See Okamoto and Matsuzaki, *Kikigaki Minamata minshūshi*, 1: 144–50, for the carters, and 2: 29–40, for the Ushio and Ōkuchi gold mines.

12. For a history of this industry focusing on Noguchi Shitagau's company, which built its factory in Minamata, see Molony, *Technology and Investment*. The definitive work on the company is Ōshio Takeshi, *Nitchitsu kontserun no kenkyū*. Both of these works, however, cover only the period through World War II. For scholarship on the postwar history of the company, see Yahagi Tadashi, "Nihon chisso hiryō (kabu) ni kan suru kenkyū"; idem, "Sengo Chisso shi, 1945–55"; idem, "Chisso shi, 1955–60: Minamatabyō"; idem, "Chisso shi, 1960–65: Goi kōjō kensetsu"; and Uno Shigeaki, "Chisso kigyō ron." Nihon chisso hiryō K.K. changed its name to Shin Nihon chisso hiryō K.K. in 1950, and to Chisso K.K. in 1965. In its first two incarnations it was usually called by the abbreviated names Nitchitsu and Shin Nitchitsu. Even the pre-1965 company is often referred to now as Chisso, although in Minamata it has from the start most often been simply "the company" (*kaisha*).

13. Shin Minamata-shi shi hensan iinkai, *Shin Minamata-shi shi*, 1: 666 and 2: 205–6; Okamoto and Matsuzaki, *Kikigaki Minamata minshūshi*, 2: 41–42; and Ui Jun, *Kōgai no seijigaku*, pp. 13–14.

14. Shin Minamata-shi shi hensan iinkai, *Shin Minamata-shi shi*, 2: 206.

15. See Okamoto and Matsuzaki, *Kikigaki Minamata minshūshi*, 2: 42; and Irokawa, "Shiranuikai minshūshi," pp. 280–81.

16. Okamoto and Matsuzaki, *Kikigaki Minamata minshūshi*, vol. 2; Maruyama Sadami, "Kigyō to chiiki keisei," p. 21. One hundred sen equaled one yen.

17. On the opprobrium shown Meiji and Taishō workers, see Thomas C. Smith, *Native Sources of Japanese Industrialization, 1750–1920*, pp. 239–41.

18. Yahagi, "Nihon chisso hiryō (kabu) ni kan suru kenkyū," p. 96.

19. Shin Minamata-shi shi hensan iinkai, *Shin Minamata-shi shi*, 2: 5–9.

20. Funaba Masatomi, "Chisso to chiiki shakai," pp. 44–45.

21. Molony, *Technology and Investment*, pp. 99–100.

22. Yahagi, "Nihon chisso hiryō (kabu) ni kan suru kenkyū," p. 67.

23. Ōshio, *Nitchitsu kontserun no kenkyū*, pp. 52–53; Yahagi, "Nihon chisso hiryō (kabu) ni kan suru kenkyū," p. 67.

24. Yahagi, "Nihon chisso hiryō (kabu) ni kan suru kenkyū," pp. 57–58, 65.

25. Ibid., pp. 58–59.

26. Ōshio, *Nitchitsu kontserun no kenkyū*, p. 121. Molony (*Technology and Investment*, p. 244) gives the number as 64.

27. Molony, *Technology and Investment*, pp. 129, 280. Japan's early postwar conservative leader, Yoshida Shigeru, was also known as "one man" (see Dower, *Empire and Aftermath*, pp. 1, 305).

28. This remark is widely known and repeated, but I have found no definitive proof that Noguchi uttered it (see Okamoto and Matsuzaki, *Kikigaki Minamata minshūshi*, 2: 165; Ui, *Kōgai no seijigaku*, p. 25).

29. Molony, *Technology and Investment*, pp. 111–12.

30. Nitchitsu's 1937 company history lists six Japanese and four pending Manchukuo patents for the production of acetaldehyde and acetic acid by processes invented wholly or partly by Hashimoto (Nihon chisso hiryō kabushiki kaisha, *Nihon chisso hiryō jigyō taikan*, pp. 145, 151).

31. Arima Sumio, "Kaisetsu," *MBJSS* 1: 9.

32. Minamatabyō kenkyūkai, ed., *Minamatabyō ni tai suru kigyō no sekinin*, pp. 123, 147; Miyazawa Nobuo, "Kaisetsu," *MBJSS* 2: 973.

33. Molony, *Technology and Investment*, p. 166.

34. A 1939 biography of Noguchi by Katagiri Ryūkichi was titled *Hantō no jigyō ō: Noguchi Shitagau* (Entrepreneurial king of the peninsula: Noguchi Shitagau). (The translation "entrepreneurial king of the peninsula" is from Molony, *Technology and Investment*, p. 156.)

35. Molony, *Technology and Investment*, pp. 168–69.

36. Yahagi, "Nihon chisso hiryō (kabu) ni kan suru kenkyū," p. 70.

37. Ibid., p. 65.

38. Onitsuka Iwao, interview, Dec. 6, 1993. See Okamoto and Matsuzaki, *Kikigaki Minamata minshūshi*, vol. 5, for accounts of life and work in Korea.

39. Okamoto and Matsuzaki, *Kikigaki Minamata minshūshi*, 4: 281, 290–91.

40. Ibid., p. 308.

41. Molony, *Technology and Investment*, p. 236.

42. Ibid., pp. 241–42.

43. Ibid., p. 156.

44. Ibid., pp. 246, 254–57; Yamada Ryōzō, "Kigyō annai," in Fukumoto Kunio, ed., *Noguchi Shitagau wa ikite iru*, pp. 235–37. Nihon kōei was headed by Kubota Yutaka, who had directed the Yalu River dam project. Shortly after its founding, Nihon kōei produced a promotional film, *Chōsen ni okeru dai suiryoku hatsuden kaihatsu no kiroku*, based on a documentary of the Yalu project. The new narration removed references to locations in Korea as being in "our country."

45. Molony, *Technology and Investment*, pp. 227, 225.

46. Ibid., pp. 231, 227 (quoting Noguchi).

47. Shin Minamata-shi shi hensan iinkai, *Shin Minamata-shi shi*, 2: 206; Yahagi, "Nihon chisso hiryō (kabu) ni kan suru kenkyū," pp. 65–66.

48. Ishimure Michiko, *Kugai jōdo*, pp. 240–41. This and subsequent quotes are from the English translation by Livia Monnet, *Paradise in the Sea of Sorrow*, pp. 283–85.

49. Nihon chisso hiryō kabushiki kaisha, *Nihon chisso jigyō gaiyō*, unpaginated. This section is reprinted in *MBJSS*, 1: 52–54. It is not clear whether the censorship was self-censorship or not. In some places several lines are blank, in others numerals have been replaced with circles, and in still others characters have been blacked out.

Chapter 2

1. See Kikuchi Masanori, "Chisso rōdō kumiai to Minamatabyō," p. 517.

2. Maruyama Sadami, "Kigyō to chiiki keisei," p. 24; Shinohara Miyohei, *Kojin shohi shishutsu*, pp. 12, 135; *Asahi Shinbun Japan Almanac 1997*, p. 275.

3. Ishida Takeshi, "Minamata ni okeru yokuatsu to sabetsu no kōzō," pp. 55–56.

4. Shin Minamata-shi shi hensan iinkai, *Shin Minamata-shi shi*, 2: 991–92, 995.

5. Irokawa, *Minamata: sono sabetsu no fūdo to rekishi*, pp. 42–44.

6. Ishimure Michiko, interview, July 12, 1994.

7. Irokawa, *Minamata: sono sabetsu no fūdo to rekishi*, p. 45.

8. Ibid., p. 48.

9. Ishida, "Minamata ni okeru yokuatsu to sabetsu no kōzō," p. 55.

10. Onitsuka Iwao, who died in 1998, was a meticulous recordkeeper, an accomplished amateur photographer and filmmaker, and one of the best sources of information on Minamata. His autobiography, *Oruga Minamata*, offers a wealth of details, especially from his own photographs and drawings. I interviewed him on Dec. 6, 1993; Jan. 1, Jan. 10, Mar. 15, July 15, and Nov. 14, 1994; and June 13, 1995, and met informally with him a number of other times.

11. See Onitsuka, *Oruga Minamata*, pp. 248–52, for a time line of Iwao's life to 1986.

12. Ibid., p. 95. See Okamoto and Matsuzaki, *Kikigaki Minamata minshūshi*, 4: 165–71, for a description of the acetylene explosion on May 28, 1937, which was one of the three biggest in the history of the factory.

13. Chō Michiaki, testimony in Kumamoto District Court, March 17, 1972; see *Hōritsu jihō* 45, no. 3 (Feb. 1973): 374.

14. Minamatabyō kenkyūkai, ed., *Minamatabyō ni tai suru kigyō no sekinin*, p. 160.

15. The chemical industry was far more dangerous than others, since the injury rate for the manufacturing industry as a whole was under 4 percent (Ōhara shakai mondai kenkyūjo, ed., *Nihon rōdō nenkan*, pp. 110–11, 113).

16. Onitsuka, *Oruga Minamata*, p. 65.

17. Okamoto and Matsuzaki, *Kikigaki Minamata minshūshi*, 4: 291–94. In 1944, there were twelve or thirteen Korean women at a brothel in Marushima in Minamata (ibid., pp. 295–99).

18. Onitsuka, *Oruga Minamata*, pp. 51–54, 59.

19. Ibid., pp. 54–55.

20. On the air raids against Minamata, see Shin Minamata-shi shi hensan iinkai, *Shin Minamata-shi shi*, 1: 853–936; and United States Strategic Bombing Survey, *Final Reports of the United States Strategic Bombing Survey 1945–1947*, Reports no. 49 and 50.

21. Shin Minamata-shi shi hensan iinkai, *Shin Minamata-shi shi*, 1: 871–72.

22. Onitsuka, *Oruga Minamata*, p. 65.

23. Shin Minamata-shi shi hensan iinkai, *Shin Minamata-shi shi*, 1: 871.

24. United States Strategic Bombing Survey, Report no. 49, pp. 55, 65; Report no. 50, p. 158. Coincidentally it was the Shōwa Electrical Industry Co., or Shōwa denkō, which owned the factory in Niigata prefecture that caused Japan's "second Minamata disease," discovered along the Agano River in 1965.

25. Some of Nitchitsu's former holdings went on to become major corporations, including Sekisui House, Sekisui Chemical, and Asahi Chemical (Molony, *Technology and Investment*, p. 318). On the breakup of the *zaibatsu*, see Bisson, *Zaibatsu Dissolution in Japan*; Burkman, ed., *The Occupation of Japan*; Hadley, *Anti-Trust in Japan*; Howard Schonberger, "Zaibatsu Dissolution and the American Restoration of Japan"; Supreme Commander for the Allied Powers (SCAP), *History of Non-Military Aspects of the Occupation of Japan* (see esp. monographs #24, "Elimination of Zaibatsu Control," and #25, "Deconcentration of Economic Power"); and U.S. Department of State, *Report of the Mission on Japanese Combines* ("The Edwards Report"), Part I, *Analytical and Technical Data* (Appendix J, pp. 208–16, plus an unnumbered page between 216 and 217, concerns Nitchitsu).

26. U.S. Department of State, *Report of the Mission on Japanese Combines*, 1: 208–10.

27. Hirohito toured Kyūshū from May 18 to June 10, 1949. On June 1 he spent 94 busy minutes in Minamata. Citizens greeted him in front of the station before he walked across the street for lunch at the Nitchitsu factory and greetings from the governor, vice governor, director of general affairs, and police commander of Kumamoto prefecture, and the governor of Kagoshima prefecture. He then toured the factory on foot (Irie Sukemasa, *Irie Sukemasa nikki*, 2: 325; Suzuki Masao, *Shōwa tennō no gojunkō*, p. 273; see also Bix, "Inventing the 'Symbol Monarchy' in Japan, 1945–52").

28. Hirohito to Crown Prince Akihito, Sept. 9, 1945, in Takahashi Hiroshi, *Shōwa tennō hatsugenroku*, p. 115.

29. Yahagi, "Sengo Chisso shi, 1945–55," p. 166.

30. Ui, *Kōgai no seijigaku*, p. 16.

31. "Eigyō kaigi ruporutāju: matareru yūki no zōsan," *Minamata kōjō shinbun*, Apr. 10, 1957; in *MBJSS*, 1: 331–32.

32. Arima Sumio, "Kaisetsu," in *MBJSS*, 1: 9–11; Ui, *Kōgai no seijigaku*, p. 17.

33. Onitsuka, *Oruga Minamata*, pp. 100–101; Kikuchi, "Chisso rōdō kumiai to Minamatabyō," p. 520.

34. Gordon, "Contests for the Workplace"; idem, *Postwar Japan as History*, p. 379.

35. Maruyama Sadami, "Kigyō to chiiki keisei," p. 24.

36. See the excerpts from the company's April 1972 pamphlet, *Kaisha annai: Chisso o shiru tame no tebiki*, reprinted in Onitsuka, *Oruga Minamata*, pp. 100–101.

37. See Gordon, "Contests for the Workplace," pp. 378–83.

38. Ishida Takeshi, "Minamata ni okeru yokuatsu to sabetsu no kōzō," pp. 51–52.

39. Maruyama Sadami, "Kigyō to chiiki keisei," p. 26.

40. Funaba, "Chisso to chiiki shakai," pp. 69, 75.

41. Ui, *Kōgai no seijigaku*, pp. 21–22.

42. See ibid., pp. 23–24, on local politics in Minamata in the 1950s.

43. Ibid., p. 25.

44. Ibid., p. 24.

45. Irokawa, "Shiranuikai minshūshi," p. 334.

46. Yamaguchi Yoshito, interview, July 15, 1994.

47. On complaints by merchants about the dominance of Suikōsha, see Shin Minamata-shi shi hensan iinkai, *Shin Minamata-shi shi*, 2: 161.

48. Yoshinaga Toshio, "Dai ni no Minamatabyō."

49. Ui, *Kōgai no seijigaku*, pp. 26–27.

50. Only 45 employees—1.1 percent of the total and less than 1.7 percent of those not in company housing—engaged in fishing as a secondary occupation (Kikuchi, "Chisso rōdō kumiai to Minamatabyō," p. 518).

51. See Saishu, *Detsuki shiki*. I have also drawn on interviews with Hamamoto on Oct. 4, 1993, Feb. 11, 1994, and Nov. 12, 1994 (this latter interview including his wife, Harue, and sister Fumiyo); on talks given by him on Nov. 3, 1994, May 7, 1995, and May 9, 1995; and on numerous informal conversations with him. There is a section on "The Hamamoto Family" in W. E. Smith and A. Smith, *Minamata*, pp. 76–81.

52. On *amimoto* and *amiko* in the Fukuoka area, see Kalland, *Fishing Villages in Tokugawa Japan*, pp. 137–41; and for the Setonaikai area, Norbeck, *Takashima*, p. 18. In Minamata as well as the Amakusa area, the *amimoto* were generally not as wealthy, and the social and economic gaps between them and the *amiko* were not as great as those suggested by Kalland and Norbeck.

53. See Shin Minamata-shi shi hensan iinkai, *Shin Minamata-shi shi*, 1: 701–6; Okamoto and Matsuzaki, *Kikigaki Minamata minshūshi*, 1: 78–84; and Onitsuka, *Oruga Minamata*, pp. 219–24, on the history of the *haze* trees (which began as a source of income for the domain in the Tokugawa period) and the lawsuit. These fields were on land originally owned directly by the Hosokawa *daimyō* and called in

Minamata *gonaikachi*, stretching from Samurai (where Onitsuka lived) through Otashiro to Detsuki.

54. Shin Minamata-shi shi hensan iinkai, *Shin Minamata-shi shi*, 2: 321.

55. Saishu, *Detsuki shiki*, p. 95.

56. Ibid.

57. See Kevin M. Doak's discussion of "internal colonialism" in the Meiji state in "What Is a Nation and Who Belongs?" pp. 288–89.

58. Irokawa Daikichi, interviewed in the series "Watashi no Minamata taiken," *Kumamoto nichinichi shinbun*, Apr. 3, 1996.

59. Okamoto Tatsuaki, "Atogaki," in Okamoto and Matsuzaki, *Kikigaki Minamata minshūshi*, 5: 344.

60. Ui, *Kōgai no seijigaku*, p. 26. Maruyama Sadami ("Kigyō to chiiki keisei," p. 33) uses the term *kigyō unmei kyōdōtai*, a "community sharing a single fate with the company." In English, Maruyama uses the term "shared destiny" (see his "Responses to Minamata Disease," p. 54).

61. The effect of the coming of a cash economy on the traditional, natural, cooperative community (*kyōdotai*) is the theme of Okamoto and Matsuzaki, *Kikigaki Minamata minshūshi*, vol. 3, *Mura no hōkai*, although its focus is on the prosperous inland farming village of Fukagawa.

62. Molony, *Technology and Investment*, p. 258.

Chapter 3

1. Onitsuka Iwao, interview, Mar. 15, 1994; Irokawa, *Minamata: sono sabetsu no fūdo to rekishi*, p. 20.

2. Ui, *Kōgai no seijigaku*, p. 146.

3. On Hosokawa, see Arima Sumio, "Hosokawa Hajime ron nōto."

4. There is very little written on Itō. One source is Ui, *Kōgai no seijigaku*, p. 7.

5. Quoted in Maruyama Sadami, "Kaisetsu," in *MBJSS*, 1: 100.

6. For the committee's records of its activities from May 28, 1956, to June 3, 1959, see "Minamata-shi kibyō taisaku iinkai nisshi," in *MBJSS*, 1: 774–95. See also Ui, *Kōgai no seijigaku*, pp. 7–9, on this committee.

7. Ui, *Kōgai no seijigaku*, p. 9.

8. Kumamoto daigaku igakubu, "Minamata chihō ni hassei seru chūshū shinkei kei shikkan ni kan suru chūkan hōkoku," Nov. 3, 1956, in *MBJSS*, 1: 799–808.

9. Tanaka Asao, "Nakigoe ga kieta," in Yamamoto Shigeo, ed., *Kanashikaru inochi idakite*, p. 13; Sugimoto Eiko, discussion at Hama Kōminkan, Minamata, July 16, 1994; Irokawa, *Minamata: sono sabetsu no fūdo to rekishi*, p. 20.

10. Miyairi used the English terms "ecology," "medical ecology," and "epidemiology" in his report, "Minamata kibyō ekigaku chōsa ni tsuite," which is in the Minamatabyō kenkyūkai Collection (MBKK).

11. "Minamata kibyō ni kan suru chōsa," in *MBJSS*, 1: 316–22. The report is also quoted at length and discussed in Ui, *Kōgai no seijigaku*, pp. 33–35.

12. Ui, *Kōgai no seijigaku*, p. 12.

13. Quoted in ibid., pp. 11–12.

14. Sugimoto Eiko (panel discussion with Hamamoto Tsuginori, Minamata Tokyo Yokayoka Matsuri, Rikkyō University, Tokyo), May 7, 1995; idem, "Watashi to Minamatabyō: kanjasan no hanashi kara," Sept. 30, 1996.

15. Ui, *Kōgai no seijigaku*, p. 42.

16. The Hiratsuka case is mentioned in the Kumamoto University research group's report of January 1957, in *MB*, p. 16.

17. On the importance of MITI, see Johnson, *MITI and the Japanese Miracle*.

18. Ui, *Kōgai no seijigaku*, p. 39.

19. Minamata shichō Hashimoto Hikoshichi, "Kibyō hasseigen ni tsuite ichi kōsatsu," Apr. 8, 1957, in *MBJSS*, 1: 360.

20. *MB*, p. 72.

21. "Minamata wan no gyohō o kinshi," in *MB*, p. 71.

22. Kōseishō kōshū eisei kyokuchō and Kumamoto-ken chiji, "Minamata chihō ni hassei shita chūshū shinkei kei shikkan ni tomonau gyōsei sochi ni tsuite," Sept. 11, 1957, in *MBJSS*, 1: 670–71.

23. See Ui, *Kōgai no seijigaku*, p. 37.

24. Ibid. The Tanigawa family is one of the two Minamata families known nationwide. (The other is the Tokutomi brothers, journalist and critic Sohō and novelist Roka.) Tanigawa Gan had written for the *Nishinippon shinbun*, and in the mid- and late-1950s was a prefectural official of the Communist party and the leader of a revolutionary literary society that included Ishimure Michiko. Tanigawa Gan's father, an ophthalmologist, headed the Minamata medical association. Gan's brother Ken'ichi was a critic, and his brother Michio was a scholar of Chinese literature (Ishimure Michiko, interview, July 12, 1994; Mishima Akio, *Nake, Shiranui no umi*, pp. 16–17; Mishima's book has been translated by Richard L. Gage and Susan B. Murata as *Bitter Sea: The Human Cost of Minamata Disease*).

25. *MB*, p. 136. Hosokawa later told Ishimure Michiko that he had read the play (Ishimure, interview, July 12, 1994). For the play, see Ibsen, *Ghosts and Other Plays*.

26. Hidaka Rokurō, "Minamata kara kangaeru 9: kyōiku," lecture, Tokyo, Oct. 9, 1996.

27. Maruyama Sadami, "Kaisetsu," in *MBJSS*, 1: 108. See W. E. Smith and A. M. Smith, *Minamata*, p. 49, for a photograph of a sedimentation pool at Hachiman.

28. McAlpine and Araki, "Minamata Disease," pp. 629–31; Hunter et al., "Poisoning by Methyl Mercury Compounds"; Hunter and Russell, "Focal Cerebral and Cerebellar Atrophy in a Human Subject Due to Organic Mercury Compounds."

29. Takeuchi Tadao, "Minamatabyō no byōrigakuteki tsuikyū no ayumi: fumei shikkan Minamatabyō kara yūki suigin chūdokubyō e," in Arima, *Minamatabyō*, pp. 34–35.

30. Ui, *Kōgai no seijigaku*, p. 40; Harada Masazumi, interview, June 8, 1995.

31. "'Minamatabyō' ni kokusaiteki mesu," *Kumamoto nichinichi shinbun*, Sept. 18, 1958; in *MB*, p. 83. The headline for this article uses the term "Minamatabyō" (Minamata disease) in quotation marks. "Minamatabyō" replaced "kibyō" (strange disease) as the standard word for the disease in newspaper reports around August 1958, although "Minamatabyō" was apparently first used in a newspaper headline in the May 5, 1957, edition of the *Nishinippon shinbun*. See Maruyama Sadami and Minamatabyō kenkyūkai, ed., *Shōwa 54 nendo Minamatabyō ni kan suru sōgōteki chōsa tehō no kaihatsu ni kan suru kenkyū hōkokusho*. This and a subsequent volume contain a list of all articles concerning Minamata disease in the major regional and national newspapers from May 8, 1956, through March 21, 1973, and are therefore an invaluable index for the researcher.

32. Kumamoto-ken eiseibu, "Nitchitsu ga Minamatabyō kenkyū ni hikyōryoku na jirei," Oct. 1959, in *MBJSS*, 1: 532.

33. Kurland, "An Epidemiological Overview of Minamata Disease and a Review of Earlier Public Health Recommendations," p. 241. See also Kurland et al., "Minamata Disease," p. 370. For summary reports of the NIH research up to the fall of 1959, see *MBJSS*, 1: 921–25.

34. "Minamata kibyō no gen'in wa Shin Nitchitsu no haikibutsu, Kōseishō kagaku han ga suitei," July 9, 1958; in *MB*, p. 79.

35. "Kumamoto-ken Minamata-shi ni hassei shita iwayuru Minamatabyō no kenkyū seika oyobi sono taisaku ni tsuite," July 7, 1958, in *MBJSS*, 1: 675–78.

36. "Minamata kibyō ni kan suru tōsha no kenkai," July 1958, in *MBJSS*, 1: 247–52.

37. *Kumamoto igakukai shi* 33, no. 3 (Mar. 1959): 639; Ui, *Kōgai no seijigaku*, pp. 49–50.

38. "Minamatabyō no gen'in wa yūki suigin," *Asahi shinbun*, July 14, 1959; in *MB*, pp. 91–92.

39. *Kumamoto igakukai shi* 34, no. 3 (Mar. 1960); in *MB*, p. 42.

40. Kitamura et al., "Minamatabyō ni kan suru kagaku dokubutsu kensaku seisaku," *Kumamoto igakukai shi* 34, no. 3 (Mar. 1960): 593 (in *MB*, p. 42; and Arima, *Minamatabyō*, p. 9); Harada, *Minamatabyō*, p. 50; Ui, *Kōgai no seijigaku*, p. 51.

41. Ui, *Kōgai no seijigaku*, p. 57.

42. "Minamatabyō no yūki suigin setsu ni hanron," *Asahi shinbun*, Aug. 6, 1959; in *MB*, p. 98. This committee had been established on July 8. In a typical attempt at balanced representation, the chairman was from Ashikita *gun*, north of Minamata, and supported mostly by fishing families; the vice chairman was a representative from Minamata who was concurrently the head of the Shin Nitchitsu labor union.

43. "Minamatabyō tokubetsu i ni nozomu," in *MB*, p. 97.

44. August 20, 1959; in *MB*, p. 97.

45. For the pamphlets, see *MBJSS*, 1: 257–60, 267–68, 275–83, 283–93. They are also discussed and reprinted, in part, in *MB*, pp. 112–16, 121–35; and summarized in Ui, *Kōgai no seijigaku*, pp. 80–87.

46. Ui, *Kōgai no seijigaku*, p. 80.

47. Arima Sumio, "Kaisetsu," in *MBJSS*, 1: 9.

48. "Minamatabyō gen'in ni tsuite," Sept. 1959, in MBKK.

49. MBKK.

50. Ui, *Kōgai no seijigaku*, p. 85.

51. Documents showing that the factory knew in 1950 that organic mercury was created in the acetaldehyde production process came to light only recently. See "Shōwa 25 nen 'yūki suigin shōjiru,'" *Nishinippon shinbun*, Jan. 3, 1995. Many more documents that would shed important light on the Minamata disease incident, such as records of executive conferences, are still held by the company. Since nearly all the court cases surrounding Minamata disease have been, and are, civil rather than criminal cases, there are many valuable documents that the company has not been required to release.

52. In Ui, *Kōgai no seijigaku*, p. 86.

53. Ibid., p. 10.

54. See ibid., pp. 35–37. Itō described his experiments in an article in *Kumamoto igakukai shi* 31, no. 2 (June 1957): 282; excerpts from this article can be found in Ui, *Kōgai no seijigaku*, p. 36. Years later, his reminiscences about the experiments were broadcast in the program *Shiranuikai, Shōwa 32 nen haru: rajio ga tsutaeta Minamatabyō jiken* in the series *Rajio anguru '94*, May 7, 1994, NHK Radio.

55. See Ui, *Kōgai no seijigaku*, pp. 86–88, on Hosokawa's experiments.

56. *MB*, p. 135.

57. Miyazawa Nobuo, "Kaisetsu," in *MBJSS*, 2: 987.

58. Ishimure Michiko, interview, July 12, 1994.

59. [Shin Nitchitsu] Gijutsu buchō (Kawasaki) to Gijutsubu jichō Ichikawa, Nov. 10, 1959, in *MBJSS*, 1: 316.

60. MBKK.

61. *Kumamoto nichinichi shinbun*, Nov. 17, 1959; Ui, *Kōgai no seijigaku*, p. 112.

62. Ui, *Kōgai no seijigaku*, p. 117; "Minamatabyō kongo no mondaiten," *Mainichi shinbun*, Nov. 17, 1959; in MBKK.

63. MBKK.

64. Kiyoura Raisaku, "Minamata wan naigai no suishitsu osen ni kan suru kenkyū," Nov. 10, 1959; in *MBJSS*, 1: 915–19.

65. "Suisanchō no gyomin taisaku," *Kumamoto nichinichi shinbun*, Nov. 14, 1959; Ui, *Kōgai no seijigaku*, p. 116. Coincidentally, Ikeda Hayato (prime minister 1960–64)

and Satō Eisaku (prime minister 1964–72 and brother of Kishi Nobusuke, who was prime minister 1957–60) both attended the Number Five Higher School in Kumamoto, which later became Kumamoto University.

66. Miyazawa Nobuo, "Kaisetsu," in *MBJSS*, 2: 973–74.

67. Hashimoto Michio, "Minamatabyō shisetsu no tenkanten de: '68 nen kōgai nintei, '74 nen minintei mondai o chūshin ni" (lecture, Jan. 24, 1995).

68. *Asahi shinbun*, Nov. 21, 1959.

69. *MBJSS*, 1: 920.

70. "Ore wa hannin ja nai?" *Mizu*, Dec. 1959; in *MB*, p. 232.

71. The Shimoyama Incident of July 1949, in which the president of Japan National Railways (JNR) was found dead on a railway track, was the first of three serious incidents in the wake of cutbacks at JNR as part of the government's retrenchment program (see Johnson, *Conspiracy at Matsukawa*).

72. "'Kaiketsu wa shita keredo . . . ,'" *Mizu*, Feb. 1960; in *MB*, p. 233.

73. "Minamata wan no gyokairui kara chūshutsu shita kōdokusei busshitsu ni tsuite." See Ui, *Kōgai no seijigaku*, p. 152. The full paper can be found in the MBKK collection. An English version, "Minamata Disease and Water Pollution," was presented to the first International Conference on Water Pollution Research in London, Sept. 3–7, 1962 (where it was criticized by B. Moore in the discussion); it can also be found in the MBKK collection.

74. Ui, *Kōgai no seijigaku*, p. 153.

75. Ibid., p. 147.

76. See ibid., pp. 154–61.

77. Documents from the committee are in *MBJSS*, 2: 1522–55. These include the minutes of its first three meetings; there are no official records of the fourth and last meeting.

78. *MB*, pp. 265–77; Ui, *Kōgai no seijigaku*, p. 157.

79. Han'ya Takahisa, lecture, Oct. 8, 1996. It is Han'ya who informed me that a company observer attended the committee meetings.

80. On the Tamiya Committee, see *MB*, pp. 277–83.

81. The report, "Minamatabyō kenkyū kondankai kenkyū keika hōkoku," can be found in *MBJSS*, 2: 1560–69.

82. Ui, *Kōgai no seijigaku*, p. 158.

83. *Geppō*, June 1960, in *MB*, p. 278; and *MBJSS*, 2: 1694.

84. *Geppō*, June 1961, in *MB*, p. 281. The June 1962 *Geppō* also makes it clear that the Tamiya Committee was created at the request of the JCIA (*MBJSS*, 2: 1694–95).

85. For the JCIA plan for the committee, see *MBJSS*, 2: 1692–93; Miyazawa Nobuo, "Kaisetsu," in *MBJSS*, 2: 975.

86. Miyazawa Nobuo, "Kaisetsu," in *MBJSS*, 2: 976.

87. Ōshima testimony quoted in Miyazawa Nobuo, "Kaisetsu," in *MBJSS*, 2: 976.

88. "Kumadai kenkyūhan, Minamatabyō no gen'in de happyō," Feb. 17, 1963, in *MB*, pp. 336–37.

89. Irukayama et al., "Studies on the Origin of the Causative Agent of Minamata Disease III."

90. "Seiryūtō haieki ni tsuite," Feb. 1962, in *MBJSS*, 2: 1149–51; "Dōbutsu jikken kekka ichiran hyō," Feb. 1962, in *MBJSS*, 2: 1178–80; Miyazawa Nobuo, "Kaisetsu," in *MBJSS*, 2: 987. The disappearance of the cats sent to the University of Tokyo is one of the most curious unsolved mysteries surrounding Minamata disease.

91. Ui, *Kōgai no seijigaku*, p. 166.

92. Miyazawa Nobuo, "Kaisetsu," in *MBJSS*, 2: 988; Ui, *Kōgai no seijigaku*, p. 166.

93. Miyazawa Nobuo, "Kaisetsu," in *MBJSS*, 2: 989. See Kotsuna Masachika, ed., *Minamatabyō*. An English version was published as Kumamoto University Study Group of Minamata, ed., *Minamata Disease* (1966).

94. Miyazawa Nobuo, "Kaisetsu," in *MBJSS*, 2: 989.

95. Nishimura Hajime, "Minamatabyō hassei gen'in no nazo ga toketa," pts. I and II; "Genryō henshin, soakuhin tsukatta," *Asahi shinbun*, Jan. 15, 1998, p. 36.

96. "Kumamoto-ken Eiseibu e no kaitō," in *MBJSS*, 2: 1495; Miyazawa Nobuo, "Kaisetsu," in *MBJSS*, 2: 989.

97. See McKean, *Environmental Protest and Citizen Politics in Japan*, pp. 46–47.

Chapter 4

1. Shin Minamata-shi shi hensan iinkai, *Shin Minamata-shi shi*, 2: 702, 703.

2. Shin Nitchitsu produced a pamphlet in September 1959 consisting of an annotated chronology of all negotiations with the Minamata Fishing Cooperative, with a collection of many documents, including all contracts between the co-op and the company; see Shin Nihon chisso hiryō K.K., *Minamata ni okeru gyogyō hoshō no enkaku*, in *MBJSS*, 1: 232–38.

3. Minamata-machi gyogyō kumiai and Nihon chisso hiryō kabushiki kaisha, "Shōsho," Apr. 30, 1926, in *MBJSS*, 1: 17. To put this in perspective, the average daily wage for agricultural workers in 1926 was 142 sen (¥1.42) for men and 110 sen for women (Andō Yoshio, ed., *Kindai Nihon keizai shi yōran*, p. 100).

4. Harada, *Minamatabyō*, pp. 9–10.

5. Minamata-machi gyogyō kyōdō kumiai and Nihon chisso hiryō kabushiki kaisha, "Keiyakusho," Jan. 10, 1943, in *MBJSS*, 1: 54–55.

6. Maeda to Fuchigami, Oct. 3, 1950, in *MBJSS*, 1: 55.

7. Harada, *Minamatabyō*, p. 10.

8. Ibid.

9. Shin Nihon chisso hiryō kabushiki kaisha and Minamata-shi gyogyō kyōdō kumiai, "Oboegaki," Aug. 22, 1951, in *MBJSS*, 1: 60.

10. Shin Nihon chisso hiryō kabushiki kaisha and Minamata-shi gyogyō kyōdō kumiai, "Keiyakusho," July 13, 1954, in *MBJSS*, 1: 66–68; and "Oboegaki," July 13, 1954, in *MBJSS*, 1: 69–70.

11. See the documents in *MBJSS*, 1: 130–47, 225–26.

12. Maruyama Sadami, "Kaisetsu," in *MBJSS*, 1: 102.

13. Minamata gyomin, "Ketsugi," in *MBJSS*, 1: 138–39; *MB*, p. 75.

14. Ui, *Kōgai no seijigaku*, p. 54.

15. Photographed by Kuwabara Shisei, in Ui, *Kōgai no seijigaku*, p. 53.

16. "Shijō atsukai no shina wa Minamatabyō no shinpai arimasen," *Nishinippon shinbun*, June 18, 1959, in *MB*, p. 88.

17. "Sakanayasan ga demo kōshin," *Kumamoto nichinichi shinbun*, June 21, 1959, in *MB*, p. 88.

18. "Minamata no sakana wa kawanu," *Nishinippon shinbun*, Aug. 1, 1959, in *MB*, p. 94.

19. *Nishinippon shinbun*, Aug. 3, 1959, in *MB*, p. 95.

20. The following account of the events of Aug. 6 is from "Ichi oku en o hoshō seyo," *Kumamoto nichinichi shinbun*, Aug. 7, 1959, in *MB*, p. 99.

21. For the Aug. 12 meeting, see "Kaitō kyō machikoshi," *Kumamoto nichinichi shinbun*, Aug. 13, 1959, in *MB*, pp. 99–100.

22. "Keiyaku de yōyaku nattoku," *Kumamoto nichinichi shinbun*, Aug. 13, 1959 (evening ed.), in *MB*, p. 100.

23. "Asu gyogyō chōsa no ue de," *Kumamoto nichinichi shinbun*, Aug. 14, 1959, in *MB*, p. 100.

24. "Hoshō 1,300 man en o kaitō," *Kumamoto nichinichi shinbun*, Aug. 18, 1959, in *MB*, pp. 101–2.

25. The events of Aug. 18 are described in "Minamata sōdō, sai aku jitai e," *Kumamoto nichinichi shinbun*, Aug. 18, 1959 (evening ed.), and "Keikantai tsui ni jitsuryoku kōshi," *Kumamoto nichinichi shinbun*, Aug. 19, 1959; both in *MB*, p. 102.

26. Ui, *Kōgai no seijigaku*, p. 69.

27. "Kōjō no heisa nado yōbō," *Kumamoto nichinichi shinbun*, Aug. 19, 1959, in *MB*, pp. 102–3.

28. Ui, *Kōgai no seijigaku*, p. 71.

29. See "Kōshō wa nankō," *Kumamoto nichinichi shinbun*, Aug. 21, 1959, in *MB*, pp. 104–5.

30. "Assen an o teiji," *Mainichi shinbun*, Aug. 27, 1959, in *MB*, p. 106.

31. "Assen an o shūsei," *Mainichi shinbun*, Aug. 28, 1959, in *MB*, p. 106.

32. Per capita GNP in 1959 was ¥143,000 ($400) (*Asahi Shinbun Japan Almanac 1997*, p. 279).

33. "Sōhō, shiodoki to handan," *Nishinippon shinbun*, Aug. 30, 1959, in *MB*, pp. 107–8.

34. "Shakkin ni kieta hoshōkin," *Asahi shinbun*, Sept. 27, 1959, in *MB*, pp. 141–42.

35. "Mō dasu maí Minamatabyō kanja," Aug. 30, 1959, in *MB*, pp. 108–9.

36. "Sappari urenu sakana," *Kumamoto nichinichi shinbun* Aug. 22, 1959, in *MB*, pp. 137–38.

37. "Shin Nitchitsu to chikaku dankō," *Kumamoto nichinichi shinbun*, Sept. 29, 1959, in *MB*, pp. 140–41.

38. Tsunagi mura, "Yōbōsho," Nov. 2, 1959, MBKK; "Minamatabyō hassei de shōgeki," *Nishinippon shinbun*, Sept. 26, 1959, in *MB*, p. 141.

39. "Shin Nitchitsu to chikaku dankō," *Kumamoto nichinichi shinbun*, Sept. 29, 1959, in *MB*, pp. 140–41.

40. "Konkyū no gyomin ni kyūen," *Kumamoto nichinichi shinbun*, Oct. 3, 1959, in *MB*, p. 142.

41. Funaba Iwazō died in 1971. Two days before his death, W. Eugene Smith and Aileen Smith photographed his hands, since "all the other patients whose hands became so terribly twisted had died years ago." For the photograph and the Smiths' recollections, see their *Minamata*, p. 73.

42. The events of Oct. 17 are described in "Gyomin 1500 nin oshikakeru," *Kumamoto nichinichi shinbun*, Oct. 18, 1959, in *MB*, p. 146.

43. Kumamoto-ken gyomin sōkekki taikai, "Ketsugi bun" and "Taikai sengen," Oct. 17, 1959, in *MBJSS*, 1: 173–74.

44. "Minamatabyō funsō," *Kumamoto nichinichi shinbun*, Oct. 21, 1959, in *MB*, p. 147; Shiranuikai suishitsu osen bōshi taisaku iinkai and Kumamoto-ken gyogyō kyōdo kumiai rengō, "Chinjōsho," Oct. 19, 1959, in *MBJSS*, 1: 174.

45. "'Gen'in kyūmei ni zenryoku sosogu,'" *Kumamoto nichinichi shinbun*, Oct. 23, 1959, in *MB*, p. 147.

46. These two laws had taken effect in March 1959, but the necessary administrative procedures had not yet been determined. Minamata Bay was not designated for investigation under these laws until 1969, after the acetaldehyde plant had been shut down (Maruyama Sadami, "Kaisetsu," in *MBJSS*, 1: 114).

47. These excerpts are taken from "'Gen'in kyūmei ni zenryoku sosogu,'" *Kumamoto nichinichi shinbun*, Oct. 23, 1959, in *MB*, p. 147. For a transcript of the hearing, see *MBJSS*, 1: 710–20. There is also a partial transcript in Baba Noboru, *Minamatabyō sanjūnen*, pp. 208–17. Baba's book includes selected transcripts of Diet proceedings concerning Minamata and a chart listing all Diet discussions of Minamata to Feb. 26, 1985.

48. "Zengaku o kokkō futan ni," *Kumamoto nichinichi shinbun*, Oct. 27, 1959, in *MB*, p. 153.

49. Nishida's letter is given in *Kuma gyoren jōhō* 15 (Nov. 1959), in *MB*, p. 152.

50. "Minamata kōjō no haisui o sokuji teishi," *Kumamoto nichinichi shinbun*, Oct. 30, 1959, in *MB*, p. 156. Conveniently for Shin Nitchitsu, readers who looked only at

the headline of this story ("Immediate Halt to Minamata Factory Wastewater") or that of the story in the *Asahi shinbun* on the same day ("Shin Nitchitsu Minamata Stopping Its Wastewater Completely"; in *MB*, p. 155) got the erroneous impression that the factory would henceforth somehow operate without discharging any wastewater at all.

51. Maruyama Sadami, "Kaisetsu," in *MBJSS*, 1: 110.

52. "Genchi de sōhō no koe kiku," *Kumamoto nichinichi shinbun*, Nov. 1, 1959, in *MB*, p. 157.

53. "Shin Nitchitsu, gyomin o kokuso," *Nishinippon shinbun*, Nov. 2, 1959, in *MB*, p. 156.

54. "Kokkai chōsa dan kimaru," *Kumamoto nichinichi shinbun*, Oct. 30, 1959, in *MB*, p. 155.

55. "Kokkai chōsa dan okoru," *Kumamoto nichinichi shinbun*, Nov. 2, 1959, in *MB*, p. 158.

56. "Ken gawa no taiman, sukunai kenkyūhi," *Mainichi shinbun*, Nov. 3, 1959, in *MB*, pp. 158–59.

57. Ishimure, *Paradise in the Sea of Sorrow*, pp. 87–90; idem, *Kugai jōdo*, pp. 85–88.

58. Komori Takeshi, "Kokumin no ishiki to undō," in Tsuru Shigeto, ed., *Gendai shihonshugi to kōgai*.

59. "Hisan na byōjō ni bōzen," *Kumamoto nichinichi shinbun*, Nov. 3, 1959, in *MB*, pp. 159–60.

60. "4 sen nin no gyomin demo," *Kumamoto nichinichi shinbun*, Nov. 2, 1959, in *MB*, p. 159.

61. "Kōjō nai ni saido rannyū," *Kumamoto nichinichi shinbun*, Nov. 3, 1959, in *MB*, pp. 160–61.

62. Ishimure, *Kugai jōdo*, p. 115; idem, *Paradise in the Sea of Sorrow*, p. 124.

63. "Shin Nitchitsu gawa no taiman," *Asahi shinbun*, Nov. 4, 1959, in *MB*, p. 163.

64. Ogura Ichirō (director of the documentary *Kibyō no kage ni*), lecture, Oct. 2, 1996.

65. Ui, *Kōgai no seijigaku*, p. 109.

66. "Monomonoshii keikai," *Kumamoto nichinichi shinbun*, Nov. 4, 1959, in *MB*, p. 164.

67. "Akushitsusha wa zen'in kenkyo," *Kumamoto nichinichi shinbun*, Nov. 5, 1959, in *MB*, p. 165.

68. Herbert Bix (*Peasant Protest in Japan*, p. 144) has noted how, in Tokugawa peasant rebellions, "the consumption of alcohol for sacral purposes increased and its intoxicating effects were enlisted in the service of the demonstration."

69. "1 nichi mo hayaku taisaku o," *Kumamoto nichinichi shinbun*, Nov. 5, 1959, in *MB*, p. 165.

70. Ishimure, *Kugai jōdo*, pp. 108–9; idem, *Paradise in the Sea of Sorrow*, p. 116.

71. *MBKK.*

72. And all three joined the new, pro-management second union when it was formed during the 1962–63 strike (*MB,* p. 166).

73. "Bōryoku higeki o uttaeru," *Kumamoto nichinichi shinbun,* Nov. 6, 1959, in *MB,* p. 166.

74. "Minamatabyō de rinji kenkai," *Kumamoto nichinichi shinbun,* Nov. 7, 1959, in *MB,* pp. 166–67.

75. "Tokubetsu i wa bunretsu jōtai," *Kumamoto nichinichi shinbun,* Nov. 7, 1959, in *MB,* p. 167.

76. "Sōgyō chūshi senu yō," *Asahi shinbun,* Nov. 6, 1959, in *MB,* p. 168. For the petition, see "Minamatabyō taisaku ni tsuite no ketsugi bun," in *MBJSS* 1: 445–46.

77. "Minamatabyō, rinji kenkai hirakazu," *Kumamoto nichinichi shinbun,* Nov. 7, 1959, in *MB,* pp. 168–69.

78. "Ketsugi bun," in *MBJSS,* 1: 935–36. See also *Sairen,* the Shin Nitchitsu union newspaper, Nov. 7, 1959, in *MBKK.*

79. Part of the resolution is given in *MB,* p. 170.

80. "Minamata kōjō, haisui teishi wa komaru," *Kumamoto nichinichi shinbun,* Nov. 8, 1959, in *MB,* p. 171.

81. "Koramu battenga," *Kumamoto nichinichi shinbun,* Nov. 9, 1959, in *MB,* p. 171.

82. "Kibyō no saki wa dō naru" and "Nitchitsu kōjō no heisa ka?" *Minamata taimusu,* Oct. 28, 1959, in *MB,* pp. 171–72.

83. "Gyomin taisaku nado kyōka," *Kumamoto nichinichi shinbun,* Nov. 12, 1959, in *MB,* p. 174.

84. "Jimintō no Minamatabyō tokubetsu i hossoku," *Nishinippon shinbun,* Nov. 29, 1959, in *MB,* p. 175.

85. "Tenki o mukaeta Minamatabyō taisaku," *Asahi shinbun,* Nov. 14, 1959, in *MB,* pp. 181–82.

86. "Minamatabyō kongo no mondaiten," *Mainichi shinbun,* Nov. 17, 1959, in *MB,* p. 182.

87. "Kaisha gawa, shimon i o kibō," *Kumamoto nichinichi shinbun,* Nov. 15, 1959, in *MB,* pp. 182–83.

88. "Kenchō kanbu, kongetsu idō," *Mainichi shinbun,* Nov. 20, 1959, in *MB,* p. 185.

89. "Minamatabyō chōtei i kimaru" and "Sankō katei," *Nishinippon shinbun,* Nov. 25, 1959, in *MB,* p. 189.

90. "Minamata chōtei i hatsu no kaigō," *Kumamoto nichinichi shinbun,* Nov. 27, 1959, in *MB,* p. 190.

91. "Tōka made ni ketsuron," *Kumamoto nichinichi shinbun,* Dec. 3, 1959, in *MB,* pp. 194–95.

92. "Zero ni chikai kaitō," *Kumamoto nichinichi shinbun,* Dec. 6, 1959, in *MB,* pp. 195–96.

93. "Minamatabyō, purankuton no jōtai mo kōryo shite, mō ichi do sōgō kenkyū o," *Mainichi shinbun*, Dec. 3, 1959, in *MB*, p. 195.

94. "Minamatabyō funsō chōtei okureru," *Nishinippon shinbun*, Dec. 8, 1959, in *MB*, p. 196.

95. "Teramoto chiji, Minamata funsō de kenkai," *Kumamoto nichinichi shinbun*, Dec. 13, 1959, in *MB*, p. 197.

96. "16, 7 nichi goro ni dai 3 iinkai o," *Mainichi shinbun*, Dec. 15, 1959, in *MB*, p. 197.

97. "Yūki ni kawaru keika wakaru," *Kumamoto nichinichi shinbun*, Dec. 16, 1959, in *MB*, p. 198.

98. *MB*, p. 198.

99. "Minamatabyō funsō, chōtei an o teiji," *Kumamoto nichinichi shinbun*, Dec. 17, 1959, in *MB*, p. 199.

100. JCP, Kumamoto-ken iinkai, *Minamatabyō tōsō no tōmen no mondaiten to kongo no hōkō*, in *MBJSS*, 1: 930.

101. "Kaiketsu shita Minamata no gyogyō hoshō," *Asahi shinbun*, Dec. 19, 1959, in *MB*, pp. 201–2. For this revised agreement, signed on Dec. 25, 1959, see *MBJSS*, 1: 657–58.

102. JCP, Kumamoto-ken iinkai, *Minamatabyō tōsō no tōmen no mondaiten to kongo no hōkō*, in *MBJSS*, 1: 929–33.

103. The only comprehensive source for information on the Mutual Aid Society and all the many other patients' organizations established later is Kumamoto daigaku bungakubu chiiki kagakuka shakaigaku kenkyūshitsu Minamatabyō kanja dantai kenkyūhan, ed., *Minamatabyō kanja dantai ni kan suru chōsa*.

104. On Watanabe, see Irokawa Daikichi, "Kumamoto Minamatabyō saiban genkokudan daihyō Watanabe Eizō no kiroku."

105. Some of Watanabe's drawings and journals are in the possession of Irokawa Daikichi at Tokyo keizai daigaku; others are in the Minamatabyō kenkyūkai collection (MBKK) in the office of Maruyama Sadami at Kumamoto University.

106. JCP, Kumamoto-ken iinkai, *Minamatabyō tōsō no tōmen no mondaiten to kongo no hōkō*, in *MBJSS*, 1: 929–33.

107. Ishimure, *Paradise in the Sea of Sorrow*, pp. 240–44; idem, *Kugai jōdo*, pp. 214–16.

108. Mishima, *Bitter Sea*, pp. 90, 93–94; idem, *Nake, Shiranui no umi*, pp. 86, 89–90.

109. See Ohnuki-Tierney, *Rice as Self*.

110. Irokawa, *Minamata: sono sabetsu no fūdo to rekishi*, p. 30.

111. Ibid., pp. 22–23.

112. "Mina ga kuraseru yō ni," *Kumamoto nichinichi shinbun*, Nov. 17, 1959, in *MB*, pp. 186–87. Actions by the Mutual Aid Society from Sept. 17 to Dec. 30, 1959 (when the solatium agreement was signed) are summarized in notes kept by Takeshita Bukichi: see "Takeshita Memo I," in *MBJSS*, 1: 121–29.

113. "Kanja no hoshō ga senketsu," *Kumamoto nichinichi shinbun*, Nov. 22, 1959, in *MB*, p. 187. For the petition they presented, see Minamatabyō katei gojokai, "Chinjōsho," Nov. 21, 1959, in *MBJSS*, 1: 129.

114. "Hoshō 300 man en (hitori atari) harae," *Kumamoto nichinichi shinbun*, Nov. 26, 1959, in *MB*, p. 187. For the demand as submitted in writing, see Minamatabyō katei gojokai to factory manager Nishida Eiichi, "Ketsugi bun," Nov. 25, 1959, in *MBJSS*, 1: 130.

115. "Minamatabyō no utagai nōkō," *Kumamoto nichinichi shinbun*, Nov. 26, 1959, in *MB*, pp. 187–88. Ogata Fukumatsu was the father of Ogata Masato (see Chapter 9).

116. "Sakusen ni toho jōkyō chinjō," Nov. 27, 1959, in *MB*, p. 191.

117. On the Ashio case, see the articles by Kenneth Pyle, F. G. Notehelfer, and Alan Stone in "Symposium: The Ashio Copper Mine Pollution Incident," *Journal of Japanese Studies* 1.2 (1975), pp. 347–407; and Shōji Kichirō and Sugai Masurō, "The Ashio Copper Mine Pollution Case." On Tanaka Shōzō, see Kenneth Strong, *Ox Against the Storm*. Both Irokawa Daikichi (*Minamata: sono sabetsu no fūdo to rekishi*, pp. 73–75, 79–83) and Frank Upham (*Law and Social Change in Postwar Japan*, pp. 69–76) have compared the 1959 events in Minamata with the Ashio case, especially the Kawamata Incident of 1900, when farmers marching toward Tokyo clashed with police. On the Kawamata Incident, see Notehelfer, "Japan's First Pollution Incident," pp. 376–80.

118. "Gojokai in ga suwarikomi," *Kumamoto nichinichi shinbun*, Nov. 29, 1959, in *MB*, pp. 191–92.

119. "Minamatabyō de futari shinu," *Kumamoto nichinichi shinbun*, Nov. 29, 1959 (evening ed.), in *MB*, p. 192.

120. *MBJSS* 1: 239.

121. Ui, *Kōgai no seijigaku*, p. 120.

122. "Minamatabyō kanja gojokai ga demo," *Kumamoto nichinichi shinbun*, Nov. 30, 1959, in *MB*, p. 192.

123. "Chiji assen taishō e," *Nishinippon shinbun*, Dec. 1, 1959, in *MB*, pp. 192–93.

124. "Settoku de ochitsuku," *Nishinippon shinbun*, Dec. 1, 1959, in *MB*, p. 193.

125. "Kumamoto kenchō e chinjō demo," *Mainichi shinbun*, Dec. 2, 1959, in *MB*, p. 193.

126. "Gaitō de shikin kanpa," *Kumamoto nichinichi shinbun*, Dec. 5, 1959, in *MB*, pp. 193–94.

127. "Takeshita Memo I," in *MBJSS*, 1: 123, 125; "Minamata wan dan," *Minamata taimusu*, Dec. 10, 1959, in *MBJSS*, 1: 965; "Minamatabyō kanja katei ni kifu," *Kumamoto nichinichi shinbun*, Dec. 7, 1959, in *MB*, p. 194; "Minamatabyō kanja gojokai ni mimaikin," *Kumamoto nichinichi shinbun*, Dec. 11, 1959, in *MB*, p. 194.

128. "Kumamoto, Yatsushiro de yobikake," *Nishinippon shinbun*, Dec. 10, 1959, in *MB*, p. 194.

129. "Minamatabyō funsō, chōtei an o teiji," *Kumamoto nichinichi shinbun,* Dec. 17, 1959, in *MB,* p. 199.

130. "Kuniku no saku 'tachiagari shikin,'" *Kumamoto nichinichi shinbun,* Dec. 17, 1959, in *MB,* p. 200.

131. "Ryōshō dekinu shiharai hōhō," *Kumamoto nichinichi shinbun,* Dec. 18, 1959, in *MB,* p. 209.

132. "Minamata shigikai tokubetsu i," *Nishinippon shinbun,* Dec. 12, 1959, in *MB,* p. 209.

133. "Kaiketsu shita Minamata no gyogyō hoshō," *Asahi shinbun,* Dec. 19, 1959, in *MB,* pp. 201–2.

134. "Minamata shigikai tokubetsu i," *Nishinippon shinbun,* Dec. 12, 1959, in *MB,* p. 209.

135. "Takeshita Memo I," in *MBJSS,* 1: 127.

136. Ui, *Kōgai no seijigaku,* p. 134.

137. "Suwarikomi o toku," *Kumamoto nichinichi shinbun,* Dec. 28, 1959, in *MB,* pp. 209–10.

138. "Hoshō chōin owaru," *Asahi shinbun,* Dec. 30, 1959, in *MB,* p. 210; "Hanashiai wa nankō," *Kumamoto nichinichi shinbun,* Dec. 30, 1959, in *MB,* p. 210.

139. For the full text of the agreement and its accompanying documents, see *MBJSS,* 1: 241–43.

140. "Minamatabyō hoshōkin, ikkagetsu buri chōin," *Kumamoto nichinichi shinbun,* Dec. 31, 1959, in *MB,* pp. 210–11.

141. Maruyama Sadami, "Kaisetsu," in *MBJSS,* 1: 118.

142. Miyazawa Nobuo, "Kaisetsu," in *MBJSS,* 2: 977.

143. Harada, *Minamatabyō,* p. 59. Several years after the factory stopped using mercury, Eugene Smith filled a glass with water from the Cyclator and was stopped by his factory tour guides before he could drink it (see W. E. Smith and A. Smith, *Minamata,* p. 55; see also ibid., p. 48, for a photograph of the Cyclator).

144. Gotō Takanori, *Chinmoku to bakuhatsu,* p. 101.

145. In Minamatabyō kenkyūkai, ed., *Minamatabyō ni tai suru kigyō no sekinin,* p. 239.

146. Miyazawa Nobuo, "Kaisetsu," in *MBJSS,* 2: 978; Irukayama Katsurō, "Minamata wan shunsetsu ni tsuite no kaitō," July 19, 1963, in *MBJSS,* 2: 1495–96.

147. Much of the following discussion of the role of the media is based on a self-critical article in the *Asahi shinbun,* "Minamatabyō shinbun no sekinin wa . . . ," Mar. 25, 1994.

148. Bix, *Peasant Protest in Japan,* p. xix.

149. On the supposed Japanese cultural aversion to litigation, see Upham, "Weak Legal Consciousness as Invented Tradition"; and Haley, "The Myth of the Reluctant Litigant."

150. See the chapter "Environmental Tragedy and Response," Upham, *Law and Social Change in Postwar Japan*, pp. 28–77; and idem, "Unplaced Persons and Movements for Place."

151. Upham, *Law and Social Change in Postwar Japan*, p. 73.

152. Upham, "Unplaced Persons and Movements for Place," p. 340.

153. See McKean, *Environmental Protest and Citizen Politics in Japan*.

154. Allinson, "The Structure and Transformation of Conservative Rule," p. 135.

Chapter 5

EPIGRAPH: Ishimure, *Paradise in the Sea of Sorrow*, p. 282; idem, *Kugai jōdo*, p. 246.

1. Both terms have been used by Irokawa Daikichi, the former in an interview, Nov. 2, 1993; the latter in "Kumamoto Minamatabyō saiban genkokudan daihyō Watanabe Eizō no kiroku," p. 267. Gotō Takanori refers to the "ten years of silence" in his *Chinmoku to bakuhatsu*, p. 93; the word *chinmoku* (silence) in his book's title refers to this period.

2. "Gyoren issei teire," *Kumamoto nichinichi shinbun*, Dec. 20, 1959, in MB, p. 213.

3. See MB, pp. 213–14.

4. "Minamata jiken, gyomin 5 nin o taiho" and "Sara ni futari o taiho," *Kumamoto nichinichi shinbun*, Jan. 13, 1960, in MB, p. 214.

5. "Gyomin 6 nin o taiho," *Kumamoto nichinichi shinbun*, Jan. 16, 1960 (evening ed.), in MB, p. 214.

6. "Sōsa wa ichi danraku, Minamata jiken," *Kumamoto nichinichi shinbun*, Jan. 16, 1960, in MB, pp. 214–15.

7. "Kenkei honbuchō, Minamata jiken chinjō dan ni genmei," *Nishinippon shinbun*, Jan. 27, 1960, in MB, p. 215.

8. See MB, pp. 216–17. For legal documents from the case, including written statements by those interrogated, and the court decision, see MBJSS, 2: 1453–83.

9. Irokawa, *Minamata: sono sabetsu no fūdo to rekishi*, p. 81.

10. "Izumi no kanja mo shinsei," *Kumamoto nichinichi shinbun*, Feb. 4, 1960, in MB, pp. 296–97.

11. "1,500 man en de chōin," *Yomiuri shinbun*, May 24, 1960, in MB, p. 308. For the contract and memorandum of understanding, see MBJSS, 2: 1104–6.

12. Ui, *Kōgai no seijigaku*, p. 23.

13. "Minamatabyō ni yochi hō," *Kumamoto nichinichi shinbun*, Feb. 8, 1960, in MB, p. 297.

14. When Minamata disease broke out in Niigata, women with a concentration of over 50 ppm of mercury in their hair were warned not to become pregnant and encouraged to get abortions if they were already pregnant. Very roughly, levels of 50 to 100 ppm are often associated with nerve damage that impairs sensory and motor

functions, and levels of 500 to 1,000 ppm with hearing loss and even death (see Minamatabyō sentā sōshisha, *Sūji kara miru Minamatabyō*, pp. 23–24).

15. *Minamata shi gikai gijiroku*, Mar. 12, 1960, in *MBJSS*, 2: 1242–44; "Minamatabyō taisaku no chinjō dan kaeru," *Mainichi shinbun*, Mar. 10, 1960, in *MB*, p. 298.

16. "Minamatabyō kankei higai hoshō yōkyū ni tsuite," in *MBJSS*, 2: 1018–20.

17. "Shi gyokyō ga hoshō yōkyū," *Kumamoto nichinichi shinbun*, Feb. 24, 1960, in *MB*, p. 302; "Hoshō wa chokusetsu kōshō de," *Kumamoto nichinichi shinbun*, Mar. 22, 1960, in *MB*, p. 303; "Demo kōshin de kisei," *Kumamoto nichinichi shinbun*, Mar. 29, 1960, in *MB*, p. 303.

18. "Minamatabyō gyogyō hoshō yōkyū shui," in *MBJSS*, 2: 1020–21.

19. "Suwarikomi 20 nichi kosu," *Yomiuri shinbun*, Apr. 10, 1960, in *MB*, p. 304; "Chūkai i de kaiketsu seyo," *Nishinippon shinbun*, Apr. 14, 1960, in *MB*, pp. 304–5.

20. Former JCIA head Ōshima's testimony in the first Niigata Minamata disease trial, quoted in Miyazawa Nobuo, "Kaisetsu," in *MBJSS*, 2: 975.

21. "Kiyoura kyōju ni tsumeyoru," *Asahi shinbun*, Apr. 16, 1960, in *MB*, p. 305.

22. *Minamata shi gikai gijiroku*, Apr. 30, 1960, in *MBJSS*, 2: 1244–46.

23. "Gyogyō hoshō assen irai oboegaki memo," Apr. 20, 1960, in *MBJSS*, 2: 1020; "Minamatabyō, kaiketsu no medo tsuku," *Nishinippon shinbun*, Apr. 21, 1960, in *MB*, pp. 305–6; *Minamata shi gikai gijiroku*, Apr. 30, 1960, in *MBJSS*, 2: 1244–46.

24. See *MB*, p. 308; "Chiji, getsumatsu ni assen," *Yomiuri shinbun*, May 15, 1960, in *MB*, p. 308.

25. "Minamatabyō (koramu)," *Mainichi shinbun*, June 24, 1960, in *MB*, pp. 308–9.

26. "Ikinayamu gyogyō hoshō," *Nishinippon shinbun*, Aug. 6, 1960, in *MB*, p. 310.

27. For the committee's announcement, see *MBJSS*, 2: 1403–5.

28. "Assen uchikiru," *Kumamoto nichinichi shinbun*, Aug. 14, 1960, in *MB*, p. 311.

29. "Migoroshi ni hitoshii taido," *Nishinippon shinbun*, Aug. 15, 1960, in *MB*, pp. 311–12.

30. The following account of the actions of Satō Takeharu and Kawamoto Teruo is taken from Gotō, *Chinmoku to bakuhatsu*, pp. 106–15. I have also relied on interviews with Kawamoto on Feb. 15, 1994, and June 3, 1995, and on talks given by Kawamoto on Jan. 21, 1994, and Oct. 1, 1996.

31. For the minutes of the meeting, see *MBJSS*, 2: 1027–32.

32. "Kōjō e no shūrō kibōsha o jomei," *Kumamoto nichinichi shinbun*, Aug. 14, 1960, in *MB*, p. 312.

33. In *MB*, p. 324.

34. "Chiji, sai assen o kyohi," *Mainichi shinbun*, Aug. 19, 1960, in *MB*, pp. 312–13.

35. "Gyomin gawa ni jōho no kūki," *Nishinippon shinbun*, Aug. 24, 1960, in *MB*, p. 313.

36. "Issai o hakushi inin," *Nishinippon shinbun*, Aug. 27, 1960, in *MB*, p. 313.

37. "Shi Nitchitsu o dō toku," *Nishinippon shinbun*, Aug. 29, 1960, in *MB*, pp. 313–14.

38. "Kaisetsu: kumiai bunretsu no kiki sukuu," *Asahi shinbun*, Aug. 29, 1960, in *MB*, p. 314; "Shin Nitchitsu ni mo dōchō tanomu," *Kumamoto nichinichi shinbun*, Aug. 31, 1960, in *MB*, p. 313.

39. "Shin Nitchitsu, jijitsujō no zero kaitō," *Nishinippon shinbun*, Sept. 4, 1960, in *MB*, pp. 314–15.

40. "Minamata wan shūhen ni futatabi shutsugyo," *Asahi shinbun*, Sept. 17, 1960, in *MB*, p. 316.

41. "Rentai hoshō sho," Aug. 12, 1961, in *MBJSS*, 2: 1076.

42. "Genkin hoshō ni wa fukumi," *Nishinippon shinbun*, Sept. 21, 1960, in *MB*, p. 317.

43. "Gyogyō kumiaiin no minasan," in *MBJSS*, 2: 1032; "Genkin hoshō ni wa fukumi," *Nishinippon shinbun*, Sept. 21, 1960, in *MB*, p. 317.

44. "Minamatabyō to Minamata shimin," *Kumamoto nichinichi shinbun*, Sept. 21, 1960, in *MB*, pp. 317–18.

45. "Gyogyō chōtei i wa fushin no koe," *Minamata taimusu*, Sept. 11, 1960, in *MBJSS*, 2: 1713.

46. "Ichi ryōjitsu chū ni assen an," *Asahi shinbun*, Oct. 12, 1960, in *MB*, pp. 318–19.

47. "Chōtei an judaku mitōshi," *Mainichi shinbun*, Oct. 13, 1960, in *MB*, p. 319.

48. "Isseki nichō no Shin Nitchitsu," *Nishinippon shinbun*, Oct. 21, 1960, in *MB*, pp. 319–20.

49. "Hatsuka ni seishiki chōin," *Kumamoto nichinichi shinbun*, Oct. 18, 1960, in *MB*, pp. 320–21.

50. "Minamatabyō o otazune, heika, Teramoto Kumamoto-ken chiji ni," Oct. 22, 1960. I have only a photocopy of this newspaper article, with the date but not the title of the newspaper, from the document collection at the Minamatabyō center sōshisha. Since the headline refers to "Governor Teramoto of Kumamoto," it is almost certainly not the *Kumamoto nichinichi shinbun*. My guess is that it is from the *Nishinippon shinbun*, since the national dailies would have been far less likely to carry such an article.

51. For the agreement and accompanying memorandum of understanding, see *MBJSS*, 2: 1106–7.

52. "Minamata hoshō kesa chōin," *Kumamoto nichinichi shinbun*, Oct. 25, 1960, in *MB*, p. 321.

53. "Gyomin o fumitsuketa," *Minamata taimusu*, Oct. 17, 1960, in *MBJSS*, 2: 358.

54. "Minamatabyō, gyogyō kumiai ni tai suru hoshō chōtei i jinin seyo," *Minamata taimusu*, Oct. 22, 1960, in *MBJSS*, 2: 1713–14.

55. See *MB*, pp. 323–24.

56. Shin Minamata-shi shi hensan iinkai, *Shin Minamata-shi shi*, 1: 30, 72.

57. "Minamata no gyogyō shinkō kaisha setsuritsu furidashi e," *Asahi shinbun*, Apr. 11, 1961, in *MB*, p. 328.

58. "Gyomin kyūsai ni yōshoku jigyō, Minamata," *Kumamoto nichinichi shinbun*, July 15, 1961, in *MB*, pp. 328–29.

59. Hiyoshi Fumiko, interview, July 9, 1994; Yamaguchi Yoshito, interview, July 15, 1994.

60. See *MB*, p. 430.

61. Gotō, *Chinmoku to bakuhatsu*, p. 210.

62. Ibid., pp. 115–16.

63. Ibid., pp. 117–18.

64. "Seikatsu hogo sai tekiyō ga zōka," *Nishinippon shinbun*, Mar. 21, 1960, in *MB*, pp. 298–99.

65. Harada, *Minamatabyō*, p. 156.

66. See *MB*, p. 329.

67. "Saranu 'Minamatabyō' no kyōfu," *Asahi shinbun*, May 16, 1961, in *MB*, pp. 329–30.

68. "Neko hatsubyō de gakkuri," *Kumamoto nichinichi shinbun*, May 20, 1961, in *MB*, p. 330.

69. "Gen'in wa jikken yō no yūdoku sakana," *Kumamoto nichinichi shinbun*, June 6, 1961, in *MB*, pp. 330–31.

70. As early as 1958, it had been noticed that there were a number of children born in the areas most affected by Minamata disease who seemed to have such severe cerebral palsy that they were never able to hold their heads up (Harada, *Minamatabyō*, p. 49).

71. "Yūki suigin to kankei aru, Minamata no nōsei shōni mahi," *Nishinippon shinbun*, June 13, 1961, in *MB*, p. 331.

72. "Sōgō kenkyū kara dantei," *Kumamoto nichinichi shinbun*, Nov. 30, 1962, in *MB*, pp. 333–34.

73. "Minamatabyō, taiji mo kansen," *Mainichi shinbun*, July 11, 1961, in *MB*, pp. 331–32.

74. "Minamatabyō ni 'taiji hatsubyō,'" *Mainichi shinbun*, Aug. 9, 1961, in *MB*, pp. 331–32.

75. Harada, *Minamatabyō*, pp. 81–85; "Seijin Minamatabyō to onaji, Minamata no nōsei shōni mahi," *Nishinippon shinbun*, Nov. 26, 1962, in *MB*, p. 332; "Nōsei shōni mahi wa 'Minamatabyō,'" *Kumamoto nichinichi shinbun*, Nov. 30, 1962, in *MB*, p. 333.

76. "Fūdo byō," *Nishinippon shinbun*, Sept. 22, 1963, in *MB*, p. 341.

77. See *MB*, p. 341.

78. For the full text of the agreement, see *MBJSS*, 2: 1111–12.

79. "Arigatō Sapporo no onēsan," *Kumamoto nichinichi shinbun*, Feb. 15, 1963, in *MB*, pp. 335–36.

80. "Ichi nichi mo hayai zenkai o inorimasu," *Nishinippon shinbun*, Mar. 23, 1963, in *MB*, pp. 339–40.

81. "Hokkoku kara suzuran," *Kumamoto nichinichi shinbun*, June 2, 1963 (evening ed.), in *MB*, p. 340.

Chapter 6

1. On Akasaki, see Mishima, *Bitter Sea*, pp. 28, 33–37, 52, 58, 61–63, 69; and idem, *Nake, Shiranui no umi*, pp. 20, 27–33, 51–52, 57–60, 65, 67, 77. Mishima's main source was Ishimure Michiko. Ishimure discussed Akasaki in an interview I conducted with her on July 12, 1994.

2. Much to Ishimure's disappointment, Mishima Akio centered his 1977 book *Nake, Shiranui no umi* (loosely translated into English in 1992 as *Bitter Sea: The Human Cost of Minamata Disease*) on Ishimure. She has written an autobiography of her young childhood, *Tsubaki no umi no ki* (translated into English by Livia Monnet and published in 1983 as *Story of the Sea of Camellias*), and tells a great deal about herself in *Kugai jōdo* and several other of her books. Other information on Ishimure is taken from my interviews with her on July 9, 1994, and July 12, 1994, a panel discussion including her on Feb. 20, 1994, and lectures by her on May 14, 1994, and Sept. 28, 1996.

3. In discussing Tanigawa, J. Victor Koschmann ("Intellectuals and Politics," p. 410) translates *kōsakusha* as "facilitator or fabricator."

4. *Kugai jōdo: waga Minamatabyō* has been translated into English by Livia Monnet and published as *Paradise in the Sea of Sorrow: Our Minamata Disease*. The second part of the trilogy, *Kugai jōdo dai ni bu*, was serialized in the journal *Henkyō*; the third part, *Ten no uo*, was published in 1974 by Chikuma shobō.

5. Most of the writings by those who worked with Ishimure in the local and prefectural groups supporting Minamata disease patients share her general outlook; see the works listed in the bibliography by Gotō Takanori, Harada Masazumi, Maruyama Sadami, Miyazawa Nobuo, Onitsuka Iwao, and Togashi Sadao.

Irokawa Daikichi's "people's history" approach to Minamata is quite similar to Ishimure's narrative, although for him the struggle is specifically against the ideology of the state and pollution by corporations, both of which symbolize attempts to destroy or take over the community. Irokawa led an "academic research group" that studied Minamata from 1976 to 1980, and published its reports in 1983 (Irokawa, ed., *Minamata no keiji: Shiranuikai sōgō chōsa hōkoku*, 2 vols.; reissued in one volume, without medical and scientific chapters, as *Shinpen Minamata no keiji: Shiranuikai sōgō chōsa hōkoku*). In his version of the Minamata story, he lays great stress on the importance of people he calls "small leaders," who resemble those he finds in the "world renewal" (*yonaoshi*) popular rebellions of the Tokugawa period, in the Freedom and Popular Rights movement of the early Meiji, and in the 1900 Kawamata incident in the Ashio copper mine pollution case (Irokawa, *Minamata: sono sabetsu no fūdo to rekishi*, pp. 75–79, 90). For Irokawa, it is these small leaders and the strength of their communities that resist the state and the corporation.

6. Ishimure, *Paradise in the Sea of Sorrow*, pp. 138–39; idem, *Kugai jōdo*, pp. 125–26.

7. Afterword, *Paradise in the Sea of Sorrow*, p. 377; *Kugai jōdo*, p. 292.

8. Kuwabara Shisei, *Shashinshū: Minamatabyō*.

9. Ishimure, *Paradise in the Sea of Sorrow*, pp. 293–94; *Kugai jōdo*, pp. 253–54.

10. Ishimure Michiko, interview, July 12, 1994.

11. Hiyoshi Fumiko, interview, July 9, 1994.

12. Ishimure, *Paradise in the Sea of Sorrow*, p. 297; *Kugai jōdo*, p. 256.

13. W. E. Smith and A. M. Smith, *Minamata*, p. 88.

14. Harada Masazumi, lecture, "40 nen me no Minamatabyō igaku," Oct. 10, 1996.

15. There were a total of seven children born in Yudō with congenital Minamata disease, and ten who developed the disease as infants.

16. Harada, *Minamatabyō*, pp. 73–75; interview, June 8, 1995. The younger brother who had congenital Minamata disease was Kaneko Yūji.

17. Harada, *Minamatabyō*, pp. 89–96.

18. Harada Masazumi, Maruyama Sadami, Togashi Sadao (all Kumamoto University professors and founding members of the Minamatabyō kenkyūkai), interview, July 13, 1994.

19. For a brief description in English of Ui Jun and his career, see Suzuki and Oiwa, *The Other Japan*, pp. 220–25.

20. Ui Jun, *Nihon no mizu o kangaeru*, p. 56.

21. A copy of the photograph is in the *MBKK* collection.

22. Mishima, *Bitter Sea*, pp. 59–60; idem, *Nake, Shiranui no umi*, pp. 62–63.

23. Arima Sumio, "Minamatabyō ni kan suru chōsa," in idem, *Minamatabyō*, p. 272.

24. Ui Jun, interview, Oct. 3, 1996.

25. Tomita Hachirō (pen name for Ui Jun), *Minamatabyō: Minamatabyō kenkyūkai shiryō*; abbreviated here as MB.

26. See Ui Jun, *Gappon kōgai genron*; and idem, ed., *Kōgai jishu kōza 15 nen*. In addition to running Jishu kōza, Ui also published *Kōgai: The Newsletter from Polluted Japan*.

27. *MB*, pp. 433, 435.

28. John W. Dower, "The Useful War," p. 14.

29. Data compiled by Yahagi Tadashi, Urawa Junior College, for Minamata Tōkyō ten Seminar No. 5, Dec. 14, 1994.

30. Yahagi, "Chisso shi, 1960–65: Goi kōjō kensetsu," p. 40.

31. Chisso sekiyu kagaku, *Goi kōjō kensetsu kiroku*, p. 60; quoted in Yahagi, "Chisso shi, 1960–65: Goi kōjō kensetsu," pp. 45–46.

32. Egashira was the maternal grandfather of Ōwada Masako, who married the crown prince in 1993 after discussions within the Imperial Household Agency over whether her grandfather's association with the Minamata disease incident should disqualify her.

33. Data compiled by Yahagi Tadashi, Urawa Junior College, for Minamata Tō-kyō ten Seminar No. 5, Dec. 14, 1994.

34. Gordon, "Contests for the Workplace," pp. 382–83.

35. On the development of more docile, cooperative unionism, see Gordon, *The Wages of Affluence.*

36. For strike-related documents, see *MBJSS,* 2: 1198–205, 1668–72, 1699–709. For union demands and flyers, company responses, workers' reminiscences, and a chronology of the strike, see Onitsuka, *Oruga Minamata,* pp. 111–17, 126–28, 133.

37. "Chin age nado ni kan suru ken," in *MBJSS,* 2: 1198–99.

38. Gotō, *Chinmoku to bakuhatsu,* pp. 118–19.

39. Kikuchi, "Chisso rōdō kumiai to Minamatabyō," p. 542.

40. For the agreements ending the strike, see *MBJSS,* 2: 1202–5. The average wage increase for 1962 would be ¥2,600 ($7.22) per month. For 1963, the increase would be ¥500 ($1.39) more than the average of the increases at the six major chemical companies with the highest increases. For 1964, wages would be worked out through the mediation of the prefectural labor commission.

41. Onitsuka, *Oruga Minamata,* p. 133.

42. Kikuchi, "Chisso rōdō kumiai to Minamatabyō," p. 540.

43. "Antei chingin ni tsuite," Nov. 30, 1962, in *MBJSS,* 2: 1708–9.

44. Kikuchi Masanori discusses the Minamata Cultural Collective in "Chisso rōdō kumiai to Minamatabyō," pp. 540–44. For several of its flyers, see *MBJSS,* 2: 1699–704.

45. "Shimin no minasama," Aug. 6, 1962, in MBKK.

46. "Nihon no kuroi kiri: bōryoku ni tsuite," Aug. 19, 1962, in MBKK.

47. Onitsuka, *Oruga Minamata,* p. 164.

48. For Onitsuka's recollections of the "persuasion" process, see ibid., pp. 166–69. He also discussed this in interviews on Dec. 6, 1993, and Mar. 15, 1994.

49. Onitsuka, *Oruga Minamata,* pp. 166–67.

50. The No. 1 union chronicled some of this discrimination soon after the strike ended in "Hidoi kōjōnai no sabetsu atsukai," in *MBJSS* 2: 1671–72.

51. Onitsuka, *Oruga Minamata,* pp. 170–75; interviews, Dec. 6, 1993, Mar. 15, 1994.

52. Kikuchi, "Chisso rōdō kumiai to Minamatabyō," p. 549.

53. Ibid., pp. 539, 552, 556; Onitsuka, *Oruga Minamata,* p. 177.

54. Quoted in Miyazawa Nobuo, "Kaisetsu," in *MBJSS,* 2: 990.

55. Irokawa relates the Hiranoya story in "Shiranuikai minshūshi," pp. 281–82, 316–21; and in *Shōwa shi sesō hen,* pp. 274–82. For other recollections of "Hiranoya no danna," see Okamoto and Matsuzaki, *Kikigaki Minamata minshūshi,* 1: 71–78.

56. *Asahi Shinbun Japan Almanac, 1995,* pp. 25, 26.

57. For the Mar. 6, 1968, contract between the Mutual Aid Society and the com-

pany, see *MBJSS*, 2: 1114. Per capita GNP in 1968 was ¥523,000; in 1959 it was ¥143,000 (*Asahi Shinbun Japan Almanac, 1997*, p. 279).

58. McKean, "Equality," pp. 202, 217.

59. Ibid., p. 206.

60. Murakami, "The Age of New Middle Mass Politics."

61. Ivy, *Discourses of the Vanishing*, pp. 29–65; idem, "Formations of Mass Culture," pp. 251–52.

62. On the Narita struggle, see Apter and Sawa, *Against the State: Politics and Social Protest in Japan*.

63. For a brief discussion of Beheiren, see Koschmann, "Intellectuals and Politics," pp. 414–16.

64. On citizens' groups and environmental issues, see McKean, *Environmental Protest and Citizen Politics in Japan*; and Ellis S. Krauss and Bradford L. Simcock, "Citizens' Movements: The Growth and Impact of Environmental Protest in Japan."

65. Lewis, "Civic Protest in Mishima."

66. On Niigata Minamata disease, see Saitō Hisashi, *Niigata Minamatabyō*.

Chapter 7

1. For a handy summary of events in the Minamata disease incident, see the detailed chronology in Arima, *Minamatabyō*, pp. 818–936; pp. 874–915 chronicle the events described in this chapter, from 1968 through 1973.

2. The Minamatabyō taisaku shimin kaigi changed its name on August 7, 1980, to Minamatabyō shimin kaigi.

3. For a convenient chronology of the Niigata Minamata disease incident, see Aga ni ikiru seisaku iinkai, *Aga sōshi*, 4: 130–215.

4. For some of Matsumoto's letters. see *MBJSS*, 2: 1641–46, 1648; for a reply from Bandō Katsuhiko, lawyer for the Niigata victims, see *MBJSS*, 2: 1662–64.

5. Yamashita Yoshihiro ("Zenkan"), interview, July 10, 1994.

6. Ishimure, interview, July 9, 1994; Matsumoto, interview, May 8, 1995.

7. McKean, *Environmental Protest and Citizen Politics in Japan*, p. 127.

8. "Minamatabyō taisaku shimin kaigi," membership form, 1968; in MBKK.

9. Ishimure, *Paradise in the Sea of Sorrow*, p. 315; idem, *Kugai jōdo*, p. 265.

10. Ishimure, *Paradise in the Sea of Sorrow*, p. 320; idem, *Kugai jōdo*, p. 270.

11. Ishimure, interview, July 9, 1994.

12. On Sept. 20, 1967, Mutual Aid Society president Nakatsu Miyoshi had written to the Minsuitai, thanking them for some pamphlets they had sent and explaining that he was sending a ¥10,000 donation from the members of the Mutual Aid Society (see *MBJSS*, 2: 1001–2).

13. Ishimure, *Paradise in the Sea of Sorrow*, p. 333; idem, *Kugai jōdo*, pp. 276–77.

14. "Kyōdō seimei," Jan. 24, 1968, in *MBJSS*, 2: 1002.

15. *Silent Spring* was first published in Japanese translation in 1964.

16. "Taikai ketsugi," in *MBJSS*, 2: 1674. The declaration is also reprinted in *Sairen* (the No. 1 union's newsletter), Aug. 31, 1968 (in the MBKK collection); and in Onitsuka, *Oruga Minamata*, pp. 202–3.

17. "'Minamatabyō' kyūmei ni shin jijitsu," *Asahi shinbun*, Aug. 27, 1968.

18. Miyazawa Nobuo, "Kaisetsu," in *MBJSS*, 2: 993.

19. Hiyoshi, interview, July 9, 1994.

20. "Futatabi yūki suigin no fuan, Chisso Minamata," *Kumamoto nichinichi shinbun*, Sept. 5, 1968.

21. Ishimure, *Kugai jōdo*, p. 289; idem, *Paradise in the Sea of Sorrow*, p. 351. Ishimure changes Murano's name to Sakagami Yuki.

22. Irokawa, *Minamata: sono sabetsu no fūdo to rekishi*, pp. 65–66.

23. "Minamatabyō no gen'in wa kōjō haieki," *Asahi shinbun*, Sept. 8, 1968.

24. For the official conclusions, see Kōseishō, "Minamatabyō ni kan suru kenkai to kongo no sochi," Sept. 26, 1968, in *MBJSS*, 2: 1412–13 (for Minamata); and Kōseishō, "Aganogawa suigin chūdoku jiken ni kan suru seifu kenkai," Sept. 26, 1968, in *MBJSS*, 2: 1415 (for Niigata; a summary actually prepared by the Science and Technology Agency).

25. Kagaku gijutsuchō, "Shōwa 40 nendo Kagaku gijutsuchō tokubetsu kenkyū sokushin chōseihi ni yoru 'Niigata suigin chūdoku ni kan suru tokubetsu kenkyū' ni tsuite no gijutsuteki kenkai," Sept. 26, 1968, in *MBJSS*, 2: 1423–24.

26. Minamatabyō kanja oyobi iryō sochi nado," Sept. 26, 1968, in *MBJSS*, 2: 1413–14.

27. MITI, "Kōjō ni okeru suigin no toriatsukai ni tsuite," July 28, 1965, in *MBJSS*, 2: 1416; MITI, "Suigin shiyō kōjō ni okeru haisui no toriatsukai ni tsuite," Sept. 25, 1968, in *MBJSS*, 2: 1416.

28. Sonoda, "Kōgaibyō no nintei ni atatte," in Baba, *Minamatabyō sanjūnen*, pp. 414–15.

29. Gotō, *Chinmoku to bakuhatsu*, pp. 98–99.

30. See ibid., pp. 99–104.

31. Saitō explained in response to questions in the Diet on Mar. 19, 1969, that he had asked representatives of the Mutual Aid Society to submit a written promise to abide by binding arbitration because "the people who arbitrate will refuse to do so if you do not promise to abide by their decisions" (Baba, *Minamatabyō sanjūnen*, p. 394).

32. For the testimony, see Baba, *Minamatabyō sanjūnen*, p. 397.

33. Hamamoto Tsuginori, lecture, "Uchi naru Minamata ni mimi o katamukeru," May 8, 1995.

34. This translation is from a copy of the form signed by Mutual Aid Society President Yamamoto Matayoshi. This copy, and another unsigned copy of the form, can be found in the MBKK collection. The text differs slightly from that given in Baba, *Minamatabyō sanjūnen*, p. 396. The request as printed in Baba's book adds the words "without complaint" after "we promise to accept," and does not have the words "by sufficiently investigating conditions in Minamata."

35. For the English translation of the name Minamatabyō o kokuhatsu suru kai, I am following that of Richard L. Gage and Susan B. Murata in their translation of Mishima Akio's *Bitter Sea*. This group is usually referred to in Japanese as Kokuhatsu suru kai, or simply Kokuhatsu.

36. *Kokuhatsu* was published by the Kumamoto Association to Indict from June 1969 to August 1973. Since the September 1973 issue, its title has been "*Minamata*": *kanja to tomo ni*.

37. Hiyoshi Fumiko, interview, July 9, 1994.

38. For the text of the complaint they filed against Chisso, see Minamatabyō kenkyūkai, ed., *Minamatabyō ni tai suru kigyō no sekinin*, pp. 335–38.

39. Baba, *Minamatabyō sanjūnen*, p. 399.

40. "Soshō kyūjo mitomerareru," *Kokuhatsu*, Aug. 25, 1969.

41. My information on the Minamata Disease Research Group comes mainly from interviews: Harada Masazumi, June 8, 1995; Ishimure Michiko, July 9 and July 12, 1994; Matsuura Toyotoshi (a member of the Association to Indict and the owner of Karigari, a coffee shop and bar where the Research Group often met), Feb. 25, 1994; Togashi Sadao, Mar. 17, 1994, Nov. 9, 1994, June 6, 1995, and Oct. 16, 1996; Yamashita Yoshihiro, Oct. 16, 1993, and July 10, 1994; Maruyama Sadami, Nov. 9, 1994; Harada Masazumi, Maruyama Sadami, Matsuura Toyotoshi, and Togashi Sadao (interviewed together), July 13, 1994.

42. "Minamatabyō assen i, raigetsuchū ni wa ketsuron, shori i no Chigusa kaichō kataru," *Kumamoto nichinichi shinbun*, March 8, 1970.

43. "Minamatabyō hoshō shori i ni kōgi bun, Shimin kaigi to Kanja gojokai soshōha," *Kumamoto nichinichi shinbun*, Apr. 7, 1970; "Mimai de naku hoshō o, Minamatabyō kanja gawa shori i ni kōgi bun," *Nishinippon shinbun*, April 7, 1970.

44. "Wareware wa sonzai o kakete shori i kaitō o soshi suru," May 13, 1970, in MBKK. The flyer was reprinted as an article in *Kokuhatsu*, May 25, 1970.

45. "Saikō gaku wa sen kyū hyaku man en," *Asahi shinbun* (evening ed.), May 25, 1970.

46. Mishima, *Bitter Sea*, pp. 115–16; idem, *Nake, Shiranui no umi*, pp. 114–15.

47. Mishima, *Bitter Sea*, p. 117; idem, *Nake, Shiranui no umi*, pp. 116–17.

48. For the union's call for the strike, see the special edition of its newsletter *Sairen*, May 26, 1970, in MBKK.

49. "Minamatabyō kanja ni wa tsumetaku," *Asahi shinbun*, June 5, 1970.

50. For Kawamoto's story up to his October 6, 1971, certification, see Gotō, *Chinmoku to bakuhatsu*, pp. 119–27, 130–31, 135–37, 150–71.

51. The Civil Liberties Bureau (Jinken yōgo kyoku) of the Ministry of Justice appoints citizens throughout the country as civil liberties commissioners, under the Civil Liberties Commissioners Law passed in 1949 during the Occupation.

52. Gotō, *Chinmoku to bakuhatsu*, p. 121.

53. Ibid., p. 123.

54. Sugimoto Eiko, lecture, July 16, 1994; idem, lecture, "Watashi to Minamatabyō," Sept. 30, 1996.

55. Arima, *Minamatabyō*, p. 884.

56. Gotō, *Chinmoku to bakuhatsu*, p. 134.

57. Miyazawa Nobuo, "Jittai kyūmei no hōhōron to nintei shinsa seido," in Arima, *Minamatabyō*, pp. 746–48.

58. Gotō, *Chinmoku to bakuhatsu*, pp. 135–36.

59. Arima, *Minamatabyō*, p. 886. For the minutes of this meeting, see Gotō, *Chinmoku to bakuhatsu*, p. 160.

60. The document submitted to the Ministry of Health and Welfare on March 1, 1971, was published by the Tōkyō Minamatabyō o kokuhatsu suru kai on May 10, 1971, under the title *Minamatabyō ni tai suru Chisso, gyōsei, igaku no sekinin: "minintei kanja" wa tsukurareta*. It was reissued, together with photographs, related documents, explanations, and a chronology, on April 10, 1972, by the Minamatabyō kenkyūkai under the title *Nintei seidō e no chōsen: Minamatabyō ni tai suru Chisso, gyōsei, igaku no sekinin*.

61. Miyazawa Nobuo, *Minamatabyō jiken yonjū nen*, pp. 403–14. Prefectural officials suggested that the data had probably been lost in moving to new offices, but Miyazawa discovered that one of the researchers, Matsushima Giichi, had kept copies of the reports of mercury levels in hair. See also Gotō, *Chinmoku to bakuhatsu*, pp. 157–58.

62. Miyazawa, *Minamatabyō jiken yonjū nen*, pp. 403–6.

63. For the official announcement, see Minamatabyō kenkyūkai, *Nintei seidō e no chōsen*, pp. 155–58.

64. "Hirogaru shien undō," *Asahi shinbun*, Oct. 27, 1969.

65. "Tokyo Minamatabyō o kokuhatsu suru kai kessei taikai rejume," *Kankyō hakai* 1, no. 3 (Aug. 1970), p. 34. The English word "hegemony," written in *katakana*, is used.

66. Mishima, *Bitter Sea*, p. 118; idem, *Nake, Shiranui no umi*, pp. 118–19.

67. Fourteen Association to Indict groups are listed in Tōkyō Minamatabyō o kokuhatsu suru kai, *Shukusatsuban Kokuhatsu zokuhen* (Tokyo: Tokyo Minamatabyō

o Kokuhatsu Suru Kai, 1974), from Asahikawa in Hokkaidō to Kagoshima at the southern end of Kyūshū, and there were undoubtedly more.

68. "Tsumetai bankoku haku," *Asahi shinbun*, July 7, 1970.

69. Mishima, *Bitter Sea*, p. 120; idem, *Nake, Shiranui no umi*, p. 122.

70. Sunada Emiko, interviews, Jan. 27 and Feb. 13, 1994.

71. Kuwabara's books on Minamata are *Shashinshū: Minamatabyō* (1965), *Minamatabyō: shashin kiroku, 1960–1970* (1970), *Minamata, Kankoku, Betonamu* (1982), *Minamata: owari naki 30 nen—genten kara tensei e* (1989), and *Minamata no hitobito: haha to ko de miru* (1998). Kusa no ne shuppankai began the publication of a multivolume collection of Kuwabara's complete works (*Kuwabara Shisei shashin zenshū*) in 1998.

72. Shiota Takeshi, *Minamata '68–'72, fukaki fuchi yori: Shiota Takeshi shashin hōkoku.*

73. Some of my information on W. Eugene and Aileen Smith is from an interview with Aileen Smith, July 14, 1995.

74. Smith's best-known photographic essays for *Life* include "Country Doctor" (Sept. 20, 1948), "Spanish Village" (April 9, 1951), "Nurse Midwife" (Dec. 3, 1951), and "A Man of Mercy" (on Albert Schweitzer, Nov. 15, 1954) (see W. W. Johnson, *W. Eugene Smith*).

75. W. E. Smith and A. M. Smith, *Minamata*. Their photographic essay "Death-Flow from a Pipe" appeared in the June 2, 1972, issue of *Life*. For the most complete selection of their Minamata photographs published in a journal, see "Special Feature: Minamata, Japan; An Essay on the Tragedy of Pollution and the Burden of Courage," in *Camera 35* 18, no. 2 (Apr. 26, 1974).

76. "Shinobu: To Gather a Life," in W. E. Smith and A. M. Smith, *Minamata*, pp. 150–69. See also W. E. Smith and A. M. Smith, photographs; Ishimure Michiko, text, *Sakamoto Shinobu-chan no koto*.

77. English and French versions of *Minamata: kanjasan to sono sekai* were also produced. For Tsuchimoto's films through early 1987, see Nemoto, *Tsuchimoto Noriaki firumogurafi*. For Tsuchimoto's own recollections of his work concerning Minamata, see *Minamata eiga henreki*. I interviewed Tsuchimoto on May 16 and Nov. 12, 1994.

78. On the Eight Millimeter Group, see Onitsuka, *Oruga Minamata*, pp. 188–204. He discussed the group in interviews on Dec. 6, 1993, Jan. 1, 1994, and March 15, 1994. At Onitsuka's request I translated, and dubbed in English, the scripts of *Minamatabyō I, Ikarenai sekai* (A world incapable of anger), and *Hyakken kiroku 20 nen* (Hyakken: a record of 20 years).

79. On the one share movement, see Gotō, *Chinmoku to bakuhatsu*, pp. 138–49.

80. For the lawyers' official statement of their objections, "'Hito kabu undō' ni kan suru bengodan kenkai," see Ishimure, *Waga shimin: Minamatabyō tōsō*, pp. 301–2.

The Kumamoto Association to Indict printed the statement, and responded to it, in an article entitled "Kanja, sōkai shusseki o ketsui," in the Oct. 25, 1970, issue of *Kokuhatsu*.

81. Gotō, *Chinmoku to bakuhatsu*, pp. 143–44.

82. The script of *Minamata: kanjasan to sono sekai* gives a good description of the shareholders' meeting and the events of the days preceding it; see *Shin Nihon bungaku* 288 (July 1971): 6–47.

83. See Kaplan and Dubro, *Yakuza*.

84. The English translation of this "hymn" is taken from Mishima, *Bitter Sea*, p. 124.

85. Script, *Minamata: kanjasan to sono sekai, Shin Nihon bungaku* 288 (July 1971): 46. For an abridged and slightly different translation of Hamamoto Fumiyo's words to Egashira, see Upham, *Law and Social Change in Postwar Japan*, p. 42.

86. See Berg and Berg, "Stockholders' Corral."

Chapter 8

1. "Yōbōsho" (by the Tokutomi group), Oct. 21, 1971; in MBKK.

2. "Kōkai shitsumon jō"; in MBKK.

3. "Kōkai shitsumon jō (sono 2)"; in MBKK.

4. No date; in MBKK.

5. "Minamatabyō mondai ni tsuite," Aug. 1971; in MBKK.

6. Quoted in Gotō, *Chinmoku to bakuhatsu*, p. 178.

7. "Suwarikomi tento ni, Nihon ken? motta otoko, kanja ra ni iyagarase tsuzuku, Minamatabyō," *Asahi shinbun*, Nov. 12, 1971.

8. Shimin yūshi ichidō, "Shomei (shimin undō) ni kyōryoku shite doko ga warui to iu no ka!"; in MBKK.

9. Shimin yūshi ichidō, "Kanjasan, kaisha o funsai shite Minamata ni nani ga nokoru to iu no desu ka!"; in MBKK. The translation is taken from Mishima, *Bitter Sea*, p. 161 (emphasis in original).

10. Minamata shimin kōgai taisaku kyōgikai, "Shin nintei kanja no minasan ni kokoro kara okotae mōshiagemasu"; MBKK.

11. Shimin yūshi ichidō, "Shomei shita ni man sū sen no shimin wa han taisei undō ya shakaishugi kaikaku o yume miru mono o rikai suru koto wa dekimasen"; in MBKK.

12. "'Minamata o akaruku suru shimin taikai' e kesshū shimashō!"; in MBKK.

13. Minamata o akaruku suru shimin renraku kyōgikai, "Shimin no minasama, Minamatabyō kanja e atatakai enjo no te o sashinobemashō," Nov. 17, 1996; in MBKK.

14. Arima, *Minamatabyō*, p. 897.

15. Gotō, *Chinmoku to bakuhatsu*, p. 185.

16. Their undated written notice of their refusal, addressed to Sasaki Saburō, president of Chisso's Minamata subsidiary, can be found in the MBKK collection.

17. Togashi, interview, June 6, 1995.

18. The best account of the direct negotiations in Tokyo is Gotō, *Chinmoku to bakuhatsu*, pp. 190–218. Except where otherwise noted, this is the source of the following section on the direct negotiations in Tokyo.

19. "Kanja, kesshi no chokusetsu kōshō," *Kokuhatsu* 31 (Dec. 25, 1971): 1.

20. Kawamoto saiban shiryōshū henshū iinkai, *Minamatabyō jishu kōshō Kawamoto saiban shiryōshū*, p. 393.

21. These numbers come from a count of articles listed in Maruyama Sadami and Minamatabyō kenkyūkai, ed., *Shōwa 55 nendo Minamatabyō ni kan suru sōgōteki chōsa tehō no kaihatsu ni kan suru kenkyū hōkokusho*. This valuable resource lists all articles related to Minamata disease in the major national and regional newspapers from Sept. 28, 1968, through March 21, 1973.

22. "Kōgi seimei," Dec, 25, 1971; in MBKK.

23. Harada Naō later established the publishing house Komichi shobō, which published a collection of letters received by Nagasaki Mayor Motoshima Hitoshi after he stated his view in December 1988, while Hirohito lay dying, that the emperor bore some responsibility for the war. Motoshima was later shot by a rightist in an assassination attempt (see Field, *In the Realm of a Dying Emperor*).

24. Harada Masazumi, panel discussion, with Yanagida Kunio, "Minamata kara mieru 2: iryō, igaku," Sept. 30, 1996.

25. A copy of the petition can be found in the MBKK collection.

26. W. E. Smith and A. M. Smith, *Minamata*, pp. 94–95.

27. Gotō, *Chinmoku to bakuhatsu*, p. 200.

28. The "Statement of Protest" (Kōgibun) issued by the 37 people who called the meeting can be found in the MBKK collection.

29. "Tokyo ni shin meisho shutsugen—Chisso dōbutsuen," Jan. 11, 1972; in MBKK.

30. See Gotō, *Chinmoku to bakuhatsu*, pp. 205–7.

31. Kawamoto, interview, June 3, 1995.

32. Gotō, *Chinmoku to bakuhatsu*, p. 215.

33. "Jishu kōshōha to sono 'shien' no jittai," July 1972; in MBKK.

34. Arima, *Minamatabyō*, p. 906.

35. The following account of the forged documents incident is based mainly on Gotō, *Chinmoku to bakuhatsu*, pp. 218–24.

36. Ibid., p. 220.

37. Part of the following discussion of the Minamata Disease Research Group

and its report is based on interviews with Togashi Sadao on Nov. 9, 1994, and June 6, 1995; and on a joint interview with Harada Masazumi, Maruyama Sadami, Matsuura Toyotoshi, and Togashi Sadao on July 13, 1994.

38. Ui's extensively annotated collection of newspaper articles and other documents is *Minamatabyō: Minamatabyō Kenkyūkai shiryō*; cited in these notes as *MB*.

39. Togashi has written far more about Minamata disease than any other legal scholar. Eighty articles he published from November 1969 to October 1995 are listed in his *Minamatabyō jiken to hō*, pp. 477–81, which reprints 45 of these articles.

40. Minamatabyō kenkyūkai, *Minamatabyō ni tai suru kigyō no sekinin*, pp. 115–16.

41. Togashi, interview, Nov. 9, 1994.

42. Taketani Mitsuo, *Gensuibaku jikken*. Taketani had proposed in 1952 the principles that became the foundation of Japan's nuclear energy policy: that its use be peaceful, open, and under government control.

43. Mishima, *Nake, Shiranui no umi*, pp. 148, 150; idem, *Bitter Sea*, pp. 133, 134.

44. Arima, *Minamatabyō*, p. 886.

45. For a transcript of Hosokawa's testimony, see *Hōritsu jihō* 45, no. 3 (Feb. 1973): 358–72.

46. Chisso kabushiki kaisha, sōmubu, "Minamatabyō ni tsuite," July 1970, pp. 11–12; in MBKK.

47. Arima, ed., *Minamatabyō*, p. 903.

48. Ibid., p. 904.

49. Minamata Disease Center Sōshisha, *Illustrated Minamata Disease*, pp. 78, 161.

50. Aileen Smith, interview, July 14, 1995.

51. These excerpts are from the translation in Gresser et al., *Environmental Law in Japan*, pp. 86–103.

52. "Minamatabyō bengodan o kyūdan suru," March 20, 1973; in MBKK.

53. See Gotō, *Chinmoku to bakuhatsu*, p. 230.

54. The following account of the Tokyo negotiations is based on the annotated and abbreviated transcripts in Ishimure, *Ten no yamu*; on Gotō, *Chinmoku to bakuhatsu*, pp. 227–53; on Tsuchimoto Noriaki's documentaries *Minamatabyō: sono nijū nen* (1976) and *Minamata's Message to the World* (1976; a slightly modified English version of the former); and on Mishima, *Nake, Shiranui no umi*, pp. 231–40; idem, *Bitter Sea*, pp. 197–202.

55. "Kaisha seiyakusho," in Ishimure, *Ten no yamu*, pp. 304–5.

56. Gotō, *Chinmoku to bakuhatsu*, p. 231.

57. For the full text of the agreement, see Togashi, *Minamatabyō jiken to hō*, pp. 459–63; and Ishimure, *Ten no yamu*, pp. 309–13.

58. Per capita GNP in 1973 was ¥1,036,000 ($3,700) (*Asahi Shinbun Japan Almanac, 1997*, p. 279).

59. On the importance to the patients of this moral victory, see Frank K. Upham, "Litigation and Moral Consciousness in Japan."

60. Gotō, *Chinmoku to bakuhatsu*, pp. 252–53.

Chapter 9

1. Minamatabyō kanja yūshi, "Hongan no sho," Mar. 2, 1994.

2. Quoted in Yoshinaga Toshio, "Konna setsubi wa iranai!" *Gonzui* 39 (Mar. 25, 1997): 17.

3. Ishimure, interview, July 12, 1994.

4. Irokawa, ed., *Minamata no keiji*.

5. The lawyers' newsletter from the first trial, *Bengodan dayori*, gives a good sense of their view of the meaning of the Minamata disease incident. Issues 1 through 30 (April 1, 1971, to June 15, 1972) were reprinted in book form by the Minamatabyō soshō bengodan and the Manaki hōritsu jimusho in Minamata in June 1972; a compilation of issues 31 to 54 (July 1, 1972, to June 15, 1973) followed in July 1973.

6. On Irokawa's romanticization of the traditional village community, see Scheiner, "The Japanese Village."

7. For a summary of events since 1973, see Gotō, *Chinmoku to bakuhatsu*, pp. 256–66. The most detailed chronology can be found in Arima, *Minamatabyō*, pp. 915–36, but this covers only through 1976. "Minamatabyō no genzai," the supplement included with the Japanese translation of W. E. Smith and A. M. Smith, *Minamata*, includes a supplementary chronology covering events through November 1991, and a summary of events from July 1973 to November 1991 written by Togashi Sadao. A chronology by Arima Sumio covering through October 1995, "Minamatabyō jiken ryaku nenpyō," is included with Togashi, *Minamatabyō jiken to hō*. Miyazawa, *Minamatabyō jiken yonjū nen*, includes a chronology covering through July 1997.

8. Hamamoto Tsuginori, "Chiryō mo suru shi koshite mita," in Akutagawa and Yanagida, *Minamata*, p. 46.

9. On the Kawamoto case, see Kawamoto saiban shiryōshū henshū iinkai, *Minamatabyō jishu kōshō Kawamoto saiban shiryōshū*; Gotō, *Chinmoku to bakuhatsu*, pp. 258–59; and Upham, *Law and Social Change in Postwar Japan*, pp. 48–53.

10. Arima, *Minamatabyō*, p. 915.

11. Ibid., p. 922.

12. Gotō, *Chinmoku to bakuhatsu*, p. 260.

13. Mita Munesuke, lecture, "Minamatabyō no gendaiteki imi o yomitoku," Apr. 21, 1995.

14. An unpublished chart of Minamata disease-related court cases, produced by a former assistant to Gotō Takanori, is the most useful listing; see Jitsukawa Yūta, "Minamatabyō kankei soshō ichiran," Sept. 5, 1994.

15. For the court's January 7, 1993, proposal, "Wakai kijitsu chōsho," see SKKS1, pp. 145–47.

16. See Jiyū Minshutō, "Minamatabyō mondai ni tsuite no memo," Sept. 29, 1994, in SKKS1, p. 181.

17. For the Cabinet resolution, "Minamatabyō mondai no kaiketsu ni tsuite," see SKKS1, pp. 155–56.

18. "Minamatabyō mondai no kaiketsu ni atatte naikaku sōridaijin danwa," in SKKS1, p. 156.

19. Kawamoto, "A Shameful Retreat," p. 38.

20. Nishi, "Despite My Convulsions, I Haven't Applied."

21. Ishimure's call for the construction of the center is included in a six-page section of the Oct. 15, 1972, edition of Kokuhatsu describing the need for the center and soliciting donations and support.

22. Sakamoto Fujie, "A Family Tragedy," pp. 32–33.

23. Tsuchimoto Noriaki produced a documentary on the Marukis and their Minamata mural in 1981, Minamata no zu, monogatari. The Marukis also illustrated an award-winning children's book for which Ishimure wrote the words, Mina-mata—umi no koe. Their Hiroshima murals are discussed in Dower and Junkerman, The Hiroshima Murals. Dower and Junkerman also produced a documentary film on the Marukis' murals, Hellfire: A Journey from Hiroshima, in 1985.

24. Kinjō produced a similar statue for Nagasaki's peace memorial park and guided residents of the village of Yomitanson in Okinawa in sculpting a memorial to villagers who died, many of them by group suicide, in a nearby cave near the end of the war. Some of the donations that helped pay for the Okinawa memorial came from Minamata (see Field, In the Realm of a Dying Emperor, p. 74).

25. Hamamoto Tsuginori, lecture, "Uchi naru Minamata ni mimi o katamu-keru," May 8, 1995.

26. Araki Yōko, lecture, "Watashi to Minamata—kanjasan no hanashi kara," Oct. 1, 1996.

27. For Ogata's story, see his autobiography, compiled by Tsuji Shin'ichi, Tokoyo no fune o kogite. In English, see D. Suzuki and Oiwa, The Other Japan, pp. 225–37. I have also relied on interviews with Ogata on Feb. 20, 1994, July 18, 1994, and June 10, 1995, and on talks by Ogata on Feb. 20, 1994, Sept. 28, 1996, and Oct. 5, 1996.

28. The English translation is from Oiwa Keinosuke, "Field Notes: Visiting Ogata Masato," p. 43. For the full text of the letter, see Ogata and Tsuji, Tokoyo no fune o kogite, pp. 222–25.

29. Ogata Masato, "Watashitachi wa ima doko ni iru no ka."

30. For this speech and the controversy surrounding it, I have drawn on Mita-mura Takeshi, "Ore a ikitakatta," which includes the full text of the speech, as well as other related documents; Ishida, "Minamata ni okeru yokuatsu to sabetsu no

kōzō," pp. 63–67; and Hidaka Rokurō, lecture, "Minamata kara kangaeru 9: kyōiku," Oct. 9, 1996.

31. See Ishida, "Minamata ni okeru yokuatsu to sabetsu no kōzō," pp. 64–66; Mitamura, "Ore a ikitakatta."

32. For records of these meetings and copies of the demands, questions, and replies, see Mitamura, "Ore a ikitakatta," pp. 29–33.

33. Quoted in ibid., p. 31.

34. The congenital patients' efforts and the concert itself are chronicled in a documentary film by Tsuchimoto Noriaki, *Waga machi waga seishun: Ishikawa Sayuri Minamata nesshō*. See also Irokawa, *Minamata: sono sabetsu no fūdo to rekishi*, pp. 87–89.

35. Tsurumi Kazuko, "Tahatsu buraku no kōzō henka to ningen gunzō," p. 161.

36. Irokawa Daikichi discusses some of the attempts to recover and rebuild in "Kōgai toshi Minamata ni okeru ningen to shizen no kyōsei no mondai."

37. The group was initially called the Minamata Disease Issues Study Group (Minamatabyō mondai kenkyūkai).

38. Minamata shiritsu Minamatabyō shiryōkan and Minamatabyō rekishi kō-shōkan, "Minamatabyō 10 no chishiki"; trans. Timothy S. George and Jane Ellen George and published in English as Minamata Disease Municipal Museum and Minamata Disease Museum, "Ten Things to Know About Minamata Disease."

39. Yoshinaga, "Konna setsubi wa iranai!" p. 18.

40. I interviewed Yoshii, then speaker of the city council, on Oct. 14, 1993.

41. The city distributed the text of Yoshii's speech, which is also reprinted in SKKS1, pp. 193–94.

Conclusion

EPIGRAPH: Maruyama Masao, "Gendai ni okeru taido kettei" (1960), 8: 315.

1. White, "The Dynamics of Political Opposition," p. 440.

2. On the Narita struggle, see Apter and Sawa, *Against the State*.

3. Steinhoff, "Protest and Democracy," p. 178.

4. On the Kanemi rice-oil poisoning case, see Reich, *Toxic Politics*. Reich is also the co-author of the first full treatment of the Minamata story in English, the chapter entitled "Tragedy at Minamata" in Huddle and Reich, *Island of Dreams*.

5. Aileen Smith has been very active in the anti–nuclear power movement from her home in Kyoto.

6. Matsumoto, interview, Oct. 18, 1996. There has been a great deal of discussion recently among political scientists of "deliberative democracy"; see, e.g., Benhabib, "Toward a Deliberative Model of Democratic Legitimacy."

7. One of the few people to write in English about this distinction between "form" and "spirit" in postwar democracy is John Dower ("The Useful War," p. 27). And the neo-Marxist Watanabe Osamu, although his work is in part a rejection of

Maruyama, also accepts this distinction when he depicts a postwar ruling class that uses democratic structures and ideology for undemocratic purposes. Watanabe, like Norma Field, sees postwar conservative political rulership and corporate society as inseparable from the emperor system (Watanabe, *Sengo seiji shi no naka no tennōsei*). His view is a critique of both the Marxist and modernist views of postwar democracy. Both were wrong, he says, in expecting that economic development would bring political progress, be it a revolution or the development of autonomous individuals. Such views, says Watanabe, not only underestimate the depth of the already existing democratic commitment by the Japanese populace but also ignore the ability of the ruling class to use democratic ideals and structures for decidedly undemocratic purposes (*Kigyō shihai to kokka*, pp. 148–49).

Like T. J. Pempel, Kent Calder, and Gary Allinson, Watanabe believes there was an important change in the 1970s but sees it as the ruling class's acceptance of both the infrastructure and the ideology of parliamentary democracy—unavoidable because democratic ideals had truly taken root among the people—in order to strengthen what was in fact a "contemporary imperialist state" (*Kigyō shihai to kokka*, pp. 183–84). Democratic ideology could be, and was, turned on its head and used to "suppress the demands and rights of 'minorities' and to restrict civil and political liberties in the name of 'majority opinion'" (ibid., p. 184). For example, says Watanabe, such arguments were used to prohibit strikes and political activity by public servants, reinstitute the imperial era name system, pass a law to protect state secrets, allow government officials to worship in their public capacity at the Yasukuni Shrine to the war dead, and argue for amending the constitution to allow Japan to remilitarize (ibid., pp. 184–85).

8. For an example of this view of democracy, see Huntington, *The Third Wave*. For a recent example in Japanese studies, see Richardson, *Japanese Democracy*.

9. This is the sort of definition implied, in different ways, by Maruyama Masao, Watanabe Osamu, and John Dower. Sheldon S. Wolin, although he was not speaking of Japan, expressed a similar idea: "Democracy needs to be reconceived as something other than a form of government: as a mode of being that is conditioned by bitter experience, doomed to succeed only temporarily, but is a recurrent possibility as long as the memory of the political survives" ("Fugitive Democracy," p. 43).

10. See, e.g., Upham, *Law and Social Change in Postwar Japan*; and Pharr, *Losing Face*. I thank Susan Pharr for helping me clarify these definitions of democracy.

Epilogue

EPIGRAPH: "'Hongan no Kai' hossoku ni atatte," Jan 29, 1995, in Ogata and Tsuji, *Tokoyo no fune o kogite*, p. 229.

1. Kurihara Akira (lecture, "Minamata kara kangaeru 11—inori," Oct. 12, 1996) compared Sugimoto Eiko's role in this ceremony and others to that of a *goze*, the

blind female singers and *shamisen* players who wandered Japan from the sixteenth century on. In addition to folk songs, *goze* often performed long chants and recitations with Buddhist or Shintō themes and were sometimes considered to have supernatural powers. Sugimoto, too, has come to be considered to have a special ability to speak with or for the souls of the dead. She has also long been thought to have inherited her father's almost magical ability to know when and where fish can be caught.

2. Follow-up "Minamata Exhibitions" have been held in other cities since the Minamata Tokyo Exhibition. There were exhibitions in Toyohashi and Tsukuba in 1998, in Takahata, Osaka, Okinawa, and Hamamatsu in 1999, and again in Tokyo in 2000.

3. Tsuchimoto Noriaki, interview, Nov. 12, 1994.

4. Tsuchimoto, lecture, "Minamata kara kangaeru 10—hyōgen, kiroku," Oct. 10, 1996.

Bibliography

Interviews

Bandō Katsuhiko 坂東克彦. May 4, 1995.

Gotō Takanori 後藤孝典. Sept. 9, 1993; May 9, 1994.

Hamamoto Tsuginori 浜元二徳. Oct. 4, 1993; Feb. 11, 1994; Nov. 3, 1994; Nov. 12, 1994.

Hannaga Kazumitsu 半永一光. Jan. 27, 1994; Mar. 19, 1994.

Harada Masazumi 原田正純. Feb. 20, 1994; June 8, 1995.

Harada Masazumi 原田正純, Maruyama Sadami 丸山定巳, Matsuura Toyotoshi 松浦豊敏, Togashi Sadao 富樫貞夫, and Yoshinaga Toshio 吉永利夫. July 13, 1994.

Hatano Hideto 旗野秀人. May 3, 1995.

Hiyoshi Fumiko 日吉フミコ. July 9, 1994.

Irokawa Daikichi 色川大吉. Nov. 2, 1993; June 22, 1994.

Ishimure Michiko 石牟礼道子. July 9, 1994; July 12, 1994.

Iwamoto Hiroki 岩本広喜. June 11, 1995.

Kanzaki Yōko 神崎陽子. Nov. 3, 1994.

Kawakami Tsugiyoshi 川上次吉. Jan. 21, 1994.

Kawamoto Teruo 川本輝夫. Feb. 15, 1994; June 3, 1995.

Koga Katsutoshi 古賀勝利. Jan. 27, 1994.

Maruyama Sadami 丸山定巳. Nov. 9, 1994.

Matsumoto Tsutomu 松本勉. May 8, 1995; Oct. 18, 1996.

Matsuura Toyotoshi 松浦豊敏. Feb. 25, 1994.

Nagai Isamu 長井勇. Nov. 5, 1994; Nov. 11, 1994.

Ogata Masato 緒方正人. Feb. 20, 1994; July 18, 1994; June 10, 1995.

Onitsuka Iwao 鬼塚巖. Dec. 6, 1993; Jan. 1, 1994; Jan. 10, 1994; Mar. 15, 1994; July 15, 1994; Aug. 14, 1994; June 13, 1995.

Onitsuka Yūji 鬼塚勇治. Jan. 27, 1994; Mar. 19, 1994; Nov. 5, 1994.

Ori Arisa 小里アリサ and Yoshinaga Toshio 吉永利夫. Nov. 14, 1994.

Saishu Satoru 最首悟. May 16, 1994.

Sakamoto Shinobu 坂本しのぶ. Oct. 11, 1993.

Smith, Aileen. July 14, 1995.

Sunada Emiko 砂田エミコ. Jan. 27, 1994; Feb. 13, 1994; June 6, 1995.

Takakura Shirō 高倉史郎 and Yanagida Kōichi 柳田耕一. Nov. 2, 1994.

Tani Yōichi 谷洋一. Oct. 18, 1996.

Tanoue Yoshiharu 田上義春. July 9, 1994.

Togashi Sadao 富樫貞夫. Mar. 17, 1994; Nov. 9, 1994; June 6, 1995, Oct. 16, 1996.

Tsuchimoto Noriaki 土本典昭. May 16, 1994; Nov. 12, 1994.

Ui Jun 宇井純. Oct. 12, 1992; Oct. 3, 1996.

Yamaguchi Yoshito 山口義人. July 15, 1994; July 18, 1994.

Yamashita Yoshihiro ("Zenkan") 山下善寛. Oct. 16, 1993; July 10, 1994.

Yoshii Masazumi 吉井正澄. Oct. 14, 1993.

Lectures and Panel Discussions

Akutagawa Jin 芥川仁 and Satō Makoto 佐藤真. Panel discussion. Tsuitō shūkai: "Aga no kishibe ni te: Aga ni ikita hitotachi o shinobu tsudoi '95" 追悼集会：「阿賀の岸辺にて：阿賀に生きた人達を偲ぶ集い '95. Yasuda-machi chūō kōminkan, Niigata-ken. May 4, 1995.

Araki Yōko 荒木洋子. Lecture to students from Kikuyō Chūbu Elementary School 菊陽中部小学校, Kumamoto prefecture. Minamatabyō sentā sōshisha, Minamata. Nov. 14, 1994.

―――. "Watashi to Minamata—kanjasan no hanashi kara" 私と水俣―患者さんの話から. Lecture. Minamata Tōkyō ten 水俣東京展. Shinagawa, Tokyo. Oct. 1, 1996.

Gotō Takanori 後藤孝典. "Minamatabyō tōsō no chōten: jishu kōshō to wa nani ka" 水俣病闘争の頂点：自主交渉とは何か. Lecture. Dai 8-kai Minamata ten seminā 第8回水俣展セミナー. Bunkyō Kumin Sentā, Tokyo. March 28, 1995.

Hagimine Tadanobu 萩嶺唯信, Hamamoto Tsuginori 浜元二徳, Harada Masazumi 原田正純, Hashiguchi Saburō 橋口三郎, Kawamoto Teruo 川本輝夫, Matsumoto Mitsuyoshi 松本満良, Sawai Seiji 沢井誠司, and Torii Isamu 鳥居勇. "Minamatabyō no keika to genjō o fumaete kankyō mondai e no torikumi ni tsuite" 水俣病の経過と現状を踏まえて環境問題への取り組みについて. Panel discussion. Dai 25 kai chihō jichi kenkyū zenkoku shūkai—hi no kuni kenkyū—pure jichi ken Minamata shū-kai 第 25 回地方自治研究全国集会一火の国研究ープレ自治研水俣集会. Minamata-shi bunka kaikan, Minamata. Oct. 18, 1993.

Hamamoto Tsuginori 浜元二徳. Lecture to visitors. Shiritsu Minamatabyō shiryōkan 市立水俣病資料館, Minamata, Nov. 3, 1994.

———. "Uchi naru Minamata ni mimi o katamukeru" ウチなる水俣に みみを傾ける. Lecture. Gakuseibu seminā: "Kankyō to seimei: kyōsei no shiten to watakushitachi no seikatsu" 学生部セミナ：「環境と生命一供生 の視点と私たちの生活」. Rikkyō University, Tokyo. May 9, 1995.

Hamamoto Tsuginori 浜元二徳 and Sugimoto Eiko 杉本栄子. Panel discussion. Minamata Tōkyō yokayoka matsuri 水俣東京よかよか祭. Rikkyō University, Tokyo. May 7, 1995.

Haneda Sumiko 羽田澄子. "Minamata—kanjasan no hanashi kara" 水俣ー 患者さんの話から. Lecture. Minamata Tōkyō ten 水俣東京展. Shina-gawa, Tokyo. Sept. 28, 1996.

Han'ya Takahisa 半谷高久. Lecture. Kataribe kōnā 語り部コーナー, Mina-mata Tōkyō ten 水俣東京展. Shinagawa, Tokyo. Oct. 8, 1996.

Harada Masazumi 原田正純. "Minamata kara sekai to Ajia e no kankyō" 水俣から世界とアジアへの環境. Lecture. Dai 25 kai chihō jichi kenkyū zenkoku shūkai—hi no kuni kenkyū—pure jichi ken Minamata shūkai 第25回地方自治研究全国集会一火の国研究ープレ自治研水俣集会. Minamata-shi bunka kaikan, Minamata. Oct. 18, 1993.

Harada Masazumi 原田正純. "Minamata kara mieru sekai" 水俣から みえる世界. Lecture. Dai 2 ki Minamata ten seminā, dai 1 kai 第2期 水俣展セミナー第1回. Shibuya kuritsu shōkō kaikan shōhisha sentā, To-kyo. June 23, 1995.

Harada Masazumi 原田正純. "40 nen me no Minamatabyō igaku" 40 年目 の水俣病医学. Lecture. Minamata Tōkyō ten 水俣東京展. Shinagawa, Tokyo. Oct. 10, 1996.

Harada Masazumi 原田正純, Ishimure Michiko 石牟礼道子, and Ogata Ma-sato 緒方正人. Panel discussion. Gonzui Minamata Seminā "Totte oki no hanashi" in Fukuoka ごんずい水俣セミナー「とっておきの話」 in 福岡. Kirisutokyō Kaikan, Fukuoka. Feb. 20, 1994.

Harada Masazumi 原田正純 and Yanagida Kunio 柳田邦男. "Minamata kara kangaeru 2: iryō, igaku" 水俣から考える 2: 医療・医学. Panel dis-cussion. Minamata Tōkyō ten 水俣東京展. Shinagawa, Tokyo. Sept. 30, 1996.

Hashiguchi Saburō 橋口三郎 and Katō Osamu 加藤修. "Minamatabyō to tomo ni ikite" 水俣病とともに生きて. Lecture. Dai 4 kai Minamatabyō o kataru shimin kōza 第4回水俣病を語る市民講座. Minamata-shi rōdō seishōnen hōmu, Minamata. March 4, 1994.

Hashimoto Michio 橋本道夫. "Minamatabyō shisetsu no tenkanten de: '68 nen kōgai nintei, '74 nen minintei mondai o chūshin ni" 水俣病施設の転換点で—'68年公害認定'74年未認定問題を中心に. Lecture. Dai 6 kai Minamata ten seminā 第6回水俣展セミナー. Bunkyō kumin sentā, Tokyo. Jan. 24, 1995.

Hidaka Rokurō 日高六郎. "Minamata kara kangaeru 9: kyōiku" 水俣から考える9: 教育. Lecture. Minamata Tōkyō ten 水俣東京展. Shinagawa, Tokyo. Oct. 9, 1996.

Hiraguchi Yoshio 平口吉夫. Lecture. Minamata no saisei o kangaeru shimin no tsudoi: sorosoro moyainaoshi hajimemba 水俣の再生を考える市民の集い: そろそろもやい直しはじめんば. Minamata-shi bunka kaikan, Minamata. Nov. 12, 1994.

Hirakida Rimiko 開田理巳子. Lecture. Minamata no saisei o kangaeru shimin no tsudoi: sorosoro moyainoshi hajimemba 水俣の再生を考える市民の集い: そろそろもやい直しはじめんば. Minamata-shi bunka kaikan, Minamata. Nov. 12, 1994.

Ishida Masaru 石田勝. "Minamatabyō to watakushi" 水俣病と私. Lecture. Dai 2 kai Minamatabyō o kataru shimin kōza 第2回水俣病を語る市民講座. Minamata-shi kōminkan, Minamata. Sept. 27, 1993.

Ishimure Michiko 石牟礼道子. Minamata Tōkyō ten, jikkō iinkai hossoku no tsudoi, kinen kōen 水俣東京展実行委員会発足の集い記念講演. Lecture. Nihon toshi sentā, Tokyo. May 14, 1994.

———. "Watashitachi wa doko e iku no ka—Minamata kara" 私たちはどこへ行くのか—水俣から. Lecture. Minamata Tōkyō ten 水俣東京展. Shinagawa, Tokyo. Sept. 28, 1996.

Kanahashi Tsutomu 金橋功. Lecture. Minamata no saisei o kangaeru shimin no tsudoi: sorosoro moyainoshi hajimemba 水俣の再生を考える市民の集い—そろそろもやい直しはじめんば. Minamata-shi bunka kaikan, Minamata. Nov. 12, 1994.

Kawamoto Teruo 川本輝夫. "Kawamoto Teruo shi, kutō no rekishi o kataru" 川本輝夫氏, 苦闘の歴史を語る (also titled "Minamatabyō jiken ni mananda koto" 水俣病事件に学んだこと). Lecture. Dai 3 kai

Minamatabyō o kataru shimin kōza 第 3 回水俣病を語る市民講座. Minamata-shi kōminkan, Minamata. Jan. 21, 1994.

Kawamoto Teruo 川本輝夫 and Irokawa Daikichi 色川大吉. "Minamata kara kangaeru 3: tatakai, undō" 水俣から考える 3: たたかい・運動. Panel discussion. Minamata Tōkyō ten 水俣東京展. Shinagawa, Tokyo. Oct. 1, 1996.

Kinoshita Reiko 木下レイ子, Ishimure Michiko 石牟礼道子, and Tatematsu Wahei 立松和平. "Watashi to Minamata—kanjasan no hanashi kara" 私と水俣―患者さんの話から. Panel discussion. Minamata Tōkyō ten 水俣東京展. Shinagawa, Tokyo. Oct. 8, 1996.

Kurihara Akira 栗原彬. "Minamata kara kangaeru 13: inori" 水俣から考える 13: 祈り. Lecture. Minamata Tōkyō ten 水俣東京展. Shinagawa, Tokyo. Oct. 12, 1996.

Maruki Toshi 丸木俊. Lecture. Minamata Tōkyō ten 水俣東京展. Shinagawa, Tokyo. Oct. 5, 1996.

Matsumura Hayato 松村敏人. Lecture. Minamata no saisei o kangaeru shimin no tsudoi: sorosoro moyainoshi hajimemba 水俣の再生を考える市民の集い―そろそろもやい直しはじめんば. Minamata-shi bunka kaikan, Minamata. Nov. 12, 1994.

Mita Munesuke 見田宗介. "Minamatabyō no gendaiteki imi o yomitoku: tamashii no arawareru basho: gendai shakai no kokkaku no kōzō to deguchi" 水俣病の現代的意味を読み解く：魂の洗われる場所―現代社会の骨格の構造と出口. Lecture. Dai 9 kai Minamata ten seminā 第 9 回水俣展セミナー. Bunkyō kumin sentā, Tokyo. April 21, 1995.

Mita Munesuke 見田宗介. Lecture. Minamata Tōkyō ten 水俣東京展. Shinagawa, Tokyo. Oct. 7, 1996.

Nagata Yasushi 永田靖. Lecture. Minamata no saisei o kangaeru shimin no tsudoi: sorosoro moyainoshi hajimemba 水俣の再生を考える市民の集い―そろそろもやい直しはじめんば. Minamata-shi bunka kaikan, Minamata. Nov. 12, 1994.

Nakamura Miyoko 仲村妙子 and Kure Tomofusa 呉智英. "Minamata kara kangaeru 8: sabetsu" 水俣から考える 8: 差別. Panel discussion. Minamata Tōkyō ten 水俣東京展. Shinagawa, Tokyo. Oct. 7, 1996.

Ogata Masato 緒方正人. "Watashi to Minamata—kanjasan no hanashi kara" 私と水俣―患者さんの話から. Lecture. Minamata Tōkyō ten 水俣東京展. Shinagawa, Tokyo. Sept. 28, 1996.

Ogata Masato 緒方正人 and Sumiya Mikio 隅谷三喜男. "Minamata kara kangaeru 7: wakai, kyūsai" 水俣から考える 7: 和解・救済. Panel discussion. Minamata Tōkyō ten 水俣東京展. Shinagawa, Tokyo. Oct. 5, 1996.

Ogura Ichirō 小倉一郎. Lecture. Minamata Tōkyō ten 水俣東京展. Shinagawa, Tokyo. Oct. 2, 1996.

Ōharu Kōnosuke 大治浩之輔. Lecture. Minamata Tōkyō ten 水俣東京展. Shinagawa, Tokyo. Sept. 30, 1996.

Okamoto Tatsuaki 岡本達明. "Chisso no kagai kōi to Minamata minshūzō" チッソの加害行為と水俣民衆像. Lecture. Dai 7 kai Minamata ten seminā 第 7 回水俣展セミナー. Bunkyō kumin sentā, Tokyo. Feb. 23, 1995.

Ōmure Tomie 大村トミエ and Hagio Moto 萩尾望都. "Watashi to Minamata—kanjasan no hanashi kara" 私と水俣ー患者さんの話から. Panel discussion. Minamata Tōkyō ten 水俣東京展. Shinagawa, Tokyo. Oct. 9, 1996.

Sakamoto Shinobu 坂本しのぶ. Lecture to students from Arisa Elementary School 有佐小学校, Yatsushiro-shi 八代市, Kumamoto prefecture. Minamatabyō sentā sōshisha, Minamata. Nov. 11, 1994.

Senba Shigekatsu 千場茂勝. "Minamatabyō mondai no keika to genjō: gyōsei to kōgai" 水俣病問題の経過と現状ー行政と公害. Lecture. Dai 25 kai chihō jichi kenkyū zenkoku shūkai—hi no kuni kenkyū—pure jichi ken Minamata shūkai 第 25 回地方自治研究全国集会ー火の国研究ープレ自治研水俣集会. Minamata-shi bunka kaikan, Minamata. Oct. 18, 1993.

Smith, Aileen, Akutagawa Jin 芥川仁, and Nagakura Hiromi 長倉洋海. "Dokyumentarī foto to wa nani ka: Yūjin Sumisu no hito to shigoto o tōshite" ドキュメンタリーフォトとは何かーユージン・スミスの人と仕事を通して. Panel discussion. Minamata Tōkyō ten 水俣東京展. Shinagawa, Tokyo. Sept. 29, 1996.

Sugimoto Eiko 杉本栄子. Lecture. Hama kōminkan, Minamata. July 16, 1994.

———. "Watashi to Minamatabyō: kanjasan no hanashi kara" 私と水俣病ー患者さんの話から. Lecture. Minamata Tōkyō ten 水俣東京展. Shinagawa, Tokyo. Sept. 30, 1996.

Sugimoto Takeshi 杉本雄. Lecture. Minamata no saisei o kangaeru shimin no tsudoi: sorosoro moyainoshi hajimemba 水俣の再生を考える

市民の集い―そろそろもやい直しはじめんば. Minamata-shi bunka kaikan, Minamata. Nov. 12, 1994.

Tanoue Yoshiharu 田上義春. Minamata Tōkyō ten, jikkō iinkai hossoku no tsudoi 水俣東京展実行委員会発足の集い. Lecture. Nihon toshi sentā, Tokyo. May 14, 1994.

Togashi Sadao 富樫貞夫 and Sataka Makoto 佐高信. "Minamata kara kangaeru 4: gyōsei, kigyō" 水俣から考える 4: 行政・企業. Panel discussion. Minamata Tōkyō ten 水俣東京展. Shinagawa, Tokyo. Oct. 2, 1996.

Tsuchimoto Noriaki 土本典昭. "Minamata kara kangaeru 10: hyōgen, kiroku" 水俣から考える 10: 表現・記録. Lecture. Minamata Tōkyō ten 水俣東京展. Shinagawa, Tokyo. Oct. 10, 1996.

Yahagi Tadashi 矢作正. "Nihon no kagaku kōgyō to Chisso no shihon no ayumi" 日本の化学工業とチッソの資本の歩み. Lecture. Dai 5 kai Minamata ten seminā 第 5 回水俣展セミナー. Bunkyō kumin sentā, Tokyo. Dec. 14, 1994.

Yoshii Masazumi 吉井正澄. Lecture. Minamata no saisei o kangaeru shimin no tsudoi: sorosoro moyainoshi hajimemba 水俣の再生を考える市民の集い―そろそろもやい直しはじめんば. Minamata-shi bunka kaikan, Minamata. Nov. 12, 1994.

Yoshinaga Toshio 吉永利夫. Lecture to volunteers with Nihon seinen hōshi kyōkai 日本青年奉仕協会 (JYVA). Minamatabyō sentā sōshisha, Minamata. Oct. 15, 1993.

―――. Lecture to members of Peace, Health, and Human Development (PHD) group. Minamatabyō sentā sōshisha, Minamata. Jan. 26, 1994.

―――. Lecture to visitors from Hyūga 日向. Minamatabyō sentā sōshisha, Minamata. June 3, 1995.

Films, Film Scripts, and Television and Radio Documentaries

Chōsen ni okeru dai suiryoku hatsuden kaihatsu no kiroku 朝鮮における大水力発電開発の記録. Nihon Kōei kabushiki kaisha / Nihon sangyō saiken gijutsu kyōkai 日本工営株式会社 / 日本産業再建技術協会. No date given in titles; Nihon Kōei was established in 1946 by former executives of Nitchitsu-related companies in Korea and Manchukuo. Black & white, 18 min. A modified version of *Ōryokkō dai suiryoku hatsuden kōji: kōji kiroku eiga* (see below).

Hellfire: A Journey from Hiroshima. John W. Dower and John Junkerman. 1985. 60 min. On the murals by Maruki Iri and Maruki Toshi.

Hyakken kiroku nijū nen: Minamatabyō sanjūgo nen, ima, Minamata wa 百間記録二十年: 水俣病三十五年，いま，水俣は. Onitsuka Iwao, 1991. 8 mm, color, 18 min. Script in author's possession.

Igaku to shite no Minamatabyō 医学としての水俣病. 3 parts. Dir. Tsuchimoto Noriaki 土本典昭. Seirinsha 青林舎, 1974-75. 16mm, color, 1 hr. 22 min., 1 hr. 43 min., 1 hr. 31 min. Script in *Gekkan tōfū*, 3 pts., 38 (May 1975), pp. 64-83; 39 (June 1975), pp. 56-78; 41 (Aug. 1975), pp. 68-88. English version: *Minamata Disease: A Trilogy.*

Ikarenai sekai 怒れない世界. Shin Nihon chisso rōsō 8 miri gurūpu/Minamatabyō shimin kaigi 新日本窒素労組八ミリグループ/水俣病市民会議, 1970. 8mm, black & white, 22 min. Script in Onitsuka Iwao, *Oruga Minamata* おるが水俣 (Tokyo: Gendai Shokan, 1986), pp. 205-11. Script in author's possession.

Kanjin 勧進. Dir. Koike Hiroko 小池裕子. Shiguro/Seirinsha/Kirokusha シグロ/青林舎/記録社, 1971. 16mm, black & white, 24 min.

Kegasareta Shiranuikai: tsuikyū sareru 17 nin no shiin 汚された不知火海・追及される 17 人の死因. In *Toki no ugoki* 時の動き series. Apr. 1957. NHK Radio.

Kibyō no kage ni 奇病の陰に. #99 in *Nihon no sugao* 日本の素顔 series. Dir. Ogura Ichirō 小倉一郎. Nov. 1959. NHK Television.

Kūhaku no 20 nen 空白の 20 年. Dir. Ōharu Kōnosuke 大治浩之輔. Mar. 22, 1979. NHK Television.

Minamatabyō I 水俣病 I. Shin Nitchitsu rōso 8 miri gurūpu/Minamatabyō shimin kaigi 新日窒労組八ミリグループ / 水俣病市民会議, 1968. 8mm, black & white, 20 min. Script in author's possession.

Minamatabyō bideo Q &A 水俣病ビデオ Q &A. Produced by Satō Makoto 佐藤真. Minamata Tōkyō ten jikkō iinkai 水俣東京展・実行委員会, 1996. Video, color, 30 min.

Minamatabyō: sono 20 nen 水俣病―その 20 年. Dir. Tsuchimoto Noriaki 土本典昭. Seirinsha 青林舎, 1976. 16mm, color, 43 min.

Minamatabyō: sono 30 nen 水俣病―その30年. Dir. Tsuchimoto Noriaki 土本典昭. Seirinsha/Shiguro 青林舎/シグロ, 1987. 16mm, color, 45 min. Script in author's possession.

Minamata: kanjasan to sono sekai 水俣―患者さんとその世界. Dir. Tsuchimoto Noriaki 土本典昭. Higashi purodakushon 東プロダクション,

1971. 35mm/16mm, black & white, 2 hr. 47 min. (2 hr. version also produced). Script in *Shin Nihon bungaku* 新日本文学 288 (July 1971), pp. 6–47. English version: *Minamata: The Victims and Their World.* 1972.

Minamata no zu, monogatari 水俣の図・物語. Dir. Tsuchimoto Noriaki 土本典昭. Seirinsha 青林舎, 1981. 35mm/16mm, color, 1 hr. 51 min.

'*Minamata' o tsutaetai: taijisei kanja wa ima* 「水俣」を伝えたい：胎児性患者は今. *Kurashi no jānaru* くらしのジャーナル, Oct. 6, 1993. NHK Television. Color, 33 min.

Minamata's Message to the World. Dir. Tsuchimoto Noriaki 土本典昭. Seirinsha 青林舎/Radio Quebec, 1976. 16mm, color, 45 min. Based on *Minamatabyō: sono 20 nen.*

Muko naru umi 無辜なる海. Dir. Katori Naotaka 香取直孝. Firumu kōbō フィルム工房, 1982. 16mm, color/black & white, 1 hr. 21 min.

Ōryokkō dai suiryoku hatsuden kōji: kōji kiroku eiga 鴨緑江大水力発電工事・工事記録映画. Chōsen Ōryokkō suiryoku hatsuden kabushiki kaisha/Manshū Ōryokkō suiryoku hatsuden kabushiki kaisha 朝鮮鴨緑江水力発電株式会社/満州鴨緑江水力発電株式会社. No date given in titles; chronicles the Yalu River dam project, begun in 1937 and completed in 1942. Black & white, 46 min.

Shimin no michi 死民の道. Dir. Minamata eiga han 水俣映画班. Shiguro/Seirinsha/Kirokusha シグロ/青林舎/記録社, 1972. 16mm, black & white, 40 min.

Shiranuikai 不知火海. Dir. Tsuchimoto Noriaki 土本典昭. Seirinsha 青林舎, 1975. 16mm, color, 2 hr. 33 min. Script in *Geijutsu undō* 芸術運動 28 (4, no. 1) (Feb. 1975): 2–55.

Shiranuikai, Shōwa 32 nen haru: rajio ga tsutaeta Minamatabyō jiken 不知火海・昭和32年春—ラジオが伝えた水俣病事件. In *Rajio anguru '94* ラジオアングル'94 series. May 7, 1994. NHK Radio.

Umi to otsukisamatachi 海とお月さまたち. Dir. Tsuchimoto Noriaki 土本典昭. Nihon kiroku eiga kenkyūjo 日本記録映画研究所, 1980. 35mm/16mm, color, 50 min.

Uzumoreta hōkoku 埋もれた報告. Dir. Ōharu Kōnosuke 大治浩之輔. Dec. 18, 1976. NHK Television.

Waga machi waga seishun: Ishikawa Sayuri Minamata nesshō わが町わが青春：石川さゆり水俣熱唱. Dir. Tsuchimoto Noriaki 土本典昭. Seirinsha 青林舎, 1978 (video), 1981 (film). Video/16mm, color, 43 min.

All Other Sources

Aga ni ikiru seisaku iinkai 阿賀に生きる制作委員会, ed. *Aga sōshi* 阿賀草紙. Vol. 1. *Aganogawa to kawamichi no hensen* 阿賀野川と河道の変遷 (July 1, 1990). Vol. 2. *Aganogawa no sen'un* 阿賀野川の船運 (Nov. 15, 1990). Vol. 3. *Aganogawa no kawazakana* 阿賀野川の川魚 (June 1, 1991). Vol. 4: *Aganogawa to Niigata Minamatabyō* 阿賀野川と新潟水俣病 (Dec. 1, 1992). Niigata-shi: Aga ni ikiru seisaku iinkai, 1990–92.

Akutagawa Jin 芥川仁, photographs, and Yanagida Kōichi 柳田耕一, text. *Minamata: genson suru fūkei—Akutagawa Jin shashinshū* 水俣・厳存する風景―芥川仁写真集. Minamata: Minamatabyō sentā sōshisha, 1980.

Allinson, Gary. "The Structure and Transformation of Conservative Rule." In Andrew Gordon, ed., *Postwar Japan as History*, pp. 123–44. Berkeley: University of California Press, 1993.

AMPO: Japan Asia Quarterly Review (journal).

Andō Yoshio 安藤良雄, ed. *Kindai Nihon keizai shi yōran* 近代日本経済史要覧. 2d ed. Tokyo: Tōkyō daigaku shuppankai, 1979.

Apter, David E., and Nagayo Sawa. *Against the State: Politics and Social Protest in Japan.* Cambridge, Mass.: Harvard University Press, 1984.

Arima Sumio 有馬澄雄. "Hosokawa Hajime ron nōto" 細川一論ノート. 3 pts. *Kuragō* 暗河 2 (Winter 1974): 88–99; 5 (Fall 1974): 122–35; 9 (Fall 1975): 46–61.

Arima Sumio 有馬澄雄, ed. *Minamatabyō—nijū nen no kenkyū to konnichi no kadai* 水俣病―20年の研究と今日の課題. Tokyo: Seirinsha, 1979.

Asahi shinbun 朝日新聞 (newspaper).

Asahi Shinbun Japan Almanac 朝日新聞ジャパン・アルマナック *1995, 1997,* and *1999* (bilingual, in both English and Japanese). Tokyo: Asahi shinbun, 1994, 1996, 1998.

Aston, W. G., trans., *Nihongi: Chronicles of Japan from the Earliest Times to A.D. 697.* London: George Allen & Unwin, 1956 (reprint of 1896 ed.).

Baba Noboru 馬場のぼる [昇]. *Minamatabyō sanjūnen: kokkai kara no shōgen* 水俣病三十年・国会からの証言. Tokyo: Eideru kenkyūjo, 1986.

Bank of Japan, Statistics Department 日本銀行統計局. *Meiji ikō honpō shuyō keizai tōkei* 明治以降本邦主要経済統計 *Hundred-Year Statistics of the Japanese Economy* (bilingual, in both English and Japanese). Tokyo, 1966.

Benhabib, Seyla. "Toward a Deliberative Model of Democratic Legitimacy." In idem, ed., *Democracy and Difference: Contesting the Boundaries of the Political*, pp. 67–94. Princeton: Princeton University Press, 1996.

Benhabib, Seyla, ed. *Democracy and Difference: Contesting the Boundaries of the Political*. Princeton: Princeton University Press, 1996.

Berg, Lisa, and Lasse Berg. "Stockholders' Corral." *AMPO* 9–10 (1971): 54–55.

Bisson, T. A. *Zaibatsu Dissolution in Japan*. Berkeley: University of California Press, 1954.

Bix, Herbert P. "Inventing the 'Symbol Monarchy' in Japan, 1945–52." *Journal of Japanese Studies* 21, no. 2 (Summer 1995): 319–63.

———. *Peasant Protest in Japan, 1590–1884*. New Haven: Yale University Press, 1986.

Burkman, Thomas W., ed. *The Occupation of Japan: Economic Policy and Reform*. Norfolk, Va.: MacArthur Memorial, 1978.

Calder, Kent E. *Crisis and Compensation: Public Policy and Political Stability in Japan, 1949–1986*. Princeton: Princeton University Press, 1988.

Camera 35 (journal).

Chisso kabushiki kaisha, Minamata kōjō チッソ株式会社水俣工場. *Chisso Minamata* チッソ水俣. (Newspaper; successor to *Minamata kōjō shinbun*.)

Doak, Kevin M. "What Is a Nation and Who Belongs? National Narratives and the Ethnic Imagination in Twentieth-Century Japan," *American Historical Review* 102, no. 2 (Apr. 1997): 282–309.

Dower, John W. *Empire and Aftermath: Yoshida Shigeru and the Japanese Experience, 1878–1954*. Cambridge, Mass.: Harvard University, Council on East Asian Studies, 1979.

———. "The Useful War." In idem, *Japan in War and Peace: Selected Essays*. New York: New Press, 1993.

Dower, John W., and John Junkerman, eds. *The Hiroshima Murals: The Art of Iri Maruki and Toshi Maruki*. Tokyo: Kōdansha International, 1985.

Field, Norma. *In the Realm of a Dying Emperor: Japan at Century's End*. New York: Pantheon, 1991.

Fukumoto Kunio 福本邦雄, ed. *Noguchi Shitagau wa ikite iru: jigyō supiritto to sono tenkai* 野口遵は生きている―事業スピリットとその展開. Tokyo: Fuji intānashonaru konsarutanto, 1964.

Funaba Masatomi 船場正富. "Chisso to chiiki shakai" チッソと地域社会. In Miyamoto Ken'ichi 宮本憲一, ed., *Kōgai toshi no saisei: Minamata*

公害都市の再生・水俣. Kōza chiiki kaihatsu to jichitai 講座地域開発と自治体. Tokyo: Chikuma shobō, 1977, pp. 38–97.

Garon, Sheldon. *Molding Japanese Minds: The State in Everyday Life*. Princeton: Princeton University Press, 1997.

————. *The State and Labor in Modern Japan*. Berkeley: University of California Press, 1987.

Garon, Sheldon, and Mike Mochizuki. "Negotiating Social Contracts." In Andrew Gordon, ed., *Postwar Japan as History*, pp. 145–66. Berkeley: University of California Press, 1993.

Gluck, Carol. *Japan's Modern Myths: Ideology in the Late Meiji Period*. Princeton: Princeton University Press, 1985.

————. "The People in History: Recent Trends in Japanese Historiography." *Journal of Asian Studies* 38, no. 1 (Nov. 1978): 25–50.

Gonzui ごんずい. Journal of Minamatabyō sentā sōshisha 水俣病センター相思社.

Gordon, Andrew. "Contests for the Workplace." In idem, ed., *Postwar Japan as History*, pp. 373–94. Berkeley: University of California Press, 1993.

————. *Labor and Imperial Democracy in Prewar Japan*. Berkeley: University of California Press, 1991.

————. *The Wages of Affluence: Labor and Management in Postwar Japan*. Cambridge, Mass.: Harvard University Press, 1998.

Gordon, Andrew, ed. *Postwar Japan as History*. Berkeley: University of California Press, 1993.

Gotō Takanori 後藤孝典. *Chinmoku to bakuhatsu: dokyumento "Minamatabyō jiken"* 沈黙と爆発：ドキュメント「水俣病事件」. Tokyo: Shūeisha, 1995.

Gresser, Julian; Kōichirō Fujikura; and Akio Morishima. *Environmental Law in Japan*. Cambridge, Mass.: MIT Press, 1981.

Hadley, Eleanor M. *Anti-Trust in Japan*. Princeton: Princeton University Press, 1970.

Haley, John O. "The Myth of the Reluctant Litigant." *Journal of Japanese Studies* 4 (1978): 359–90.

Hamamoto Tsuginori, "Our Environment and Healthy Bodies Will Never Be Restored." *AMPO* 27, no. 3 (1997): 34–35.

Harada Masazumi 原田正純. *Minamatabyō* 水俣病. Tokyo: Iwanami shoten, 1972.

————. *Minamatabyō wa owatte inai* 水俣病は終わっていない. Tokyo: Iwanami shoten, 1985.

Hōritsu jihō 法律時報 (journal).

Huddle, Norie, and Michael Reich, with Nahum Stiskin. *Island of Dreams: Environmental Crisis in Japan.* New York: Autumn Press, 1975; Cambridge, Mass.: Schenkman Books, 1987.

Hunter, Donald; Richard R. Bomford; and Dorothy S. Russell. "Poisoning by Methyl Mercury Compounds." *Quarterly Journal of Medicine* 33 (1940): 193–13.

Hunter, Donald, and Dorothy S. Russell. "Focal Cerebral and Cerebellar Atrophy in a Human Subject Due to Organic Mercury Compounds." *Journal of Neurology, Neurosurgery, and Psychiatry* 17 (Nov. 1954): 235–41.

Huntington, Samuel P. *The Third Wave: Democratization in the Late Twentieth Century.* Norman: University of Oklahoma Press, 1991.

Ibsen, Henrik. *A Public Enemy* (usually trans. *An Enemy of the People*). In *Ghosts and Other Plays.* Trans. Peter Watts. London: Penguin, 1964.

Irie Sukemasa 入江相政. *Irie Sukemasa nikki* 入江相政日記, vol. 2. Ed. Asahi shinbunsha 朝日新聞社; supervising ed., Irie Tametoshi 入江為年. Tokyo: Asahi shinbunsha, 1990.

Irokawa Daikichi 色川大吉. "Kōgai toshi Minamata ni okeru ningen to shizen no kyōsei no mondai" 公害都市水俣における人間と自然の共生の問題. *Tōkyō keidai gakkaishi* 東京経大学会誌 190 (Jan. 1995): 159–73.

————. "Kumamoto Minamatabyō saiban genkokudan daihyō Watanabe Eizō no kiroku" 熊本水俣病裁判原告団代表渡辺栄蔵の記録. *Tōkyō keidai gakkaishi* 東京経済大学会誌 158 (Nov. 1988): 268–43 (page order inverted).

————. *Minamata: sono sabetsu no fūdo to rekishi* 水俣—その差別の風土と歴史. Minamata: Han kōgai Minamata Kyōtō kaigi jimukyoku, 1980.

————. "Shiranuikai minshūshi: Minamatabyō jiken shi josetsu" 不知火海民衆史：水俣病事件史序説. In idem, ed., *Shinpen Minamata no keiji: Shiranuikai sōgō chōsa hōkoku* 新編水俣の啓示—不知火海総合調査報告. Tokyo: Chikuma shobō, 1995.

————. *Shōwa shi sesō hen* 昭和史世相篇. Tokyo: Shōgakukan, 1994.

————. "The Survival Struggle of the Japanese Community." *Japan Interpreter* 9, no. 4 (1975): 466–94. Reprinted in J. Victor Koschmann, ed., *Authority and the Individual in Japan: Citizen Protest in Historical Perspective,* pp. 250–82. Tokyo: University of Tokyo Press, 1978.

Irokawa Daikichi 色川大吉, ed. *Minamata no keiji: Shiranuikai sōgō chōsa hōkoku* 水俣の啓示―不知火海総合調査報告. 2 vols. Tokyo: Chikuma shobō, 1983. Reissued in one volume, without the medical and scientific chapters, as *Shinpen Minamata no keiji: Shiranuikai sōgō chōsa hōkoku* 新編水俣の啓示―不知火海総合調査報告. Tokyo: Chikuma shobō, 1995.

Irukayama Katsurō et al. "Studies on the Origin of the Causative Agent of Minamata Disease, III: Industrial Wastes Containing Mercury Compounds from Minamata Factory." *Kumamoto Medical Journal* 15, no. 2 (June 30, 1962): 57–68.

Ishida Takeshi 石田雄. *Japanese Political Culture: Change and Continuity.* New Brunswick, N.J.: Transaction Books, 1983.

————. "Minamata ni okeru yokuatsu to sabetsu no kōzō" 水俣における抑圧と差別の構造. In Irokawa Daikichi 色川大吉, ed., *Shinpen Minamata no keiji: Shiranuikai sōgō chōsa hōkoku* 新編水俣の啓示―不知火海総合調査報告, pp. 39–90. Tokyo: Chikuma shobō, 1995.

————. "Sengo shakai kagaku to sonraku shi kenkyū: Ōishi Kaichirō, Nishida Yoshiaki hen *Kindai Nihon no gyōsei mura kōhan no imi*" 戦後社会科学と村落史研究：大石嘉一郎・西田美昭編「近代日本の行政村」公判の意味. *Tochi seido shigaku* 土地制度史学 134 (Jan. 1992): 34–43.

Ishida Takeshi and Ellis S. Krauss, eds. *Democracy in Japan.* Pittsburgh: University of Pittsburgh Press, 1989.

Ishimure Michiko 石牟礼道子. *Kugai jōdo: waga Minamatabyō* 苦海浄土―わが水俣病. Tokyo: Kōdansha, 1969. Trans. Livia Monnet, *Paradise in the Sea of Sorrow: Our Minamata Disease.* Kyoto: Yamaguchi Publishing House, 1990.

————. *Tsubaki no umi no ki* 椿の海の記. Tokyo: Asahi shinbunsha, 1976. Trans. Livia Monnet, *Story of the Sea of Camellias.* Kyoto: Yamaguchi Publishing House, 1983.

Ishimure Michiko 石牟礼道子, ed. *Ten no uo* 天の魚. Tokyo: Chikuma shobō, 1974.

————. *Ten no yamu: jitsuroku Minamatabyō tōsō* 天の病む：実録水俣病闘争. Fukuoka: Ashi shobō, 1974.

————. *Waga shimin: Minamatabyō tōsō* わが死民―水俣病闘争. Tokyo: Gendai hyōronsha, 1972.

Ishimure Michiko 石牟礼道子, story; Maruki Toshi 丸木俊 and Maruki Iri 丸木位里, pictures. *Minamata—umi no koe* 水俣—海のこえ. Tokyo: Komine shoten, 1982.

Ivy, Marilyn. *Discourses of the Vanishing: Modernity, Phantasm, Japan.* Chicago: University of Chicago Press, 1995.

————. "Formations of Mass Culture." In Andrew Gordon, ed., *Postwar Japan as History,* pp. 239–58. Berkeley: University of California Press, 1993.

Japan: An Illustrated Encyclopedia. Tokyo: Kōdansha, 1993.

Japan, Kankyōchō 環境庁, ed. *Kankyō hakusho (sōsetsu)* 環境白書 (総説) and *Kankyō hakusho (kakuron)* 環境白書 (各論). 1993, 1994, 1995.

Johnson, Chalmers. *Conspiracy at Matsukawa.* Berkeley: University of California Press, 1972.

————. *MITI and the Japanese Miracle: The Growth of Industrial Policy, 1925–1975.* Stanford: Stanford University Press, 1982.

Johnson, William. *W. Eugene Smith: A Chronological Bibliography, 1934–1980.* 2 pts. plus addendum. Tucson: University of Arizona, Center for Creative Photography, 1980 (Pts. I & II), 1984 (addendum).

Kalland, Arne. *Fishing Villages in Tokugawa Japan.* Honolulu: University of Hawaii Press, 1995.

Kankyō hakai 環境破壊 (journal).

Kankyō sōzō minamata jikkō iinkai 環境創造みなまた実行委員会, ed. *Saisei suru Minamata* 再生する水俣. Fukuoka: Ashi shobō, 1995.

Kaplan, David E., and Alec Dubro. *Yakuza: The Explosive Account of Japan's Criminal Underworld.* Reading, Mass.: Addison-Wesley, 1986.

Kasza, Gregory James. *The State and the Mass Media in Japan, 1918–1945.* Berkeley: University of California Press, 1988.

Katagiri Ryūkichi 片桐龍吉. *Hantō no jigyō ō: Noguchi Shitagau* 半島の事業王: 野口遵. Tokyo: Tōkai shuppansha, 1939.

Kawamoto saiban shiryōshū henshū iinkai 川本裁判資料集編集委員会, ed. *Minamatabyō jishu kōshō Kawamoto saiban shiryōshū* 水俣病自主交渉川本裁判資料集. Tokyo: Gendai jānarizumu shuppankai, 1981.

Kawamoto Teruo. "A Shameful Retreat." *AMPO* 27, no. 3 (1997): 37–38.

Kersten, Rikki. *Democracy in Postwar Japan: Maruyama Masao and the Search for Autonomy.* London and New York: Routledge, 1996.

Kikuchi Masanori 菊地昌典. "Chisso rōdō kumiai to Minamatabyō" チッセ労働組合と水俣病. In Irokawa Daikichi 色川大吉, ed., *Shinpen*

Minamata no keiji: Shiranuikai sōgō chōsa hōkoku 新編水俣の啓示— 不知火海総合調査報告, pp. 509–71. Tokyo: Chikuma shobō, 1995.

Kōgai: The Newsletter from Polluted Japan. Special issues: *Mercury Pollution Problem, 1* (1975); *Mercury Pollution Problem, 2: Mercury Pollution in Canada* (1975); *Mercury Pollution Problem, 3: Reports from HESC Conference* (1975); *Mercury Pollution Problem, 4: The Newest Results in Japan and Canada* (1976).

Kokuhatsu 告発. Journal of the Minamatabyō o kokuhatsu suru kai 水俣病を告発する会 (Kumamoto). June 14, 1969–Aug. 25, 1973. Reprinted in Tōkyō Minamatabyō o kokuhatsu suru kai 東京水俣病を告発する会, ed., *Shukusatsuban kokuhatsu* 縮刷版告発 (1971), and *Shukusatsuban kokuhatsu zokuhen* 縮刷版告発続編 (1974). Tokyo: Tōkyō Minamatabyō o kokuhatsu suru kai. Replaced by *Minamata: kanja to tomo ni*.

Komori Takeshi 小森武. "Kokumin no ishiki to undō" 国民の意識と運動. In Tsuru Shigeto 都留重人, ed., *Gendai shihonshugi to kōgai* 現代資本主義と公害. Tokyo: Iwanami shoten, 1968.

Koschmann, J. Victor. "Intellectuals and Politics." In Andrew Gordon, ed., *Postwar Japan as History*, pp. 395–423. Berkeley: University of California Press, 1993.

———. *Revolution and Subjectivity in Postwar Japan.* Chicago: University of Chicago Press, 1996.

Kotsuna Masachika 忽那将愛, ed. *Minamatabyō: Yūki suigin chūdoku ni kan suru kenkyū* 水俣病: 有機水銀中毒に関する研究. Kumamoto: Kumamoto daigaku, Igakubu, Minamatabyō kenkyūhan, 1966. English version: Kumamoto University Study Group of Minamata, ed. *Minamata Disease.* 1968.

Krauss, Ellis S., and Bradford L. Simcock. "Citizens' Movements: The Growth and Impact of Environmental Protest in Japan." In Kurt Steiner, Ellis S. Krauss, and Scott C. Flanagan, eds., *Political Opposition and Local Politics in Japan*, pp. 187–227. Princeton: Princeton University Press, 1980.

Kugai 苦海. Journal of Tokyo Minamatabyō o kokuhatsu suru kai.

Kumamoto Daigaku, Bungakubu, Chiiki kagakuka shakaigaku kenkyūshitsu, Minamatabyō kanja dantai kenkyūhan 熊本大学文学部地域科学科社会学研究室水俣病患者団体研究班 ed. *Minamatabyō kanja dantai ni kan suru chōsa* 水俣病患者団体に関する調査. Kumamoto: Kumamoto daigaku, Bungakubu, Chiiki kagakuka shakaigaku kenkyūshitsu, Minamatabyō kanja dantai kenkyūhan, 1994.

Kumamoto nichinichi shinbun 熊本日日新聞 (newspaper).

Kurland, Leonard T. "An Epidemiological Overview of Minamata Disease and a Review of Earlier Public Health Recommendations." In Tsuru Shigeto et al., eds., *Minamatabyō jiken ni okeru shinjitsu to seigi no tame ni— Minamatabyō kokusai fōramu (1988 nen) no kiroku* 水俣病事件における真実と正義のために―水俣病国際フォーラム (1988 年) の記録/*For Truth and Justice in the Minamata Disease Case: Proceedings of the International Forum on Minamata Disease 1988* (bilingual, in both English and Japanese). Tokyo: Keisō Shobō, 1989.

Kurland, Leonard, et al. "Minamata Disease." *World Neurology* 1 (May 1960): 370.

Kuwabara Shisei 桑原史成. *Minamatabyō: shashin kiroku 1960–1970* 水俣病―写真記録 1960–1970. Tokyo: Asahi shinbun, 1970.

———. *Minamata, Kankoku, Betonamu* 水俣・韓国・ベトナム. Tokyo: Banseisha, 1982.

———. *Minamata no hitobito: haha to ko de miru* 水俣の人びと：母と子でみる. Tokyo: Kusa no ne shuppankai, 1998.

———. *Minamata: owari naki 30 nen—genten kara tensei e* 水俣：終りなき30年―原点から転生へ. 2d ed.. Tokyo: Aki shobō, 1989.

———. *Shashinshū: Minamatabyō* 写真集―水俣病. Tokyo: San'ichi shobō, 1965.

Lewis, Jack G. "Civic Protest in Mishima: Citizens' Movements and the Politics of the Environment in Contemporary Japan." In Kurt Steiner, Ellis S. Krauss, and Scott C. Flanagan, eds. *Political Opposition and Local Politics in Japan*, pp. 274–313. Princeton: Princeton University Press, 1980.

Life (journal).

Maruyama Masao 丸山真男. "Gendai ni okeru taido kettei" 現代における態度決定. In *Maruyama Masao shū* 丸山真男集, 8: 301–17. Tokyo: Iwanami shoten, 1995–97.

———. "Theory and Psychology of Ultranationalism." In idem, *Thought and Behavior in Modern Japanese Politics*. Trans. Ivan Morris. Oxford: Oxford University Press, 1963. This essay was first published in *Sekai* in May 1946.

Maruyama Sadami 丸山定巳. "Kigyō to chiiki keisei: Chisso (kabu) to Minamata" 企業と地域形成―チッソ(株)と水俣. *Bungakubu ronsō* [Kumamoto daigaku bungaku kai] 文学部論叢 [熊本大学文学会] 16 (Apr. 1985): 19–37.

————. "Responses to Minamata Disease." In James K. Mitchell, ed., *The Long Road to Recovery: Community Responses to Industrial Disaster*, pp. 41–59. Tokyo: United Nations University Press, 1996.

Maruyama Sadami 丸山定巳 and Minamatabyō kenkyūkai 水俣病研究会, eds. *Shōwa 54 nendo Minamatabyō ni kan suru sōgōteki chōsa tehō no kaihatsu ni kan suru kenkyū hōkokusho (Shōwa 54 nendo Kankyōchō kōgai bōshi nado chōsa kenkyū itakuhi ni yoru hōkokusho)* 昭和 54 年度水俣病に関する総合的調査手法の開発に関する研究報告書(昭和 54 年度環境庁公害防止等調査研究委託費による報告書). Nihon kōshū eisei kyōkai, Mar. 31, 1980.

————. *Shōwa 55 nendo Minamatabyō ni kan suru sōgōteki chōsa tehō no kaihatsu ni kan suru kenkyū hōkokusho (Shōwa 55 nendo Kankyōchō kōgai bōshi nado chōsa kenkyū itakuhi ni yoru hōkokusho)* 昭和 55 年度水俣病に関する総合的調査手法の開発に関する研究報告書 (昭和 55 年度環境庁公害防止等調査研究委託費による報告書). Nihon kōshū eisei kyōkai, Mar. 1981.

McAlpine, Douglas, and Araki Shukuro. "Minamata Disease: An Unusual Neurological Disorder Caused by Contaminated Fish." *Lancet* 2 (Sept. 20, 1958): 629–31.

McKean, Margaret A. *Environmental Protest and Citizen Politics in Japan*. Berkeley: University of California Press, 1981.

————. "Equality." In Ishida Takeshi and Ellis S. Krauss, eds., *Democracy in Japan*, pp. 201–24. Pittsburgh: University of Pittsburgh Press, 1989.

Minamatabyō kenkyūkai 水俣病研究会, ed. *Minamatabyō jiken shiryōshū 1926–1968* 水俣病事件資料集, 1926–1968. 2 vols. Fukuoka: Ashi shobō, 1996. Abbreviated in the notes as *MBJSS*. Supplemented by Minamatabyō kenkyūkai, ed. *Minamatabyō kenkyū* (q.v.).

————. *Minamatabyō kenkyū* 水俣病研究. Vol. 1: *Minamatabyō mondai no seiji kaiketsu* 水俣病問題の政治解決. Fukuoka: Ashi shobō, 1999. The first of 10 projected volumes of documents and analysis intended to supplement Minamatabyō kenkyūkai, ed., *Minamatabyō jiken shiryōshū 1926–1968* (q.v.). This volume includes a collection of 68 documents related to the third "solution" to the Minamata disease issue, "Seiji ketchaku kankei shiryō I" 政治決着関係資料 I, abbreviated in the notes as SKKS1.

————. *Minamatabyō ni tai suru kigyō no sekinin: Chisso no fuhō kōi* 水俣病に対する企業の責任— チッソの不法行為. Kumamoto: Minamatabyō o kokuhatsu suru kai, 1970.

————. *Nintei seido e no chōsen: Minamatabyō ni tai suru Chisso, gyōsei, igaku no sekinin* 認定制度への挑戦—水俣病にたいするチッソ・行政・医学 の責任. Kumamoto: Minamatabyō o kokuhatsu suru kai, 1972.

Minamatabyō sentā sōshisha 水俣病センター相思社. *Sūji kara miru Minamatabyō* 数字からみる水俣病. Minamata: Minamatabyō sentā sōshisha, 1996, 1997, 2001.

Minamatabyō soshō bengodan, Manaki hōritsu jimusho 水俣病訴訟 弁護団馬奈木法律事務所. *Bengodan dayori* 弁護団だより. 2 vols. Reprint of nos. 1 (Apr. 1, 1971)–30 (June 15, 1972), and nos. 31 (July 1, 1972)– 54 (June 15, 1973). Minamata: Minamatabyō soshō bengodan, Manaki hōritsu jimusho, 1972, 1973.

Minamata Disease Center Sōshisha 水俣病センター相思社, ed. *Illustrated Minamata Disease (E de miru Minamatabyō* 絵で見る水俣病). In English and Japanese. Yokohama: Seori shobō, 1993.

Minamata hakkō iinkai 水俣発行委員会, ed. *Gekkanshi Minamata Nos. 1–50* 月刊誌水俣 Nos. 1–50.

Minamata: kanja to tomo ni 水俣—患者とともに. Journal of Minamatabyō o kokuhatsu suru kai 水俣病を告発する会 (Kumamoto). Nos. 1–186 (Sept. 1973–Oct. 1986) reprinted in Minamatabyō o kokuhatsu suru kai 水俣病を告発する会, ed., *Shukusatsuban Minamata* 縮刷版水俣 (Kumamoto: Minamatabyō o kokuhatsu suru kai, 1986). (Successor to *Kokuhatsu*).

Minamata-shi gikai, Jimukyoku 水俣市議会事務局. *Minamata-shi gikai kaigiroku* 水俣市議会会議録. Minamata: Minamata-shi gikai, Jimukyoku, n.d.

Minamata shiritsu Minamatabyō shiryōkan 水俣市立水俣病資料館 and Minamatabyō rekishi kōshōkan 水俣病歴史考証館, "Minamatabyō 10 no chishiki" 水俣病 10 の知識. Pamphlet. 1994, rev. 1997. Trans. Timothy S. George and Jane Ellen George and published as Minamata Disease Municipal Museum and Minamata Disease Museum, "Ten Things to Know About Minamata Disease." 1995; rev. 1998.

Minamata-shi shi hensan iinkai 水俣市史編纂委員会, ed. *Minamata-shi shi* 水俣市史. Minamata: Minamata shiyakusho, 1966.

Mishima Akio 三島昭男. *Nake, Shiranui no umi: Minamata ni sasageta chinkon no tatakai* 哭け、不知火の海—水俣に捧げた鎮魂の闘い. Tokyo: San'ichi shobō, 1977. Rev. and trans. Richard L. Gage and Susan B. Murata, *Bitter Sea: The Human Cost of Minamata Disease*. Tokyo: Kosei, 1992.

Mitamura Takeshi 三田村猛司. "Ore a ikitakatta: buraku no heta ni shi-gami tsuite mo" 俺ア生きたかった一部落の端にしがみついても. *Shiranui* 不知火 6 (Spring 1977): 16–34.

Miyamoto Ken'ichi 宮本憲一, ed. *Kōgai toshi no saisei: Minamata* 公害都市の再生・水俣. Kōza chiiki kaihatsu to jichitai 講座地域開発と自治体. Tokyo: Chikuma shobō, 1977.

Miyazawa Nobuo 宮澤信雄. *Minamatabyō jiken yonjū nen* 水俣病事件四十年. Fukuoka: Ashi shobō, 1997.

Molony, Barbara. *Technology and Investment: The Prewar Japanese Chemical Industry.* Cambridge, Mass.: Harvard University, Council on East Asian Studies, 1990.

Murakami Yasusuke. "The Age of New Middle Mass Politics: The Case of Japan." *Journal of Japanese Studies* 8, no. 1 (1982): 29–72.

Nemoto Masayuki 根本正行, ed. *Tsuchimoto Noriaki firumogurafi* 土本典昭フィルモグラフィ. Tokyo: Shiguro, 1987.

Nihon chisso hiryō kabushiki kaisha 日本窒素肥料株式会社. *Jigyō gaiyō* 事業概要. Osaka: Nihon chisso hiryō kabushiki kaisha, Mar. 1930.

———. *Nihon chisso hiryō jigyō taikan* 日本窒素肥料事業大勧. Osaka: Nihon chisso hiryō kabushiki kaisha, 1937.

———. *Nihon chisso jigyō gaiyō* 日本窒素事業概要. Osaka: Nihon chisso hiryō kabushiki kaisha, 1940.

Nishi Yasunori. "Despite My Convulsions, I Haven't Applied." Trans. Hirata Aya. *AMPO* 27, no. 3 (1977): 39.

Nishimura Hajime 西村肇. "Minamatabyō hassei gen'in no nazo ga toketa" 水俣病発生原因の謎が解けた. 2 pts. *Gendai kagaku* 現代化学 323 (Feb. 1998): 60–66; 324 (Mar. 1998): 14–22.

Nishinippon shinbun 西日本新聞 (newspaper).

Nobukuni Masafumi 信国正史. *Shin Sagara shiwa* 新相良史話. 2 vols. Kumamoto: Kumamoto nichinichi shinbun kōhō bunka sentā, 1990–91.

Norbeck, Edward. *Takashima: A Japanese Fishing Village.* Salt Lake City: University of Utah Press, 1954.

Notehelfer, F. G. "Japan's First Pollution Incident." *Journal of Japanese Studies* 1, no. 2 (Spring 1975): 351–83.

Ogata Masato 緒方正人. "Watashitachi wa ima doko ni iru ka: shisutemu no naka no Minamatabyō" 私たちは今どこにいるか—システムの中の水俣病. *Gonzui* ごんずい 21 (Mar. 1994): 12–14.

Ogata Masato 緒方正人 and Tsuji Shin'ichi 辻信一. *Tokoyo no fune o kogite: Minamatabyō shishi* 常世の舟を漕ぎて：水俣病私史. Yokohama: Seori shobō, 1996.

Ōhara shakai mondai kenkyūjo 大原社会問題研究所, ed. *Nihon rōdō nenkan* 日本労働年間, vol. 26. Tokyo: Jiji tsūshinsha, 1954.

Ohnuki-Tierney, Emiko. *Illness and Culture in Contemporary Japan.* New York: Cambridge University Press, 1984.

———. *Rice as Self: Japanese Identities Through Time.* Princeton: Princeton University Press, 1993.

Oiwa Keinosuke. "Field Notes: Visiting Ogata Masato." *Kokugakuin kenkyū* 国学院研究 13 (Jan. 1995): 33–46.

Okamoto Tatsuaki 岡本達明 and Matsuzaki Tsugio 松崎次夫, eds. *Kikigaki Minamata minshūshi* 聞書水俣民衆史. Vol. 1, *Meiji no mura* 明治の村 (1990); vol. 2, *Mura ni kōjō ga kita* 村に工場が来た (1988); vol. 3, *Mura no hōkai* 村の崩壊 (1989); vol. 4, *Gōsei kagaku kōjō to shokkō* 合成化学工場と職工 (1990); vol. 5, *Shokuminchi wa tengoku datta* 植民地は天国だった (1990). Tokyo: Sōfūkan, 1988–90.

Onitsuka Iwao 鬼塚巌. *Oruga Minamata* おるが水俣. Tokyo: Gendai shokan, 1986.

Ōshio Takeshi 大塩武. *Nitchitsu kontserun no kenkyū* 日窒コンツェルンの研究. Tokyo: Nihon keizai hyōronsha, 1989.

Ōtsuka Hisao. "The Formation of Modern Man: The Popular Base for Democratization." Trans. Patricia Murray. *Japan Interpreter* 6, no. 1 (Spring 1970): 1–5.

Pempel, T. J. "The Unbundling of 'Japan, Inc.': The Changing Dynamics of Japanese Policy Formation." *Journal of Japanese Studies* 13, no. 2 (Summer 1987): 271–306.

Pharr, Susan J. *Losing Face: Status Politics in Japan.* Berkeley: University of California Press, 1990.

Pierson, John D. *Tokutomi Sohō, 1864–1957: A Journalist for Modern Japan.* Princeton: Princeton University Press, 1980.

Reich, Michael R. *Toxic Politics: Responding to Environmental Disasters.* Ithaca: Cornell University Press, 1991.

Richardson, Bradley. *Japanese Democracy: Power, Coordination, and Performance.* New Haven: Yale University Press, 1997.

Sairen さいれん. Newsletter of Gōka rōren shin Nihon chisso rōdō kumiai 合化労連新日本窒素労働組合.

Saishu Satoru 最首悟, ed. *Detsuki shiki: Hamamoto Tsuginori katari* 出月
私記—浜本二徳語り. Tokyo: Shinchōsha, 1989.

Saitō Hisashi 斎藤恒. *Niigata Minamatabyō* 新潟水俣病. Tokyo: Mainichi
shinbunsha, 1996.

Sakamoto Fujie. "A Family Tragedy." Trans. Sugihara Megumi. *AMPO* 27,
no. 3 (1997): 30–33.

Scheiner, Irwin. "The Japanese Village: Imagined, Real, Contested." In Stephen Vlastos, ed., *Mirror of Modernity: Invented Traditions of Modern Japan*,
pp. 67–78. Berkeley: University of California Press, 1998.

Schonberger, Howard. "Zaibatsu Dissolution and the American Restoration
of Japan." *Bulletin of Concerned Asian Scholars* 5, no. 2 (Sept. 1973): 16–31.

Shin Minamata-shi shi hensan iinkai 新水俣市史編さん委員会, ed. *Shin
Minamata-shi shi* 新水俣市史. 2 vols. Minamata: Minamata-shi, 1991.

Shin Nihon bungaku 新日本文学 (journal).

Shin Nihon chisso hiryō kabushiki kaisha, Minamata kōjō 新日本窒素
肥料株式会社水俣工場. *Minamata kōjō shinbun* 水俣工場新聞. (Newspaper; predecessor of *Chisso Minamata*.)

Shinohara Miyohei 篠原三代平. *Kojin shohi shishutsu* 個人蕗費支出
/*Personal Consumption Expenditures*, vol. 6 of Ohkawa Kazushi 大川一司,
Shinohara Miyohei 篠原三代平, and Umemura Mataji 梅村又次, eds.,
Chōki keizai tōkei: suikei to bunseki 長期経済統計: 推計と分析 /*Estimates
of Long-Term Economic Statistics of Japan Since 1868* (bilingual, in English
and Japanese). Tokyo: Tōkyō keizai shinpōsha, 1967.

Shiota Takeshi 塩田武史. *Minamata '68–'72, fukaki fuchi yori: Shiota Takeshi
shashin hōkoku* 水俣'68–'72, 深き淵より: 塩田武史写真報告. Fukuoka:
Nishinippon shinbunsha, 1973.

Shiranui: ima Minamata wa 不知火—いま水俣は (journal published by Sunada Akira).

Shōji Kichirō and Sugai Masurō. "The Ashio Copper Mine Pollution Case:
The Origins of Environmental Destruction." In Ui Jun, ed., *Industrial
Pollution in Japan*, pp. 18–63. Tokyo: United Nations University Press,
1992.

Smith, Thomas C. *Native Sources of Japanese Industrialization, 1750–1920*. Berkeley: University of California Press, 1988.

Smith, W. Eugene. "Special Feature: Minamata, Japan—An Essay on the
Tragedy of Pollution and the Burden of Courage." *Camera* 35 18, no. 2
(Apr. 26, 1974): 26–51.

Smith, W. Eugene, and Aileen Smith. "Death-Flow from a Pipe." *Life*, June 2, 1972, pp. 74–81.

———. *Minamata*. New York: Holt, Rinehart and Winston, 1975. Translated by Nakao Hajime 中尾ハジメ and published in Japanese as *Shashinshū Minamata* 写真集水俣. Tokyo: San'ichi shobō, 1991 (1980).

Smith, W. Eugene, and Aileen M. Smith, photographs; Ishimure Michiko 石牟礼道子, text. *Sakamoto Shinobu-chan no koto: hana bōshi* 坂本しのぶちゃんのこと：花帽子. Tokyo: Sōjusha, 1973.

Steiner, Kurt, Ellis S. Krauss, and Scott C. Flanagan, eds. *Political Opposition and Local Politics in Japan*. Princeton: Princeton University Press, 1980.

Steinhoff, Patricia G. "Protest and Democracy." In Ishida Takeshi and Ellis S. Krauss, eds., *Democracy in Japan*, pp. 171–98. Pittsburgh: University of Pittsburgh Press, 1989.

Strong, Kenneth. *Ox Against the Storm: A Biography of Tanaka Shōzō—Japan's Conservationist Pioneer*. Vancouver: University of British Columbia Press, 1987.

Supreme Commander for the Allied Powers (SCAP). *History of Non-Military Aspects of the Occupation of Japan*. 55 vols. 1945–51.

Suzuki, David, and Oiwa Keibo. *The Other Japan: Voices Beyond the Mainstream*. Golden, Colo.: Fulcrum, 1999.

Suzuki Masao 鈴木正男. *Shōwa tennō no gojunkō* 昭和天皇の御巡幸. Tokyo: Tendensha, 1992.

"Symposium: The Ashio Copper Mine Pollution Incident." Articles by Kenneth B. Pyle ("Introduction: Japan Faces Her Future," pp. 347–50), F. G. Notehelfer ("Japan's First Pollution Incident," pp. 351–83), and Alan Stone ("The Japanese Muckrakers," pp. 385–407). *Journal of Japanese Studies* 1, no. 2 (Spring 1975): 347–407.

Takahashi Hiroshi 高橋紘. *Shōwa tennō hatsugenroku: Taishō 9 nen–Shōwa 64 nen no shinjitsu* 昭和天皇発言録―大正9年―昭和64年の真実. Tokyo: Shōgakkan, 1989.

Taketani Mitsuo 武谷三男. *Gensuibaku jikken* 原水爆実験. Tokyo: Iwanami shoten, 1957.

Togashi Sadao 富樫貞夫. *Minamatabyō jiken to hō* 水俣病事件と法. Fukuoka: Sekifūsha, 1995.

Tōkyō Minamatabyō o kokuhatsu suru kai 東京水俣病を告発する会, ed. *Minamatabyō ni tai suru Chisso, gyōsei, igaku no sekinin: "minintei kanja" wa tsu-*

kurareta 水俣病にたいするチッソ・行政・医学の責任—「未認定患者」はつくられた. Tokyo: Minamatabyō o kokuhatsu suru kai, 1971.

————. *Shukusatsuban kokuhatsu* 縮刷版告発. Tokyo: Tōkyō Minamatabyō o kokuhatsu suru kai, 1971.

————. *Shukusatsuban kokuhatsu zokuhen* 縮刷版告発続編. Tokyo: Tōkyō Minamatabyō o kokuhatsu suru kai, 1974.

Tomita Hachirō (or Tonda Yarō) 富田八郎 (pen name of Ui Jun 宇井純), ed. *Minamatabyō: Minamatabyō kenkyūkai shiryō* 水俣病—水俣病研究会資料. Kumamoto: Minamatabyō o kokuhatsu suru kai, 1969. Abbreviated in the notes as *MB*.

Tsuchimoto Noriaki 土本典昭. *Minamata eiga henreki: kiroku nakereba jijitsu nashi* 水俣映画遍歴—記録なければ事実なし. Tokyo: Shinchōsha, 1988.

Tsuru Shigeto 都留重人, ed. *Gendai shihonshugi to kōgai* 現代資本主義と公害. Tokyo: Iwanami shoten, 1968.

Tsuru Shigeto 都留重人 et al., eds. *Minamatabyō jiken ni okeru shinjitsu to seigi no tame ni—Minamatabyō kokusai fōramu (1988 nen) no kiroku* 水俣病事件における真実と正義のために—水俣病国際フォーラム (1988 年) の記録. *For Truth and Justice in the Minamata Disease Case: Proceedings of the International Forum on Minamata Disease 1988* (bilingual, in both English and Japanese). Tokyo: Keisō shobō, 1989.

Tsurumi Kazuko 鶴見和子. "Man, Nature and Technology: A Case of Minamata." In idem, ed., *Aspects of Endogenous Development in Modern Japan*. Sophia University, Institute of International Relations Research Papers, Series A-38, Part III. Tokyo: Sophia University, 1979.

————. "Tahatsu buraku no kōzō henka to ningen gunzō: shizen hakai kara naihatsuteki hatten e" 多発部落の構造変化と人間群像：自然破壊から内発的発展へ. In Irokawa Daikichi 色川大吉, ed., *Shinpen Minamata no keiji: Shiranuikai sōgō chōsa hōkoku* 新編水俣の啓示—不知火海総合調査報告, pp. 155–98. Tokyo: Chikuma shobō, 1995.

Ui Jun 宇井純. *Gappon kōgai genron* 合本公害原論. Tokyo: Aki shobō, 1988.

————. *Kōgai no seijigaku: Minamatabyō o otte* 公害の政治学：水俣病を追って. Tokyo: Sanseidō, 1968.

————. *Nihon no mizu o kangaeru* 日本の水を考える. Text for NHK educational television series, 1994.

Ui Jun 宇井純, ed. *Industrial Pollution in Japan*. Tokyo: United Nations University Press, 1992.

————. *Kōgai jishu kōza 15 nen* 公害自主講座15年. Tokyo: Aki shobō, 1991.

United States, Department of State. *Report of the Mission on Japanese Combines* ("The Edwards Report"), *Part I, Analytical and Technical Data.* Department of State Publication 2628, Far Eastern Series 14. Washington, D.C., 1946.

United States, Strategic Bombing Survey. *Final Reports of the United States Strategic Bombing Survey 1945–1947.* Report No. 49, "Chemicals in Japan's War," and Report No. 50, "Chemicals in Japan's War: Appendix to the Report." Washington, D.C., n.d.

Uno Shigeaki 宇野重昭. "Chisso kigyō ron" チッソ企業論. In Irokawa Daikichi 色川大吉, ed., *Shinpen Minamata no keiji: Shiranuikai sōgō chōsa hōkoku* 新編水俣の啓示―不知火海総合調査報告, pp. 467–507. Tokyo: Chikuma shobō, 1995.

Upham, Frank K. *Law and Social Change in Postwar Japan.* Cambridge, Mass.: Harvard University Press, 1987.

————. "Litigation and Moral Consciousness in Japan: An Interpretive Analysis of Four Japanese Pollution Suits." *Law & Society Review* 10 (1976): 579–619.

————. "Unplaced Persons and Movements for Place." In Andrew Gordon, ed., *Postwar Japan as History,* pp. 325–46. Berkeley: University of California Press, 1993.

————. "Weak Legal Consciousness as Invented Tradition." In Stephen Vlastos, ed., *Mirror of Modernity: Invented Traditions of Modern Japan,* pp. 42–64. Berkeley: University of California Press, 1998.

Vlastos, Stephen. *Peasant Protests and Uprisings in Tokugawa Japan.* Berkeley: University of California Press, 1986.

Vlastos, Stephen, ed. *Mirror of Modernity: Invented Traditions of Modern Japan.* Berkeley: University of California Press, 1998.

Walthall, Anne. *Social Protest and Popular Culture in Eighteenth-Century Japan.* Tucson: University of Arizona Press, 1986.

Watanabe Osamu 渡辺治. *Kigyō shihai to kokka* 企業支配と国家. Tokyo: Aoki shoten, 1991.

————. *Sengo seiji shi no naka no tennōsei* 戦後政治史の中の天皇制. Tokyo: Aoki shoten, 1992.

Waters, Neil. *Japan's Local Pragmatists: The Transition from Bakumatsu to Meiji in the Kawasaki Region.* Cambridge, Mass.: Harvard University, Council on East Asian Studies, 1983.

White, James W. "The Dynamics of Political Opposition." In Andrew Gordon, ed., *Postwar Japan as History*, pp. 424–47. Berkeley: University of California Press, 1993.

Wolin, Sheldon S. "Fugitive Democracy." In Seyla Benhabib, ed., *Democracy and Difference: Contesting the Boundaries of the Political*, pp. 31–45. Princeton: Princeton University Press, 1996.

Yahagi Tadashi 矢作正. "Chisso shi, 1955–60: Minamatabyō" チッソ史 1955–60 水俣病. *Urawa ronsō* 浦和論叢 17 (Jan. 1997): 23–46.

———. "Chisso shi, 1960–65: Goi kōjō kensetsu" チッソ史 1960–65 五井工場建設. *Urawa ronsō* 浦和論叢 20 (June 1998): 21–60.

———. "Nihon chisso hiryō (kabu) ni kan suru kenkyū" 日本窒素 肥料(株)に関する研究. *Urawa ronsō* 浦和論叢 10 (March 1993): 55–96.

———. "Sengo Chisso shi, 1945–55" 戦後チッソ史 1945–55. *Urawa ronsō* 浦和論叢 14 (June 1995): 145–79.

Yamamoto Shigeo 山本茂雄, ed. *Kanashikaru inochi idakite: Minamata no shōgen* 愛しかる生命いだきて—水俣の証言. Tokyo: Shin Nihon shuppansha, 1976.

Yoshinaga Toshio 吉永利夫. "Dai ni no Minamatabyō" 第二の水俣病. *Keizai seminā* 経済セミナー 365 (June 1985): 88.

———. "Konna setsubi wa iranai!" こんな設備はいらない! *Gonzui* ごんずい 39 (Mar. 25, 1997): 17–18.

Young, Louise. *Japan's Total Empire: Manchuria and the Culture of Wartime Imperialism*. Berkeley: University of California Press, 1998.

Index

Ad hoc certification committee (Minamatabyō shinsa kyōgikai), Ministry of Health and Welfare, 206; Kumamoto prefecture, 206

Aganogawa kenkyūkai, *see* Agano River Research Group

Agano River, 175, 187

Agano River Research Group (Aganogawa kenkyūkai), 183

Agriculturalism, *see* Nōhonshugi

Air raids, *see* Bombing

Ajia to Minamata o musubu kai, *see* Conference Linking Minamata and Asia

Akagi Hirokatsu, 69

Akasaki Satoru, 154–55, 161, 167, 179–80, 198

Akihito, 32, 75

Akiyama Takeo, 86–87, 101

Akune, 147

Akutagawa Jin, 284, 289–90

Allinson, Gary, 299n26, 336n7

All-Japan Prefectural and Municipal Workers' Union (Zen Nihon jichi dantai rōdō kumiai; Jichirō), 184

Amakusa Islands, 134, 144, 155, 276; migration to Minamata, 14, 27–28, 35, 38, 133

Amimoto (net owners) and *amiko* (hired by *amimoto*), 38, 51, 135–36, 141, 205, 304n52

Andō Nobuo, 115

Anpo, *see* United States–Japan Mutual Security Treaty

Antiwar movement, 285. *See also* League for Peace in Vietnam; United States–Japan Mutual Security Treaty

Araki Seishi, 157

Araki Yōko, 272–73

Arbitration Group (Ichininha), 193–202 *passim*, 205, 211, 216, 225–28, 235, 250, 256

Ariake Sea, 66, 254, 266

Arirang Brigade, 30

Arita Shigeo, 5–6

Ashikita, 82, 87, 146

Ashikita Moyainaoshi Center, 278

Ashikita Village Fishing Cooperative, 82, 89

Ashio, 108, 118, 120, 127. *See also* Kawamata incident; Tanaka Shōzō

Association to Indict [Those Responsible for] Minamata Disease (Minamatabyō o kokuhatsu suru kai), 157, 161, 196–201, 211–12, 223–24, 229, 231, 237, 263, 327n35; *Kokuhatsu*

(newsletter), 155, 196–98, 200, 211,
216; nationwide affiliates, 196, 211,
215, 219, 252; split with trial lawyers,
196, 247, 249–50. *See also* Fukuoka
Association to Indict [Those Re-
sponsible for] Minamata Disease;
Minamata Disease Research
Group; Osaka Association to Indict
[Those Responsible for] Minamata
Disease; Tokyo Association to In-
dict [Those Responsible for]
Minamata Disease
Association to Protect Minamata
(Minamata o mamoru kai), 167
Atomic bomb victims (*hibakusha*), 218,
269, 275, 334*n*23, 334*n*24. *See also*
Hiroshima; *Lucky Dragon* incident;
Nagasaki
Auschwitz, 272

Bandō Katsuhiko, 191–92
Basic Law for Environmental Pollution
Control (Kōgai taisaku kihon hō),
207
Beheiren, *see* League for Peace in Viet-
nam
Bhopal, 272
Big Four pollution cases, 174–76, 206,
245. *See also* Minamata disease; Nii-
gata Minamata disease; Toyama
cadmium poisoning; Yokkaichi air
pollution
Bikini Atoll, 244
Bix, Herbert, 119, 313*n*68
Bombing (of Minamata in WWII),
30–31, 134
Buddhism, 262, 279, 337*n*1. *See also*
Shingon Buddhism; Zen
Buddhism
Burakumin, 218

Cabinet, 62, 267, 269–70
Calder, Kent, 298*n*26, 336*n*7
Carson, Rachel, 183
Cat experiments, *see under* Minamata
disease
Catholicism, *see* Christianity
Certification of patients, *see under*
Minamata disease
Changjin River, 22
Chernobyl, 272
Chigusa Tatsuo, 199–200, 202
Chihara (Shin Nitchitsu managing di-
rector), 84, 98–99, 128–32 *passim*,
137, 139
Chikuhō, 27, 38, 104, 263
Chikyūza, 212
Chisso kabushiki kaisha, 163, 276,
300*n*12; government financial sup-
port, 264, 266–67, 270, 278. *See also*
Chōsen chisso hiryō; Dentsū; Di-
rect Negotiations Group; Dredging,
landfill, and reclaimed land; Ega-
shira Yutaka; Factory workers; Goi
plant; Industrial Bank of Japan; Irie
Kanji; Kawashima Tsuneya; Kuga
Shōichi; Lawsuits and trials; "castle
town" *under* Minamata; Minamata
Fishing Cooperative; Nihon Chisso
hiryō kabushiki kaisha; Nikkeiren;
One-share movement; Shimada
Ken'ichi; Shin Nihon chisso hiryō
kabushiki kaisha; Shin Nihon ka-
gaku; *Sōkaiya*; Solatium agreement
and payments; Strikes; Tokue
Takeshi; Tokyo Building; Tokyo
Negotiations; Unions; *Wakai*
Chisso kyōgikai, *see* Nitrogen
Council
Chisso sekiyu kagaku, *see* Goi plant
Chō Michiaki, 30

Chōsen chisso hiryō, 21–23, 35–36, 47.
See also Changjin River; Hungnam;
Yalu River
Chōteiha, see Mediation Group
Christianity, 14, 252–53
Chūkanha, see Middle Group
Chūō kōgai taisaku shingikai; see
Council for Control of Environmental Pollution
Circle Village (Sākuru mura), 104–5,
154–56
Citizens' Assembly to Brighten Minamata (Minamata o akaruku suru
shimin renraku kyōgikai), 227–28
Citizens' Conference for the Development of Minamata (Minamata-shi
hatten shimin kyōgikai), 186
Citizens' Council for Minamata Disease Countermeasures (Minamatabyō taisaku shimin kaigi), 125, 179–
85, 191–92, 196–202 passim, 207, 211–
12, 216, 218, 223, 237, 241–42, 247;
founding and leadership, 125, 158,
167, 179–80, 252, 263, 276
Citizens' forums to discuss Minamata
disease (Minamatabyō o kataru
shimin kōza), 277
Citizens' Movement, 173–75
Civil liberties commissioners (jinken
yōgo iin), 203, 328n51. See also Kumamoto Prefecture Association of
Civil Liberties Commissioners
Coal mining, see Chikuhō; Miike; Mitsui Mining Company; Ōmuta;
Strikes
Comfort women, 269
Community, see Unmei kyōdōtai
Complaints against administrative
acts (gyōsei fufuku shinsa seikyū),
207–10

Conference Linking Minamata and
Asia (Ajia to Minamata o musubu
kai), 272
Confucianism, 118
Congenital Minamata disease, see under
Minamata disease
Consumer activism, 283
Council for Control of Environmental
Pollution (Chūō kōgai taisaku shin-
gikai), 223, 228–29, 233–38
Crown prince (Naruhito), 323n32
Cyclator, 114–16, 144, 186, 192, 317n143

Dannoura, 13
Democracy, 9, 10, 222, 257, 280–86, 335
Democratic Party, 287
Dentsū, 228
Detsuki, 1, 5, 27, 38, 50, 156, 220, 271,
277
Diet (national legislature), 61, 64, 82–
93, 101, 114, 130–31, 138, 193, 248, 267,
312n47, 326n31. See also Pollution
Diet; War apology
Direct Negotiations Group (Jishu kō-
shōha; later the Trial Group
[Soshōha]; formed by members of
Mutual Aid Society in April 1969;
not identical to group in next en-
try), 193–95
Direct Negotiations Group (Jishu kō-
shōha; formed by newly certified
patients led by Kawamoto Teruo in
fall 1971), 211–12, 221, 223–39, 247–
48, 250, 254, 257
Discover Japan campaign, 173
Discrimination, 26–29, 34, 41, 105–9
passim, 204, 218, 264, 270–79 passim,
290. See also Atomic bomb victims;
Burakumin; Minamata disease;
Unions

Documentaries, *see* Films and film-
    makers
Dokubutsu oyobi gekibutsu torishi-
    mari hō, *see* Law for the Control of
    Poisonous and Powerful Sub-
    stances
Dower, John, 162, 334n23, 335n7, 336n9
Dredging, landfill, and reclaimed land,
    80, 126, 139–40, 224, 261–62, 268,
    278–79

Ebara Infilco, 115. *See also* Cyclator
Economic growth, *see* Gross National
    Product
Economic Planning Agency (EPA), 66,
    84–85, 88, 129–30, 152, 189
Edogawa (river), *see* Honshū Paper
    Company
Education, 27, 29, 38, 55, 118, 134, 139,
    158, 180, 184, 280. *See also* Ministry of
    Education; Unions; *and individual
    schools by name*
Edwards Report, 31–32
Egashira Yutaka, 163, 188, 192, 216, 219–
    21, 228
Egoshita Kazuko, 5, 6
Egoshita Kazumi, 231
Eight Millimeter Group, 215–16
Electrochemical industry, 17
Emperors, empresses, and imperial
    family, 187. *See also* Imperial House-
    hold Agency; *and individuals by name*
Environment Agency, 201, 210, 224,
    234–38 *passim*, 254–55, 267–69, 288–
    89
Environmental Dispute Coordination
    Commission (Kōgai nado chōsei
    iinkai), 239–40
Exchange rates (yen-dollar), 295n5
Expo '70, 212

Factory Effluents Control Law (Kōjō
    haisui nado no kisei ni kansuru
    hōritsu), 85, 94, 185
Factory workers, 17, 20, 26–32;
    Koreans, 22, 30; pay, 2, 22, 26–28,
    30, 34, 324n40. *See also* Strikes;
    Unions
False patients (*nise kanja*), 273
Field, Norma, 296n24, 336n7
Films and filmmakers, 7, 284, 334n23.
    See also individual filmmakers by name
First Minamata Fishing Dispute, 76–
    81, 83, 102
Fisheries Agency, 66, 84, 88, 96
Fisheries Law, 53
Fishing cooperatives, *see individual coop-
    eratives by name*
Food Hygiene Investigation Commit-
    tee (Shokuhin eisei chōsakai; Min-
    istry of Health and Welfare), 61–63,
    66, 83, 85, 89, 185, 189
Food Sanitation Act (Shokuhin eisei
    hō), 53
Freedom and Popular Rights Move-
    ment (Jiyū minken undō), 282,
    297n, 322n5
Fuchigami Sueki, 73–79 *passim*, 106–12
    passim, 131, 137, 142
Fujioka Taishin, 85–86, 88
Fukami family, 15–16
Fukami Yoshitake, 73, 142
Fuke Masaki, 169, 204, 228
Fukuda Takeo, 62–63
Fukunaga Kazutomi, 84–85, 88, 92
Fukuoka, 211, 215, 227
Fukuoka Association to Indict [Those
    Responsible for] Minamata Disease
    (Fukuoka Minamatabyō o ko-
    kuhatsu suru kai), 218
Fukuoka High Court, 266, 268–69, 273

Fukuoka Minamatabyō o kokuhatsu
suru kai, *see* Fukuoka Association to
Indict [Those Responsible for]
Minamata Disease
Fukuro, 271
Fukuro Bay, 59
Fukuro Middle School, 156
Funaba Iwazō, 82, 312n41
Funaba Tōkichi, 82
Funatsu, 27
Furusato būmu (old hometown boom),
173

Garon, Sheldon, 298n25
General Council of Trade Unions of
Japan, *see* Sōhyō
Get in Touch with the Environment in
Minamata (*Kankyō fureai in Mina-
mata*) festival, 278
Gimin (martyrs), *see* Peasant protests
and rebellions
Goi plant (Chisso), 162–64, 172, 231,
233, 238. *See also* Natsume Hideo
Gojokai, *see* Minamata Disease
Patients Families Mutual Aid
Society
Gōka rōren; *see* Japanese Federation of
Synthetic Chemistry Workers
Unions
Gold mines, 16
Gordon, Andrew, 34, 164
Goshonoura, 144, 146, 209
Gotō Haruo, 93
Gotō Takanori, 115, 189, 206, 208, 216–
20, 233, 239–40, 263, 265, 318n1
Goze, 336n1. *See also* Sugimoto Eiko
Gross National Product (GNP), 171,
256–57, 269, 324n57, 332n58
Guandong (Kwantung) Army, 22
Gulf War, 272

Gyōsei fufuku shinsa seikyū, see Complaints against administrative acts

Hachiman, 74, 80, 87, 95, 137, 139; waste
settlement pools, 55, 87–88, 114–15,
134
Hainan Island, 23
Hair, mercury in, 128, 144–47, 149,
208–9, 318n14, 328n61
Halstead, Bruce, 55
Hama-chō, 27
Hamamatsu Minamata Exhibition,
337n2
Hamamoto Fumiyo, 2, 7, 108, 216, 220,
261
Hamamoto Kazunori, 7, 38
Hamamoto Matsu, 6–7, 220
Hamamoto Sōhachi, 6–7, 38–39, 220
Hamamoto Tsuginori, 1–7 *passim*, 18,
38–40, 108, 193, 207, 213, 216, 220,
229–30, 261–64 *passim*, 271–73, 277,
295n1
Hamasu Yoshitaka, 148–49
Han'ya Takahisa, 66–67
Harada Masazumi, 73, 106, 150, 158–61,
175, 198, 208, 232, 242, 247, 263–64,
272, 277
Harada Naō, 231, 331n23
Harada Takayoshi, 149–50
Hara denshi, 276
Hashiguchi Saburō, 277
Hashimoto Hikoshichi, 20, 30–31, 36,
53, 59, 134, 152–53, 157
Hashimoto Michio, 63, 188–89, 201
Haze (Japan wax) trees, 38, 193, 304n53
Hibakusha, see Atomic bomb victims
Hibiya Park, 200
Hidaka Rokurō, 54, 231
Hidden Christians, *see* Christianity
Higashi (town), 147

Higo Bank, 137

Hiranoya no danna, *see* Ogata Korenori

Hiratsuka manganese poisoning, 52

Hirohito, 24, 32–33, 140, 187, 303n27, 331n23

Hiroshima, 13, 218, 243, 269, 272, 275, 334n23. *See also* Atomic bomb victims

Hirota Sunao, 106, 136

Hito kabu undō, *see* One-share movement

HIV blood scandal, 287

Hiyoshi Fumiko, 143, 158, 161, 167, 180, 185, 211, 219, 252

Hokusei gakuen, 152–54, 158

Hometown boom, *see* Furusato būmu

Honda Keikichi, 196, 200, 217, 231

Honshū Paper Company, 87

Hosokawa (daimyō), 15–16

Hosokawa Hajime, 5, 47–51, 54, 57, 60–61, 68, 112, 150, 158, 160–61, 175, 189, 245, 289. *See also* cat experiments *under* Minamata disease

Hospitals, *see individual hospitals by name*

Hungnam (Kōnan), 21, 23

Hunter-Russell syndrome, 55, 145, 208–9, 267

Hyakken Harbor, 3, 36, 38, 54, 73, 77, 79–80, 137, 148

Hyakken waste settlement pools and outfall, 57, 95, 87, 100–101

Hydroelectric power, 16–17, 32

Ichihara Kiyo, 203

Ichininha, *see* Arbitration Group

Igarashi Yoshiaki, 240–41

Ikeda (Shin Nitchitsu executive director), 79–81

Ikeda Hayato, 61–63, 121, 173, 308n65

Ikematsu Nobuo, 224, 227

Ikki, *see* Peasant protests and rebellions

Imperial Household Agency, 323n32

Industrial Bank of Japan, 163, 254

Irie Kanji, 230

Irokawa Daikichi, 16, 28, 106, 127, 170, 187, 263, 284, 287–88, 297n, 316n117, 318n1, 322n5

Iron triangle, 280–81

Irukayama Katsurō, 68, 70, 115

Ise Bay, 175

Ishida Masaru, 223, 229–30, 235–36, 277

Ishida Takeshi, 288, 297n

Ishihara Waketake, 131, 136

Ishikawa Sayuri, 276–77

Ishimure Hiroshi, 156, 167, 262

Ishimure Michiko, 24, 27, 61, 89–90, 93, 103–5, 125, 154–58, 160–62, 167, 179–82, 187, 200, 209, 211, 222, 229–31, 262–63, 271, 284; writings, 155–57, 172, 196, 198–99, 212, 242–43, 267, 289, 322n2, 334n23

Ishimure Michio, 156

Ishino (assistant factory manager), 108–9

Itai-itai byō, *see* Toyama cadmium poisoning

Itō Hasuo, 5, 47–49, 51, 54, 60, 82, 84, 112, 148

Iwao Yutaka, 98

Iwasaka Mari, 150–51

Iwasaka Masaki, 151

Iwasaka Sueko, 150–51

Iwasaka Yoshiko, 150

Izu Tomihito, 98

Izumi, 29, 82, 128, 133, 136, 147, 206, 255

Japan Chemical Industry Association (Nihon kagaku kōgyō kyōkai), 59, 66–67, 117, 166. *See also* Ōshima

Takeji; Vinyl Chloride and Acetaldehyde Special Committee
Japan Communist Party, 34, 101, 104–5, 173, 175, 196–98, 234, 246, 282–83; in Minamata, 54, 103–4, 196, 226, 231
Japanese Federation of Synthetic Chemistry Workers Unions (Gōka rōren), 166
Japan Federation of Employers' Associations, *see* Nikkeiren
Japan Medical Association, 66–67
Japan National Railways, 173, 309*n*71. *See also* Shimoyama Incident
Japan Pediatric Association, 149
Japan Self-Defense Forces, 280
Japan Socialist Party, 97, 129, 173, 234, 269, 282–83; in Minamata, 36, 93, 158, 196, 226
Jichirō, *see* All-Japan Prefectural and Municipal Workers' Union
Jigoro (outsiders), 275
Jinken yōgo iin, see Civil liberties commissioners
Jinmu Boom, 33
Jinnai, 27, 31, 109
Jinzū River, 175
Jishu kōshōha, *see* Direct Negotiations Group
Jishu kōza, 161
Jitsukawa Wataru, 85
Jiyū minken undō, see Freedom and Popular Rights Movement
Junkerman, John, 334*n*23

Kagoshima city, 13
Kagoshima prefecture, 127–28, 134, 144, 255, 289
Kaisha-yuki (someone who "goes to the company"), *see* Factory workers

Kakure Kirishitan (hidden Christians), *see* Christianity
Kama Tsurumatsu, 156
Kamaishi, 40
Kamegatake, 146
Kamimura Tomoko, 214, 232, 271
Kamimura Yoshiko, 214, 232
Kamioka Mine, 175. *See also* Mitsui Metal Mining Company
Kaneko Naoyoshi, 235
Kanemi rice oil, 283
Kan Naoto, 287
Kankyō fureai in Minamata, see Get in Touch with the Environment in Minamata
Kanose, 176, 187
Kansai, 27
Karayuki-san, 14
Kase (of MITI Fukuoka office), 98
Kawamata incident, 118, 127, 316*n*117, 322*n*5. *See also* Ashio; Tanaka Shōzō
Kawamoto Kana, 133–34
Kawamoto Katōta, 133–35, 143–44, 203, 209, 216, 230
Kawamoto Miyako, 134, 144, 232
Kawamoto Shigeru, 134, 144
Kawamoto Teruo, 3, 133–35, 144, 164–66, 191, 203–8, 210–21 *passim*, 261–67 *passim*, 270, 277, 284; direct negotiations, 222–40 *passim*, 247; Tokyo negotiations, 251–53, 257
Kawamura Kazuo, 107–9
Kawamura Tsugiyoshi, 85, 88
Kawashima Tsuneya, 231, 233–34, 238
Kawazu Toratake, 98
Keikō, emperor, 14
Kibyō taisaku iinkai, see Strange Disease Countermeasures Committee
Kikuchi Masanori, 167
Kinjō Minoru, 272, 334*n*24

Kinki, 27

Kisarazu, 138

Kishi Nobusuke, 121, 173, 309n65

Kita Takeo, 204

Kitagawa Kinsai, 136–37

Kitakyūshū, 13, 211, 227, 283

Kitamura Shōji, 55, 57, 66

Kiyoura Raisaku, 62, 65–67, 99, 130–31

Kōgai funsō shori hō, see Law Concerning the Settlement of Environmental Pollution Disputes

Kōgai higaisha kyūsai hō, see Law
for Special Measures for Relief
from Pollution-Related Health
Damage

Kōgai nado chōsei iinkai, see Environmental Dispute Coordination
Commission

Kōgai ni kakawaru kenkō higai no
kyūsai ni kansuru tokubetsu sochi
hō, see Law for Special Measures for
Relief from Pollution-Related
Health Damage

Kōgai taisaku kihon hō, see Basic Law
for Environmental Pollution Control

Kōgai taisaku zenkoku renraku kyōgikai, see National Alliance for Pollution Countermeasures

Koiji Island, 3, 24, 50, 80, 148

Koiso Kuniaki, 22

Kojima Akikazu, 68, 160, 245

Kōjō haisui nado no kisei ni kansuru
hōritsu, see Factory Effluents Control Law

Kokuhatsu (newsletter), see under Association to Indict [Those Responsible for] Minamata Disease

Kokuritsu eisei shikenjo, see National
Hygiene Laboratory

Kokuritsu kōshū eiseiin, see National
Institute for Public Health

Kōkyō yōsuiiki no suishitsu no hozen
ni kansuru hōritsu, see Water
Quality Conservation Law

Komenotsu, 17, 82, 147

Komichi Shobō, 331n23

Komichi Tokuichi, 231

Komori Takeshi, 90, 119

Kōnan, see Hungnam

Kōnin, emperor, 15

Korea and Koreans, see Arirang Brigade; Changjin River; Chōsen
chisso hiryō; Factory workers;
Hungnam; Korean War; Prostitution; Yalu River

Korean War, 32

Kotsuna Masachika, 68–69

Koyama Osanori, 237–38

Kōyasan, 223

Kuchiberashi ("reducing the number of
mouths" to be fed), 27, 262–63

Kuga Shōichi, 226, 230–31, 235,
251–53

Kumamoto Castle, 13

Kumamoto city, 13, 110, 146

Kumamoto District Court, 194, 197,
239, 241, 247–48, 251, 266, 268. See
also Lawsuits and trials

Kumamoto igakukai, see Kumamoto
Medical Association

Kumamoto-Kagoshima Pollution Victims Certification Investigation
Committee (Kumamoto-ken-
Kagoshima-ken kōgai higaisha nintei shinsakai), 205–10, 252

Kumamoto-ken jinken yōgo iin rengōkai, see Kumamoto Prefecture Association of Civil Liberties Commissioners

Kumamoto Medical Association (Kumamoto igakukai), 60, 150
Kumamoto Minamata Disease Trial Lawyers' Group, 197
Kumamoto Prefectural Alliance of Fishing Cooperatives, 82–102 *passim*, 106, 110–20 *passim*, 126, 133, 136, 182
Kumamoto prefecture, 3, 5–6, 74, 82, 84, 87–88, 107, 112, 144, 246, 266–69, 277–79, 289; public health office in Minamata, 5, 47–48, 60, 148, 203, 205; prefectural legislature, 89, 95–102 *passim*, 138, 193, 246, 273; Commerce and Fisheries Department, 136, 139, 141. *See also* Special Committee on Minamata Disease Countermeasures
Kumamoto Prefecture Association of Civil Liberties Commissioners (Kumamoto-ken jinken yōgo iin rengōkai), 203, 205
Kumamoto University, 49, 51–70, 75, 83, 85, 87, 92, 99, 112, 115, 117, 128, 145, 148–50, 153, 155, 158–60, 189, 197–99, 209, 229, 242–43, 309*n*65; hospital, 2, 6–7; funding, 64, 70, 88–89, 152
Kurihara Akira, 336*n*1
Kurland, Leonard, 55–56, 64
Kuwabara Shisei, 157–58, 160–61, 172, 212, 284, 289
Kyōdōtai, see Unmei kyōdōtai
Kyūshū University, 66

Labor, *see* Factory workers; Strikes; Unions
Landfill, *see* Dredging, landfill, and reclaimed land
Land reform, 39, 40, 193

Law Concerning the Settlement of Environmental Pollution Disputes (Kōgai funsō shori hō), 202, 223
Law for Special Measures for Relief from Pollution-Related Health Damage (Kōgai ni kakawaru kenkō higai no kyūsai ni kansuru tokubetsu sochi hō; Kōgai higaisha kyūsai hō), 205–7
Law for the Control of Poisonous and Powerful Substances (Dokubutsu oyobi gekibutsu torishimari hō), 242, 249
Lawsuits and trials, 160, 180, 182, 190, 195–99, 237–54 *passim*, 267–73 *passim*, 277, 283–85, 308*n*51; barriers to litigation, 120, 151–52, 197; trial of fishermen for 1959 factory invasion, 126–27, 267; Niigata Minamata disease trials, 175–76, 179, 183, 246–47; March 1973 Kumamoto verdict, 222, 248–49, 263, 281; trial of Kawamoto Teruo, 238, 264–68 *passim*; trial of Chisso executives, 264, 266. *See also* Big Four pollution cases
League for Peace in Vietnam (Beheiren), 173–74, 196, 211, 221
Liberal Democratic Party, 97, 120, 129, 208, 268–69, 280–81; in Minamata, 36–37, 224, 235, 278
Liberty and Popular Rights Movement, *see* Freedom and Popular Rights Movement
Local industrial policy, 16–17
Lucky Dragon incident, 243–44

MacArthur, Douglas, 34
Maeda Eiki, 3, 17, 170
Maeda Kōzō, 73
Maeda Noriyoshi, 235, 240

Magsaysay Prize, 271
Manaki Akio, 197
Manchukuo, 22
Martyrs, see Peasant protests and rebellions
Maruki Iri, 272, 289, 334n23
Maruki Toshi, 272, 289, 334n23
Marushima fish market, 129, 137
Maruyama Masao, 280, 285, 297n, 336n7, 336n9
Maruyama Sadami, 199
Matsuda Ichijirō, 130–32, 135–36, 141–42
Matsuda Shin'ichi, 56
Matsuda Tetsuzō, 88, 92
Matsuda Tomiji, 90
Matsumoto Hideyo, 150
Matsumoto Tsutomu, 167, 179–80, 182, 276, 284
Matsunaga Kumiko, 153
May 25 Action, 211, 215
McAlpine, Douglas, 55
McKean, Margaret, 172, 180, 298n25
Mediation Group (Chōteiha), 231, 235, 239–41, 247, 250, 254, 256
Meisuien, 276–77
Meisuikai, see Mediation Group
Memorial ceremonies, 191, 278–79, 287–88, 336n1
Meshima, 107–8, 273
Middle Group (Chūkanha), 237, 247, 256
Miike, 13, 35, 104, 126, 136, 160, 164, 166, 181. See also Ōmuta; Strikes
Miki Takeo, 238, 254–56
Mimaikin, see Solatium agreement and payments
Minamata (village, town, and city), 14–16, 18, 27, 35–38, 45, 109, 191, 193, 240, 274, 277–79; immigration to,

14, 27–28, 35, 38, 133; employment, 18, 35–36, 38–39; "castle town," 26, 35, 119, 175, 277; city council, 51, 89, 93–97, 142–43, 158, 180, 199. See also Bombing; Education; Minamata Disease Countermeasures Committee; Minamata municipal hospitals; Welfare and unemployment payments
Minamata-Ashikita Regional Development Foundation, 267
Minamata Bay, 54–55, 57, 60–61, 65, 74, 77–78, 88, 90–91, 99, 115, 117, 144, 185, 261–62. See also Dredging, landfill, and reclaimed land
Minamata bunka shūdan, see Minamata Cultural Collective
Minamatabyō hōritsu mondai kenkyūkai, see Minamata Disease Legal Issues Study Group
Minamatabyō hoshō chōtei iinkai, see Minamata Disease Compensation Mediation Committee
Minamatabyō hoshō shori iinkai, see Minamata Disease Compensation Committee
Minamatabyō kanja katei gojokai, see Minamata Disease Patients Families Mutual Aid Society
Minamatabyō kanja shinsakai, see Minamata Disease Patients' Investigation Committee
Minamatabyō kanja shinsa kyōgikai, see Minamata Disease Patient Examination Commission
Minamatabyō kenkyūkai, see Minamata Disease Research Group
Minamatabyō kenkyū kondankai, see Minamata Disease Research Consultation Group

Minamatabyō o kangaeru gakusei kaigi, *see* Student Council to Think About Minamata Disease

Minamatabyō o kataru kai, *see* Minamata disease discussion groups

Minamatabyō o kataru shimin kōza, *see* Citizens' forums to discuss Minamata disease

Minamatabyō o kokuhatsu suru kai, *see* Association to Indict [Those Responsible for] Minamata Disease

Minamatabyō sentā sōshisha, *see* Minamata Disease Center Sōshisha

Minamatabyō shimin shūkai, *see* Minamata Disease Citizens' Assembly

Minamatabyō shinsa kyōgikai, *see* Ad hoc certification committee

Minamatabyō sōgō chōsa kenkyū renraku kyōgikai, *see* Minamata Disease General Investigation and Research Liaison Council

Minamatabyō soshō shien, kōgai o nakusuru kenmin kaigi, *see* Prefectural Citizens' Council to Support the Minamata Disease Trial and Eliminate Pollution

Minamatabyō taisaku shimin kaigi, *see* Citizens' Council for Minamata Disease Countermeasures

Minamatabyō tokubetsu taisaku iinkai, *see* Special Committee on Minamata Disease Countermeasures

Minamatabyō Tokyo kōshōdan, *see* Minamata Disease Tokyo Negotiations Group

Minamata Chamber of Commerce, 138, 186. *See also* Minamata Junior Chamber of Commerce

Minamata Chemical, *see* Minamata kagaku

Minamata Citizens' Pollution Countermeasures Association (Minamata shimin kōgai taisaku kyōgikai), 224, 226–27

Minamata City League for Peace (Minamata-shi heiwa dōmei), 167

Minamata Cultural Collective (Minamata bunka shūdan), 167–69, 179

Minamata disease: cause, 2, 5, 21, 49–70, 93, 95, 107–8, 112–13, 121, 130–31, 161, 180–92 *passim*, 198, 210, 220, 241, 245; effects on animals and plants, 3–5, 50, 76, 148–49; stigma and discrimination, 5, 6, 28, 49, 51; names for disease, 6, 46, 51, 224, 236, 275, 307n31; misdiagnosis, 18, 48–49; certification of patients, 49–50, 106, 111–12, 145, 203–10, 235, 237–38, 252, 264–77 *passim*, 283, 289; cat experiments; 57, 60–61, 65–66, 68, 93, 158, 160–61, 185, 245; congenital, 63–64, 69, 112, 149–51, 158–60, 204–5, 208, 214–15, 251, 264, 272, 276–77, 318n14, 321n70; government announcement of cause; 182, 185–91; third Minamata disease, 254, 266. *See also* Ad hoc certification committee; Big Four pollution cases; Discrimination; Kumamoto-Kagoshima Pollution Victims Certification Investigation Committee; Minamata Disease Patient Examination Commission; Minamata Disease Patients' Investigation Committee; Niigata Minamata disease; Strange Disease Countermeasures Committee; Uncertified patients

Minamata Disease Center Sōshisha (Minamatabyō sentā sōshisha), 271, 277–78

Minamata Disease Citizens' Assembly (Minamatabyō shimin shūkai), 233–34

Minamata Disease Compensation Committee (Minamatabyō hoshō shori iinkai), 199–202, 223

Minamata Disease Compensation Mediation Committee (Minamatabyō hoshō chōtei iinkai), 235–41, 250, 254–55

Minamata Disease Countermeasures Committee (Minamata city council), 74, 106, 111, 131, 143

Minamata disease discussion groups (Minamatabyō o kataru kai), 210–11

Minamata Disease General Investigation and Research Liaison Council (Minamatabyō sōgō chōsa kenkyū renraku kyōgikai), 66–67

Minamata Disease Legal Issues Study Group (Minamatabyō hōritsu mondai kenkyūkai), 193, 195

Minamata Disease Municipal Museum, 272–73, 278

Minamata Disease Patient Examination Commission (Minamatabyō kanja shinsa kyōgikai), 112, 145, 150

Minamata Disease Patients Families Mutual Aid Society (Minamatabyō kanja katei gojokai), 89–90, 98–118 passim, 141–42, 151, 180–83, 188, 191–94, 197, 223, 325n12, 326n31

Minamata Disease Patients' Investigation Committee (Minamatabyō kanja shinsakai), 203–6

Minamata Disease Research Consultation Group (Minamatabyō kenkyū kondankai; "Tamiya Committee"), 66–68

Minamata Disease Research Group (Minamatabyō kenkyūkai), 160, 198–99, 208, 211, 241–44, 249

Minamata Disease Tokyo Negotiations Group (Minamatabyō Tokyo kōshōdan), 250, 254–55, 271

Minamata Exhibitions, 337n2

Minamata Farmers' Association (Minamata nōminkai), 166

Minamata Fishing Cooperative, 53, 72–84 passim, 87, 92, 97–98, 101–2, 106, 113–20 passim, 126–44 passim, 148–49, 182, 236, 255, 265

Minamata Fish Retailers' Cooperative, 75–76, 137, 148, 182

Minamata Food Poisoning Subcommittee (Minamata shoku chūdoku bukai), see Food Hygiene Investigation Committee

Minamata High School, 134, 275–76, 289

Minamata Junior Chamber of Commerce, 277. See also Minamata Chamber of Commerce

Minamata kagaku (Minamata Chemical), 57

Minamata kenkyūkai, see Minamata Research Group

Minamata Memorial, 279

Minamata Moyainaoshi Center, 278

Minamata municipal hospitals, 6, 47–51 passim, 87, 89–91, 107, 109, 112, 145, 152–59 passim, 203–4

Minamata nōminkai, see Minamata Farmers' Association

Minamata o akaruku suru shimin renraku kyōgikai; see Citizens' Assembly to Brighten Minamata

Minamata o mamoru kai, see Association to Protect Minamata

Minamata Research Group (Minamata kenkyūkai), 277–78

Minamata River, 27, 54–55, 70, 80, 82, 87, 101, 115

Minamata-shi heiwa dōmei, *see* Minamata City League for Peace

Minamata shimin kōgai taisaku kyōgikai, *see* Minamata Citizens' Pollution Countermeasures Association

Minamata shoku chūdoku bukai (Minamata Food Poisoning Subcommittee), *see* Food Hygiene Investigation Committee

Minamata Tokyo Exhibition (1996), 287–91. *See also* Minamata Exhibitions

Ministry of Agriculture and Forestry, 62, 84–85, 129

Ministry of Construction, 279

Ministry of Education, 89, 267

Ministry of Health and Welfare, 5, 49, 51, 53, 56, 61–64, 66, 70, 83–86, 88, 97, 107, 111–12, 117, 129, 152, 185–94, 198–201, 203, 206–11, 215, 224, 267, 287, 289. *See also* Ad hoc certification committee; Complaints against administrative acts; Hashimoto Michio; Minamata Disease Patient Examination Commission; Watanabe Yoshio

Ministry of International Trade and Industry (MITI), 7, 53, 61–63, 66, 84–88, 97–99, 101, 114–18, 121, 129, 162, 173, 185, 187, 246

Ministry of Labor, 84

Ministry of Transport, 129

Minna no ie, 271–72

Minsuitai, *see* Niigata Prefecture Council of Democratic Groups for

Minamata Disease Countermeasures

Misawa (Shin Nihon Chisso General Affairs Section chief), 151–52

Mishima-Numazu, 174

Mission on Japanese Combines, *see* Edwards Report

Misumi, 59

Mita Munesuke, 267

Mitsubishi Heavy Industries, 221

Mitsubishi Real Estate, 234

Mitsui Metal Mining Company, 175, 182, 248. *See also* Toyama cadmium poisoning

Mitsui Mining Company, 35. *See also* Miike

Miyagawa Kuheita, 55, 65

Miyairi Masato, 49

Miyake Reiji, 3

Miyamoto Ken'ichi, 183

Miyamoto Shigemi, 212, 229–30, 284, 289

Miyazawa Kiichi, 189

Miyazawa Nobuo, 208–9

Mizoguchi Toyoko, 5, 273

Mizugami Nagayoshi, 6, 107

Mizukami Tsutomu, 202

Mochizuki, Mike, 298n25

Modō, 3, 27–28, 51, 59, 133, 149, 156, 160, 277

Morinaga Ryūzō, 136, 139, 141

Motoshima Hiroshi, 331n23

Moyainaoshi, 278

Murakami Ushita, 84

Murakami Yasusuke, 172

Murano Tamano, 187

Murayama Tomiichi, 269–70

Mutual Aid Society, *see* Minamata Disease Patients Families Mutual Aid Society

Myōjin, 159, 272

Nagano Harutoshi, 94
Nagasaki, 13, 134, 243, 269, 272, 331n23,
    334n24
Nagashima, 82, 96
Nago (landless peasants), 170
Nagure (poor immigrants), 275
Nakahashi Tokugorō, 18
Nakamura (Minamata Fishing Coop-
    erative secretary), 81, 87, 136
Nakamura Todomu, 79, 81, 88, 96–
    97, 100, 106–14 passim, 131, 136–38,
    142
Nakaoka Satsuki, 89–90
Nakatsu Miyoshi, 112, 181, 191–92, 227–
    28, 325n12
Nakatsu Yoshio, 1–2
Nanjing, 272
Narita, 281–82
Naruhito, see Crown prince (Naruhito)
National Alliance for Pollution Coun-
    termeasures (Kōgai taisaku zen-
    koku renraku kyōgikai), 183, 197
National Alliance of Fishing Coopera-
    tives (Zengyoren), see Oka
National Athletic Meet, 140
National Hygiene Laboratory (Koku-
    ritsu eisei shikenjo), 66
National Institute for Public Health
    (Kokuritsu kōshū eiseiin), 49–51, 56
National Institutes of Health (NIH;
    U.S.), 55–56, 64, 70
Natsume Hideo, 233
Natsume Sōseki, 160
New Left, 173, 175, 282, 285
News media, 5, 70, 102, 110, 116–18, 172,
    185, 231–33. See also Newspapers;
    Radio; Television

Newspapers, 37–38, 96–100 passim, 117,
    216; listings of articles on Minamata,
    307n31, 331n21
New Tokyo International Airport, see
    Narita
New zaibatsu (shinkō zaibatsu), 20
NHK, see Nihon hōsō kyōkai
Nichigetsu maru, 287–88, 290–91
Nihon Carbide, 17
Nihon Chisso hiryō kabushiki kaisha
    (Nitchitsu), 17–33, 38, 72–73,
    300n12. See also Arirang Brigade;
    Bombing; Chisso kabushiki kaisha;
    Chō Michiaki; Chōsen chisso hiryō;
    Dredging, landfill, and reclaimed
    land; Edwards Report; Electro-
    chemical industry; Factory workers;
    Hainan Island; Hashimoto Hiko-
    shichi; Hirohito; Jinmu Boom; Jin-
    nai; Local industrial policy; Maeda
    Eiki; Maeda Kōzō; "castle town"
    under Minamata; Minamata Fishing
    Cooperative; New zaibatsu; Nihon
    Carbide; Nihon kōei; Nitrogen
    Council; Nobeoka; Noguchi Shita-
    gau; Occupation; Ogata Korenori;
    Onitsuka Iwao; Shin Nihon chisso
    hiryō kabushiki kaisha; Sōgi Elec-
    tric Corporation; Southeast Asia;
    Taiwan; Taiyuan; Umedo Harbor;
    Unions; Yūshi
Nihon hōsō kyōkai (NHK), 208
Nihon kagaku kōgyō kyōkai, see Japan
    Chemical Industry Association
Nihon kōei, 23, 301n44
Nihon zeon, 160
Niigata-ken minshu dantai Minama-
    tabyō taisaku kaigi, see Niigata Pre-
    fecture Council of Democratic

Groups for Minamata Disease Countermeasures

Niigata Minamatabyō higaisha no kai, *see* Niigata Minamata Disease Victims' Association

Niigata Minamata disease, 59, 115, 161, 174–76, 179–88 *passim*, 191–92, 208–9, 216, 246–48, 255, 318n14. *See also* Agano River; Agano River Research Group; Big Four pollution cases; Kanose; Lawsuits and trials; Niigata Minamata Disease Victims' Association; Niigata Organic Mercury Poisoning Victims' Association; Niigata Prefecture Council of Democratic Groups for Minamata Disease Countermeasures; Shōwa denkō; Yasunishi Masao

Niigata Minamata Disease Victims' Association (Niigata Minamatabyō higaisha no kai), 181–183, 197

Niigata Organic Mercury Poisoning Victims' Association (Niigata yūki suigin chūdoku higaisha no kai), 181–83

Niigata Prefecture Council of Democratic Groups for Minamata Disease Countermeasures (Niigata-ken minshu dantai Minamatabyō taisaku kaigi; Minsuitai), 181–82, 325n12

Nikkeiren (Japan Federation of Employers' Associations), 166

Nise kanja, *see* False patients

Nishi Yasunori, 270

Nishida Eiichi, 57–58, 74–81 *passim*, 84–87 *passim*, 92–93, 98, 109–10, 113, 130, 245, 250, 266

Nishida Shinako, 110

Nishimura Hajime, 69

Nitchitsu, *see* Nihon Chisso hiryō kabushiki kaisha

Nitrogen Council (Chisso kyōgikai), 20

Nobeoka, 20

Noda Kaneyoshi, 5, 48

Noguchi Shitagau, 16, 17, 19–25, 169–71

Nōhonshugi (agriculturalism), 105

Nōminkai, *see* Minamata Farmers' Association

Nomura Yoshihiro, 202

Nuclear power, 283, 332n42, 335n5

Occupation, 31–32, 34, 59. *See also* Land reform; Red Purge

Oda Makoto, 174

Ogami Mitsuyoshi, 112

Ogata Fukumatsu, 107–8, 273

Ogata Korenori, 170–71

Ogata Masato, 261, 273–74, 284, 287, 287, 334n27

Ogata Shizue, 240

Oil shock, 284

Ōishi Buichi, 210, 234–35, 237

Oka (director of National Alliance of Fishing Cooperatives), 98

Okami (those above), 24, 119, 190, 249

Okamoto Tatsuaki, 69, 170

Okinawa, 182, 272, 337n2. *See also* Yomitanson

Okinawa Minamata Exhibition, 337n2

Okinawa University, 161

Ōkuchi, 16

Old hometown boom, *see* Furusato būmu

Ōmuta, 13, 16, 160, 164. *See also* Miike

One-share movement (*hito kabu undō*), 216–22, 224, 226

Onitsuka Iwao, 29–31, 166–69, 180, 185, 215, 263, 302n10

Onitsuka Shinpei, 30

Onitsuka Yoshisada, 93
Onitsuka Yūji, 277
Ōno Ichirō, 85
Osaka, 212, 218, 223, 337n2
Osaka Association to Indict [Those Responsible for] Minamata Disease (Osaka Minamatabyō o kokuhatsu suru kai), 218
Osaka Minamatabyō o kokuhatsu suru kai, *see* Osaka Association to Indict [Those Responsible for] Minamata Disease
Osaka Minamata Exhibition, 337n2
Ōshima Takeji, 59, 67
Ostracism, *see* Discrimination
Otashiro, 170
Otoku, 170–71
Otomezuka nōen, 271–72
Ōtsuka Hisao, 297n
Ōwada Masako, 323
Ozawa Fumio, 241

PCBs, *see* Kanemi rice oil
Peasant protests and rebellions, 15, 89–90, 118–20, 313n68, 322n5
Pempel, T. J., 298n26, 336n7
Pharr, Susan, 298n25, 336n10
Photographers, 284. *See also individual photographers by name*
Police, 59, 73–79 *passim*, 83, 88, 91–93, 97, 116, 126–27, 167, 217–18, 230, 238, 280
Polluter Pays Principle (PPP), 266–67
Pollution Diet, 207–8
Pollution May Day, 207
Popular Rights Movement, *see* Freedom and Popular Rights Movement
Prefectural Citizens' Council to Support the Minamata Disease Trial and Eliminate Pollution (Minama-

tabyō soshō shien, kōgai o nakusuru kenmin kaigi), 196, 207, 247, 250
Prejudice, *see* Discrimination
Prostitution, 27, 303n17
Public prosecutors, 184, 238, 266

Rachel Carson, 183
Radio, 51
Rape of Nanjing, 272
Rebellions, *see* Peasant protests and rebellions
Reclaimed land, *see* Dredging, landfill, and reclaimed land
Red Purge, 34
Riot (fishermen at factory, 1959), 61, 91–93, 101, 108, 126, 167–68, 267

Sagara family, 15
Saiban kenkyūkai (Trial Research Group), *see* Minamata Disease Research Group
Saiki Shigeru, 16
Saitō Jirō, 245, 248
Saitō Morisuke, 68
Saitō Noboru, 192, 326n31
Sakagami Yuki, 156
Sakamoto Fujie, 272
Sakamoto Shinobu, 214–15, 251, 272, 276
Sakurai Saburō, 6, 74
Sākuru mura, *see* Circle Village
Salt production in Minamata, 16, 17
Samurai (hamlet name), 29
Sapporo, 152–54, 158
Sarugō, *see* Shirahama
Sasaki Saburō, 331n16
Sashiki, 17
Satō Eisaku, 185, 189, 309n65
Satō Takeharu, 133–35, 143, 205, 207, 228–34, 236, 257, 261

Satō Yae, 232, 234

Satsuma Rebellion, 15

Sawada Issei, 210, 223–24, 232–35, 237, 255, 266

Schools, *see* Education; *and individual schools by name*

Science and Technology Agency, 185, 187

Security Treaty, *see* United States–Japan Mutual Security Treaty

Sedifloater, 115–16. *See also* Cyclator

Seikatsu hogo hō, *see* Welfare Protection Law

Seinendan, see Young people's groups

Senkō un'yu (Senkō Transport), 143

Sera Kansuke, 63–65, 67–70, 99

Shimabara, 14

Shimada Ken'ichi, 186, 228–35 *passim*, 251–53

Shimakura Chiyoko, 110

Shimazu family, 15

Shimin kaigi, *see* Citizens' Council for Minamata Disease Countermeasures

Shimotōri, 110

Shimoyama Incident, 65, 309*n*71

Shingon Buddhism, 223

Shinkō zaibatsu, see New zaibatsu

Shin Nihon chisso hiryō kabushiki kaisha (Shin Nitchitsu), 2–3, 30, 33–38, 41, 68–69, 125–26, 160, 300*n*12; hospital, 5, 47–48, 54, 68, 158, 160. *See also* Chihara; Chisso kabushiki kaisha; Cyclator; Dredging, landfill, and reclaimed land; Egashira Yutaka; Factory workers; First Minamata Fishing Dispute; Goi plant; Gotō Haruo; Hachiman; Hashimoto Hikoshichi; Hosokawa Hajime; Hyakken Harbor; Hyakken

waste settlement pools and outfall; Ikeda; Industrial Bank of Japan; Ishino; Japan Chemical Industry Association; Kawamura Kazuo; Kitagawa Kinsai; Kumamoto Prefectural Alliance of Fishing Cooperative; "castle town" *under* Minamata; cat experiments *under* Minamata disease; Minamata Fishing Cooperative; Minamata kagaku; Ministry of International Trade and Industry; Misawa; Nagano Harutoshi; Nihon chisso hiryō kabushiki kaisha; Nishida Eiichi; Onitsuka Iwao; Onitsuka Yoshisada; Riot; Sedifloater; Senkō un'yu; Shiranuikai Fishing Dispute; Solatium agreement and payments; Strikes; Unions; *Unmei kyōdōtai;* Yamataka Matanori; Yoshioka Kiichi

Shin Nihon kagaku, 35, 224. *See also* Ikematsu Nobuo

Shin Nitchitsu, *see* Shin Nihon chisso hiryō kabushiki kaisha

Shinohara Tamotsu, 91, 108

Shintō, 337*n*1. *See also* Yasukuni Shrine

Shiota Takeshi, 212, 284, 289

Shirahama (also called Sarugō, Tonton-mura), 27

Shiranuikai Fishing Dispute, 82–102

Shiranui Sea, 14, 54, 66, 83, 99, 107, 115, 127, 143, 156, 206, 254, 266, 271, 279, 287, 290

Shishijima, 82, 106

Shōda Michiko, 75

Shōji Hikaru, 183

Shokuhin eisei chōsakai, *see* Food Hygiene Investigation Committee

Shokuhin eisei hō, *see* Food Sanitation Act

Shōtoku, empress, 15, 16
Shōwa denkō, 31, 67, 115, 175–76, 179, 183, 187, 248, 255. *See also* Andō Nobuo; Yasunishi Masao
Shōwa emperor, *see* Hirohito
Single-share movement, *see* One-share movement
Smith, Aileen M., 6, 158, 212–15, 233, 247, 284, 289, 335n5
Smith, W. Eugene, 6, 158, 212–15, 232–33, 247, 271, 284, 289, 317n143
Sōgi Electric Corporation, 16, 17
Sōhyō (General Council of Trade Unions of Japan), 164, 166–67, 191, 196, 234
Sōkaiya (gangsters who extort protection money for company shareholder's meetings), 218–19, 221
Solatium agreement and payments (*mimaikin*), 72–77 passim, 83, 110–18 passim, 125, 144, 151–52, 171, 183–86, 190–92, 198, 206, 222, 225, 241, 244, 246, 248, 256, 270
Sonoda Sunao, 185–92 passim
Sōshisha, *see* Minamata Disease Center Sōshisha
Soshōha, *see* Trial Group
Southeast Asia, 23
Southern Minamata Moyainaoshi Center (Orange Hall), 278
Special Committee on Minamata Disease Countermeasures (Minamatabyō tokubetsu taisaku iinkai; Kumamoto prefectural assembly), 57–58, 76, 86, 88, 94, 145
Steinhoff, Patricia, 282
Stone statues on reclaimed land, 261–62, 278–79
Strange Disease Countermeasures Committee (Kibyō taisaku iin-

kai; Minamata city), 48–50, 206
Strikes: at Miike in 1960, 13, 164, 181; at Miike in 1953, 35; at Minamata in 1953, 28, 34; at Minamata in 1962–63, 28, 150–51, 163–69, 179, 181–82, 184, 203, 215; at Minamata in 1970, 202, 216; by public servants, 336n7
Student Council to Think About Minamata Disease (Minamatabyō o kangaeru gakusei kaigi), 197
Sugimoto Eiko, 51–52, 205, 277, 287, 336n1
Sugimoto Takeshi, 205
Sugimoto Toshi, 51
Suikōsha, 37, 110
Sunada Akira, 212, 216, 271
Sunada Emiko, 212, 271
Supreme Court, 245, 264–66, 268, 273

Taiwan, 23
Taiyuan, 23
Takahata Minamata Exhibition, 337n2
Takaono, 147
Takefuji (Ministry of Health and Welfare Pollution Section chief), 193
Taketani Mitsuo, 244, 332n42
Takeuchi Tadao, 52, 57, 60, 150, 252
Takishita Masafumi, 276–77
Tamiya Committee, *see* Minamata Disease Research Consultation Group
Tamiya Takeo, 66–67
Tanaka Asao, 49
Tanaka Jitsuko, 5, 49
Tanaka Kakuei, 237
Tanaka Shizuko, 5, 49, 289
Tanaka Shōzō, 108, 127
Tanaka Yoshiaki, 219
Tanigawa Gan, 54, 103–5, 154–56, 231, 306n24

Tanigawa Ken'ichi, 231, 306n24
Tanigawa Michio, 306n24
Tanoue Yoshiharu, 251, 257, 261, 271
Tanoura, 82, 87, 100, 146, 206
Tatetsu Seijun, 150
Teachers' unions, *see* Unions
Television, 220
Tenant unions, 282
Teramoto Hirosaku, 61–62, 78–79, 87–88, 93–100, 106–12 *passim*, 115, 126–27, 130–32, 136, 140, 185–87, 192–93, 199, 246
Terasono Katsushi, 127–28
Textbook screening, 267
Third Minamata disease, *see under* Minamata disease
Tocqueville, Alexis de, 285
Togashi Sadao, 198, 229, 242–45, 248, 263
Tōhō University, 65
Tokita Kikuji, 65, 67
Tokue Takeshi, 186
Tokuomi Haruhiko, 57, 206–10
Tokutomi Masafumi, 224–25, 227
Tokutomi Roka, 306n24
Tokutomi Sohō, 299n4, 306n24
Tokyo Association to Indict [Those Responsible for] Minamata Disease (Tokyo Minamatabyō o kokuhatsu suru kai), 211–12, 215–16, 218, 229
Tokyo Building, 229, 231–34
Tokyo District Court, 265
Tokyo High Court, 265
Tokyo Institute of Technology (Tokyo kōgyō daigaku), 62, 99, 130
Tokyo Minamatabyō o kokuhatsu suru kai, *see* Tokyo Association to Indict [Those Responsible for] Minamata Disease

Tokyo-Minamata Pilgrimage Group, 212, 216
Tokyo Negotiations, 221, 250–57, 285. *See also* Minamata Disease Tokyo Negotiations Group
Tokyo toritsu daigaku, 66
Tokyo University, *see* University of Tokyo
Tomita Hachirō, *see* Ui Jun
Tonton-mura, *see* Shirahama
Toyama cadmium poisoning (*Itai-itai byō*), 70, 174–75, 182, 189, 248. *See also* Big Four pollution cases; Kamioka Mine, Mitsui Metal Mining Company
Toyohashi Minamata Exhibition, 337n2
Toyota city, 40
Toyotomi Hideyoshi, 15
Trial Group (Soshōha), 193–97 *passim*, 200, 205, 207, 211–12, 216, 222–23, 228–29, 232, 236–39 *passim*, 247–54 *passim*. *See also* Direct Negotiations Group; Lawsuits and trials
Trial Research Group (Saiban kenkyūkai), *see* Minamata Disease Research Group
Tropical Research Institute, 55
Tsubaki Tadao, 209
Tsubodan, 1, 5, 219
Tsuchimoto Noriaki, 200–201, 214–16, 220, 251, 263, 284, 289–90, 334n23
Tsukinoura, 27–28, 50, 133, 149, 156, 213, 271, 277
Tsukuba Minamata Exhibition, 337n2
Tsukuda Tameyoshi, 275–76
Tsunagi, 29, 76, 82, 87, 96, 108, 146
Tsunagi Village Fishing Cooperative, 82, 91, 100

Tsunagi Village Women's Association, 82

Tsushima, 143

Uchida Makio, 66
Ueno Chizuko, 288
Ueno Eiko, 191
Ueno Hidenobu, 231
Ugaki Kazushige, 22
Ui Jun (pen name Tomita Hachirō), 57–59, 65, 67–68, 126, 148, 211, 242, 249; on company dominance of and support from city, 36, 92; on role of newspapers, 37; on stages of pollution incidents, 46–47, 64, 66; on fishing cooperative, 141–42; role in Minamata movement, 160–62, 172, 183, 199–201, 215; link between Minamata and Niigata, 175–76, 179, 181, 263
Umbilical cords, 149
Umedo Harbor, 17, 166
Uncertified patients, 203–10
Unemployment, see Welfare and unemployment payments
Unions, 95, 164, 280, 285; No. 1 union in Minamata, 28, 34–37, 69, 93–95, 164–69, 180–88 passim, 199, 202, 215, 223, 226, 266; government employees, 82, 96, 184; teachers, 95–96, 158, 225, 276; No. 2 union in Minamata, 164–69, 186, 224, 266; at Goi factory, 233. See also Eight Millimeter Group; Japanese Federation of Synthetic Chemistry Workers Unions; Nagano Harutoshi; Onitsuka Iwao; Red Purge; Sōhyō; Strikes; Tenant unions; Yamashita Yoshihiro
United front (to defend company and city), 92–96, 102–3

United Nations, 160–61
United States–Japan Mutual Security Treaty, 103–4, 121, 164, 173, 182, 234, 285
University of Tokyo, 68, 103, 160–61, 202, 211, 267
Unmei kyōdōtai (community sharing a single fate), 40–41, 305n60
Unzen, 14
Upham, Frank, 120–21, 316n117
Ushibuka, 133
Ushio, 16
Utasebune, 287, 290. See also Nichigetsu maru
Uto, 254

Vietnam, 272
Vinyl Chloride and Acetaldehyde Special Committee (JCIA), 67

Wakai (court-mediated out-of-court settlement), 268–71, 283, 285, 288
Wanibuchi Takeshi, 63
War apology, 269–70
Watanabe Eizō, 89–90, 102–3, 106–8, 111–14, 118, 141, 151, 191, 197, 207, 211, 216, 249
Watanabe Katsuichi, 224
Watanabe Kyōji, 157, 196, 215, 242
Watanabe Masaaki, 151
Watanabe Osamu, 335n7, 336n9
Watanabe Yoshio, 62
Water Quality Conservation Law (Kōkyō yōsuiiki no suishitsu no hozen ni kansuru hōritsu), 85, 94, 97, 130, 185
Waters, Neil, 299n7
Welfare and unemployment payments, 71–72, 134, 144, 185, 202. See also Welfare Protection Law

Welfare Protection Law (Seikatsu hogo hō), 79, 94
White, James, 281
Wolin, Sheldon S., 336n9
Women, 30, 76, 82
Workers, *see* Factory workers; Strikes; Unions

Yalu River, 22
Yamaguchi Yoshito, 143
Yamamoto Matayoshi, 188, 191–92
Yamanouchi Naso, 171
Yamashita Yoshihiro (Zenkan), 180, 199
Yamataka Matanori, 134
Yasukuni Shrine, 336n7
Yasunishi Masao, 67, 187
Yatsushiro, 14, 89, 96, 110, 275
Yawata, 13, 31
Yen-dollar exchange rates, *see* Exchange rates
Yokkaichi air pollution, 174–75, 182. *See also* Big Four pollution cases
Yokota (Kumamoto prefecture Mining and Industry Section chief), 111
Yomitanson, 334n24

Yoshii Masazumi, 261, 278–79, 289
Yoshimoto Tetsurō, 277
Yoshinaga Toshio, 277–78
Yoshioka Kiichi, 61–62, 84, 92, 97–99, 109–11, 115, 132, 137, 163, 245, 266
Yoshizawa Nagamori, 85, 88
Young people's groups (*seinendan*), 3, 41, 295n7
Yudō, 27, 50, 88, 90, 102, 153, 156, 159, 212, 214, 223, 236, 271, 277
Yunoko, 154, 170
Yunoko Tourism Association, 186
Yunokuchi, 106
Yunotsuru, 170
Yunoura, 82, 87, 107, 146
Yūshi (leading figures) of Minamata, 16–17

Zaibatsu, *see* New *zaibatsu*
Zen Buddhism, 252
Zengyoren (National Alliance of Fishing Cooperatives), *see* Oka
Zen Nihon jichi dantai rōdō kumiai (Jichirō), *see* All-Japan Prefectural and Municipal Workers' Union

Harvard East Asian Monographs

(* out-of-print)

*1. Liang Fang-chung, *The Single-Whip Method of Taxation in China*

*2. Harold C. Hinton, *The Grain Tribute System of China, 1845–1911*

3. Ellsworth C. Carlson, *The Kaiping Mines, 1877–1912*

*4. Chao Kuo-chün, *Agrarian Policies of Mainland China: A Documentary Study, 1949–1956*

*5. Edgar Snow, *Random Notes on Red China, 1936–1945*

*6. Edwin George Beal, Jr., *The Origin of Likin, 1835–1864*

7. Chao Kuo-chün, *Economic Planning and Organization in Mainland China: A Documentary Study, 1949–1957*

*8. John K. Fairbank, *Ching Documents: An Introductory Syllabus*

*9. Helen Yin and Yi-chang Yin, *Economic Statistics of Mainland China, 1949–1957*

*10. Wolfgang Franke, *The Reform and Abolition of the Traditional Chinese Examination System*

11. Albert Feuerwerker and S. Cheng, *Chinese Communist Studies of Modern Chinese History*

12. C. John Stanley, *Late Ching Finance: Hu Kuang-yung as an Innovator*

13. S. M. Meng, *The Tsungli Yamen: Its Organization and Functions*

*14. Ssu-yü Teng, *Historiography of the Taiping Rebellion*

15. Chun-Jo Liu, *Controversies in Modern Chinese Intellectual History: An Analytic Bibliography of Periodical Articles, Mainly of the May Fourth and Post–May Fourth Era*

*16. Edward J. M. Rhoads, *The Chinese Red Army, 1927–1963: An Annotated Bibliography*

17. Andrew J. Nathan, *A History of the China International Famine Relief Commission*

*18. Frank H. H. King (ed.) and Prescott Clarke, *A Research Guide to China-Coast Newspapers, 1822–1911*

19. Ellis Joffe, *Party and Army: Professionalism and Political Control in the Chinese Officer Corps, 1949–1964*

*20. Toshio G. Tsukahira, *Feudal Control in Tokugawa Japan: The Sankin Kōtai System*

21. Kwang-Ching Liu, ed., *American Missionaries in China: Papers from Harvard Seminars*

22. George Moseley, *A Sino-Soviet Cultural Frontier: The Ili Kazakh Autonomous Chou*

Harvard East Asian Monographs

23. Carl F. Nathan, *Plague Prevention and Politics in Manchuria, 1910–1931*

*24. Adrian Arthur Bennett, *John Fryer: The Introduction of Western Science and Technology into Nineteenth-Century China*

25. Donald J. Friedman, *The Road from Isolation: The Campaign of the American Committee for Non-Participation in Japanese Aggression, 1938–1941*

26. Edward LeFevour, *Western Enterprise in Late Ching China: A Selective Survey of Jardine, Matheson and Company's Operations, 1842–1895*

27. Charles Neuhauser, *Third World Politics: China and the Afro-Asian People's Solidarity Organization, 1957–1967*

28. Kungtu C. Sun, assisted by Ralph W. Huenemann, *The Economic Development of Manchuria in the First Half of the Twentieth Century*

*29. Shahid Javed Burki, *A Study of Chinese Communes, 1965*

30. John Carter Vincent, *The Extraterritorial System in China: Final Phase*

31. Madeleine Chi, *China Diplomacy, 1914–1918*

*32. Clifton Jackson Phillips, *Protestant America and the Pagan World: The First Half Century of the American Board of Commissioners for Foreign Missions, 1810–1860*

33. James Pusey, *Wu Han: Attacking the Present through the Past*

34. Ying-wan Cheng, *Postal Communication in China and Its Modernization, 1860–1896*

35. Tuvia Blumenthal, *Saving in Postwar Japan*

36. Peter Frost, *The Bakumatsu Currency Crisis*

37. Stephen C. Lockwood, *Augustine Heard and Company, 1858–1862*

38. Robert R. Campbell, *James Duncan Campbell: A Memoir by His Son*

39. Jerome Alan Cohen, ed., *The Dynamics of China's Foreign Relations*

40. V. V. Vishnyakova-Akimova, *Two Years in Revolutionary China, 1925–1927*, tr. Steven L. Levine

*41. Meron Medzini, *French Policy in Japan during the Closing Years of the Tokugawa Regime*

42. Ezra Vogel, Margie Sargent, Vivienne B. Shue, Thomas Jay Mathews, and Deborah S. Davis, *The Cultural Revolution in the Provinces*

*43. Sidney A. Forsythe, *An American Missionary Community in China, 1895–1905*

*44. Benjamin I. Schwartz, ed., *Reflections on the May Fourth Movement.: A Symposium*

*45. Ching Young Choe, *The Rule of the Taewŏngun, 1864–1873: Restoration in Yi Korea*

46. W. P. J. Hall, *A Bibliographical Guide to Japanese Research on the Chinese Economy, 1958–1970*

47. Jack J. Gerson, *Horatio Nelson Lay and Sino-British Relations, 1854–1864*

48. Paul Richard Bohr, *Famine and the Missionary: Timothy Richard as Relief Administrator and Advocate of National Reform*

49. Endymion Wilkinson, *The History of Imperial China: A Research Guide*

50. Britten Dean, *China and Great Britain: The Diplomacy of Commercial Relations, 1860–1864*

51. Ellsworth C. Carlson, *The Foochow Missionaries, 1847–1880*

Harvard East Asian Monographs

52. Yeh-chien Wang, *An Estimate of the Land-Tax Collection in China, 1753 and 1908*

53. Richard M. Pfeffer, *Understanding Business Contracts in China, 1949–1963*

54. Han-sheng Chuan and Richard Kraus, *Mid-Ching Rice Markets and Trade: An Essay in Price History*

55. Ranbir Vohra, *Lao She and the Chinese Revolution*

56. Liang-lin Hsiao, *China's Foreign Trade Statistics, 1864–1949*

*57. Lee-hsia Hsu Ting, *Government Control of the Press in Modern China, 1900–1949*

58. Edward W. Wagner, *The Literati Purges: Political Conflict in Early Yi Korea*

*59. Joungwon A. Kim, *Divided Korea: The Politics of Development, 1945–1972*

*60. Noriko Kamachi, John K. Fairbank, and Chūzō Ichiko, *Japanese Studies of Modern China Since 1953: A Bibliographical Guide to Historical and Social-Science Research on the Nineteenth and Twentieth Centuries, Supplementary Volume for 1953–1969*

61. Donald A. Gibbs and Yun-chen Li, *A Bibliography of Studies and Translations of Modern Chinese Literature, 1918–1942*

62. Robert H. Silin, *Leadership and Values: The Organization of Large-Scale Taiwanese Enterprises*

63. David Pong, *A Critical Guide to the Kwangtung Provincial Archives Deposited at the Public Record Office of London*

*64. Fred W. Drake, *China Charts the World: Hsu Chi-yü and His Geography of 1848*

*65. William A. Brown and Urgrunge Onon, translators and annotators, *History of the Mongolian People's Republic*

66. Edward L. Farmer, *Early Ming Government: The Evolution of Dual Capitals*

*67. Ralph C. Croizier, *Koxinga and Chinese Nationalism: History, Myth, and the Hero*

*68. William J. Tyler, tr., *The Psychological World of Natsume Sōseki*, by Doi Takeo

69. Eric Widmer, *The Russian Ecclesiastical Mission in Peking during the Eighteenth Century*

*70. Charlton M. Lewis, *Prologue to the Chinese Revolution: The Transformation of Ideas and Institutions in Hunan Province, 1891–1907*

71. Preston Torbert, *The Ching Imperial Household Department: A Study of Its Organization and Principal Functions, 1662–1796*

72. Paul A. Cohen and John E. Schrecker, eds., *Reform in Nineteenth-Century China*

73. Jon Sigurdson, *Rural Industrialism in China*

74. Kang Chao, *The Development of Cotton Textile Production in China*

75. Valentin Rabe, *The Home Base of American China Missions, 1880–1920*

*76. Sarasin Viraphol, *Tribute and Profit: Sino-Siamese Trade, 1652–1853*

77. Ch'i-ch'ing Hsiao, *The Military Establishment of the Yuan Dynasty*

78. Meishi Tsai, *Contemporary Chinese Novels and Short Stories, 1949–1974: An Annotated Bibliography*

*79. Wellington K. K. Chan, *Merchants, Mandarins and Modern Enterprise in Late Ching China*

80. Endymion Wilkinson, *Landlord and Labor in Late Imperial China: Case Studies from Shandong by Jing Su and Luo Lun*

*81. Barry Keenan, *The Dewey Experiment in China: Educational Reform and Political Power in the Early Republic*

*82. George A. Hayden, *Crime and Punishment in Medieval Chinese Drama: Three Judge Pao Plays*

*83. Sang-Chul Suh, *Growth and Structural Changes in the Korean Economy, 1910–1940*

84. J. W. Dower, *Empire and Aftermath: Yoshida Shigeru and the Japanese Experience, 1878–1954*

85. Martin Collcutt, *Five Mountains: The Rinzai Zen Monastic Institution in Medieval Japan*

86. Kwang Suk Kim and Michael Roemer, *Growth and Structural Transformation*

87. Anne O. Krueger, *The Developmental Role of the Foreign Sector and Aid*

*88. Edwin S. Mills and Byung-Nak Song, *Urbanization and Urban Problems*

89. Sung Hwan Ban, Pal Yong Moon, and Dwight H. Perkins, *Rural Development*

*90. Noel F. McGinn, Donald R. Snodgrass, Yung Bong Kim, Shin-Bok Kim, and Quee-Young Kim, *Education and Development in Korea*

91. Leroy P. Jones and Il SaKong, *Government, Business, and Entrepreneurship in Economic Development: The Korean Case*

92. Edward S. Mason, Dwight H. Perkins, Kwang Suk Kim, David C. Cole, Mahn Je Kim et al., *The Economic and Social Modernization of the Republic of Korea*

93. Robert Repetto, Tai Hwan Kwon, Son-Ung Kim, Dae Young Kim, John E. Sloboda, and Peter J. Donaldson, *Economic Development, Population Policy, and Demographic Transition in the Republic of Korea*

94. Parks M. Coble, Jr., *The Shanghai Capitalists and the Nationalist Government, 1927–1937*

95. Noriko Kamachi, *Reform in China: Huang Tsun-hsien and the Japanese Model*

96. Richard Wich, *Sino-Soviet Crisis Politics: A Study of Political Change and Communication*

97. Lillian M. Li, *China's Silk Trade: Traditional Industry in the Modern World, 1842–1937*

98. R. David Arkush, *Fei Xiaotong and Sociology in Revolutionary China*

*99. Kenneth Alan Grossberg, *Japan's Renaissance: The Politics of the Muromachi Bakufu*

100. James Reeve Pusey, *China and Charles Darwin*

101. Hoyt Cleveland Tillman, *Utilitarian Confucianism: Chen Liang's Challenge to Chu Hsi*

102. Thomas A. Stanley, *Ōsugi Sakae, Anarchist in Taishō Japan: The Creativity of the Ego*

103. Jonathan K. Ocko, *Bureaucratic Reform in Provincial China: Ting Jih-ch'ang in Restoration Kiangsu, 1867–1870*

104. James Reed, *The Missionary Mind and American East Asia Policy, 1911–1915*

105. Neil L. Waters, *Japan's Local Pragmatists: The Transition from Bakumatsu to Meiji in the Kawasaki Region*

106. David C. Cole and Yung Chul Park, *Financial Development in Korea, 1945–1978*

Harvard East Asian Monographs

107. Roy Bahl, Chuk Kyo Kim, and Chong Kee Park, *Public Finances during the Korean Modernization Process*

108. William D. Wray, *Mitsubishi and the N.Y.K, 1870–1914: Business Strategy in the Japanese Shipping Industry*

109. Ralph William Huenemann, *The Dragon and the Iron Horse: The Economics of Railroads in China, 1876–1937*

110. Benjamin A. Elman, *From Philosophy to Philology: Intellectual and Social Aspects of Change in Late Imperial China*

111. Jane Kate Leonard, *Wei Yüan and China's Rediscovery of the Maritime World*

112. Luke S. K. Kwong, *A Mosaic of the Hundred Days:. Personalities, Politics, and Ideas of 1898*

113. John E. Wills, Jr., *Embassies and Illusions: Dutch and Portuguese Envoys to K'ang-hsi, 1666–1687*

114. Joshua A. Fogel, *Politics and Sinology: The Case of Naitō Konan (1866–1934)*

*115. Jeffrey C. Kinkley, ed., *After Mao: Chinese Literature and Society, 1978–1981*

116. C. Andrew Gerstle, *Circles of Fantasy: Convention in the Plays of Chikamatsu*

117. Andrew Gordon, *The Evolution of Labor Relations in Japan: Heavy Industry, 1853–1955*

*118. Daniel K. Gardner, *Chu Hsi and the "Ta Hsueh": Neo-Confucian Reflection on the Confucian Canon*

119. Christine Guth Kanda, *Shinzō: Hachiman Imagery and Its Development*

*120. Robert Borgen, *Sugawara no Michizane and the Early Heian Court*

121. Chang-tai Hung, *Going to the People: Chinese Intellectuals and Folk Literature, 1918–1937*

*122. Michael A. Cusumano, *The Japanese Automobile Industry: Technology and Management at Nissan and Toyota*

123. Richard von Glahn, *The Country of Streams and Grottoes: Expansion, Settlement, and the Civilizing of the Sichuan Frontier in Song Times*

124. Steven D. Carter, *The Road to Komatsubara: A Classical Reading of the Renga Hyakuin*

125. Katherine F. Bruner, John K. Fairbank, and Richard T. Smith, *Entering China's Service: Robert Hart's Journals, 1854–1863*

126. Bob Tadashi Wakabayashi, *Anti-Foreignism and Western Learning in Early-Modern Japan: The "New Theses" of 1825*

127. Atsuko Hirai, *Individualism and Socialism: The Life and Thought of Kawai Eijirō (1891–1944)*

128. Ellen Widmer, *The Margins of Utopia: "Shui-hu hou-chuan" and the Literature of Ming Loyalism*

129. R. Kent Guy, *The Emperor's Four Treasuries: Scholars and the State in the Late Chien-lung Era*

130. Peter C. Perdue, *Exhausting the Earth: State and Peasant in Hunan, 1500–1850*

131. Susan Chan Egan, *A Latterday Confucian: Reminiscences of William Hung (1893–1980)*

132. James T. C. Liu, *China Turning Inward: Intellectual-Political Changes in the Early Twelfth Century*

Harvard East Asian Monographs

133. Paul A. Cohen, *Between Tradition and Modernity: Wang T'ao and Reform in Late Ching China*

134. Kate Wildman Nakai, *Shogunal Politics: Arai Hakuseki and the Premises of Tokugawa Rule*

135. Parks M. Coble, *Facing Japan: Chinese Politics and Japanese Imperialism, 1931–1937*

136. Jon L. Saari, *Legacies of Childhood: Growing Up Chinese in a Time of Crisis, 1890–1920*

137. Susan Downing Videen, *Tales of Heichū*

138. Heinz Morioka and Miyoko Sasaki, *Rakugo: The Popular Narrative Art of Japan*

139. Joshua A. Fogel, *Nakae Ushikichi in China: The Mourning of Spirit*

140. Alexander Barton Woodside, *Vietnam and the Chinese Model.: A Comparative Study of Vietnamese and Chinese Government in the First Half of the Nineteenth Century*

141. George Elision, *Deus Destroyed: The Image of Christianity in Early Modern Japan*

142. William D. Wray, ed., *Managing Industrial Enterprise: Cases from Japan's Prewar Experience*

143. T'ung-tsu Ch'ü, *Local Government in China under the Ching*

144. Marie Anchordoguy, *Computers, Inc.: Japan's Challenge to IBM*

145. Barbara Molony, *Technology and Investment: The Prewar Japanese Chemical Industry*

146. Mary Elizabeth Berry, *Hideyoshi*

147. Laura E. Hein, *Fueling Growth: The Energy Revolution and Economic Policy in Postwar Japan*

148. Wen-hsin Yeh, *The Alienated Academy: Culture and Politics in Republican China, 1919–1937*

149. Dru C. Gladney, *Muslim Chinese: Ethnic Nationalism in the People's Republic*

150. Merle Goldman and Paul A. Cohen, eds., *Ideas Across Cultures: Essays on Chinese Thought in Honor of Benjamin L Schwartz*

151. James Polachek, *The Inner Opium War*

152. Gail Lee Bernstein, *Japanese Marxist: A Portrait of Kawakami Hajime, 1879–1946*

153. Lloyd E. Eastman, *The Abortive Revolution: China under Nationalist Rule, 1927–1937*

154. Mark Mason, *American Multinationals and Japan: The Political Economy of Japanese Capital Controls, 1899–1980*

155. Richard J. Smith, John K. Fairbank, and Katherine F. Bruner, *Robert Hart and China's Early Modernization: His Journals, 1863–1866*

156. George J. Tanabe, Jr., *Myōe the Dreamkeeper: Fantasy and Knowledge in Kamakura Buddhism*

157. William Wayne Farris, *Heavenly Warriors: The Evolution of Japan's Military, 500–1300*

158. Yu-ming Shaw, *An American Missionary in China: John Leighton Stuart and Chinese-American Relations*

159. James B. Palais, *Politics and Policy in Traditional Korea*

160. Douglas Reynolds, *China, 1898–1912: The Xinzheng Revolution and Japan*

161. Roger Thompson, *China's Local Councils in the Age of Constitutional Reform*

162. William Johnston, *The Modern Epidemic: History of Tuberculosis in Japan*

Harvard East Asian Monographs

163. Constantine Nomikos Vaporis, *Breaking Barriers: Travel and the State in Early Modern Japan*

164. Irmela Hijiya-Kirschnereit, *Rituals of Self-Revelation: Shishōsetsu as Literary Genre and Socio-Cultural Phenomenon*

165. James C. Baxter, *The Meiji Unification through the Lens of Ishikawa Prefecture*

166. Thomas R. H. Havens, *Architects of Affluence: The Tsutsumi Family and the Seibu-Saison Enterprises in Twentieth-Century Japan*

167. Anthony Hood Chambers, *The Secret Window: Ideal Worlds in Tanizaki's Fiction*

168. Steven J. Ericson, *The Sound of the Whistle: Railroads and the State in Meiji Japan*

169. Andrew Edmund Goble, *Kenmu: Go-Daigo's Revolution*

170. Denise Potrzeba Lett, *In Pursuit of Status: The Making of South Korea's "New" Urban Middle Class*

171. Mimi Hall Yiengpruksawan, *Hiraizumi: Buddhist Art and Regional Politics in Twelfth-Century Japan*

172. Charles Shirō Inouye, *The Similitude of Blossoms: A Critical Biography of Izumi Kyōka (1873–1939), Japanese Novelist and Playwright*

173. Aviad E. Raz, *Riding the Black Ship: Japan and Tokyo Disneyland*

174. Deborah J. Milly, *Poverty, Equality, and Growth: The Politics of Economic Need in Postwar Japan*

175. See Heng Teow, *Japan's Cultural Policy Toward China, 1918–1931: A Comparative Perspective*

176. Michael A. Fuller, *An Introduction to Literary Chinese*

177. Frederick R. Dickinson, *War and National Reinvention: Japan in the Great War, 1914–1919*

178. John Solt, *Shredding the Tapestry of Meaning: The Poetry and Poetics of Kitasono Katue (1902–1978)*

179. Edward Pratt, *Japan's Protoindustrial Elite: The Economic Foundations of the Gōnō*

180. Atsuko Sakaki, *Recontextualizing Texts: Narrative Performance in Modern Japanese Fiction*

181. Soon-Won Park, *Colonial Industrialization and Labor in Korea: The Onoda Cement Factory*

182. JaHyun Kim Haboush and Martina Deuchler, *Culture and the State in Late Chosŏn Korea*

183. John W. Chaffee, *Branches of Heaven: A History of the Imperial Clan of Sung China*

184. Gi-Wook Shin and Michael Robinson, eds., *Colonial Modernity in Korea*

185. Nam-lin Hur, *Prayer and Play in Late Tokugawa Japan: Asakusa Sensōji and Edo Society*

186. Kristin Stapleton, *Civilizing Chengdu: Chinese Urban Reform, 1895–1937*

187. Hyung Il Pai, *Constructing "Korean" Origins: A Critical Review of Archaeology, Historiography, and Racial Myth in Korean State-Formation Theories*

188. Brian D. Ruppert, *Jewel in the Ashes: Buddha Relics and Power in Early Medieval Japan*

189. Susan Daruvala, *Zhou Zuoren and an Alternative Chinese Response to Modernity*

190. James Z. Lee, *The Political Economy of a Frontier: Southwest China, 1250–1850*

Harvard East Asian Monographs

191. Kerry Smith, *A Time of Crisis: Japan, the Great Depression, and Rural Revitalization*

192. Michael Lewis, *Becoming Apart: National Power and Local Politics in Toyama, 1868–1945*

193. William C. Kirby, Man-houng Lin, James Chin Shih, and David A. Pietz, eds., *State and Economy in Republican China: A Handbook for Scholars*

194. Timothy S. George, *Minamata: Pollution and the Struggle for Democracy in Postwar Japan*

195. Billy K. L. So, *Prosperity, Region, and Institutions in Maritime China: The South Fukien Pattern, 946–1368*

196. Yoshihisa Tak Matsusaka, *The Making of Japanese Manchuria, 1904–1932*